W9-BIO-292

Planning YOUR PREGNANCY and BIRTH

Third Edition

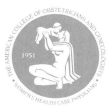

The American College of Obstetricians and Gynecologists

Planning Your Pregnancy and Birth, Third Edition, was developed by a panel of experts working in consultation with staff of the American College of Obstetricians and Gynecologists (ACOG):

Editorial Task Force

Members

Nancy C. Chescheir, MD
Bonnie J. Dattel, MD
Nathana L. Lurvey, MD
Susan F. Meade, RNC, FPNP
Susan Ramin, MD
Laura E. Riley, MD
Allan T. Sawyer, MD

ACOG staff

Gerald B. Holzman, MD, FACOG,
   ACOG Vice President, Education
Rebecca D. Rinehart, Director,
   Publications
Margo Harris, Senior Editor
Thomas P. Dineen, Manager of
   Production and Design
Mary Clark, Design

The assistance of the following ACOG staff is greatly appreciated:

Debra Hawks
Alice Kirkman
Penny Rutledge
Pamela Van Hine

Chris Briscoe/Index Stock, *Cover photograph*
Leah Hennen, *Editorial*
Jane Levine, *Photography*
Naylor Design Inc., *Design and layout*
Terese Winslow, *Illustration*

ACOG guide to planning for pregnancy, birth, and beyond.
   Planning your pregnancy and birth / American College of Obstetricians and Gynecologists.—3rd ed.
      p. cm.
      Includes index.
      ISBN 0-915473-56-9
      1. Pregnancy. 2. Childbirth. 3. Infants—Care. I. American College of Obstetricians and Gynecologists. II. Title.

RG556 .A26 2000
618.2—dc21   99-058049

Copyright © 2000, The American College of Obstetricians and Gynecologists
409 12th Street, SW, Washington, DC 20024-2188

ISBN 0-915473-56-9

Designed as an aid to patients, *Planning Your Pregnancy and Birth* sets forth current information and opinions on subjects related to women's health and reproduction. The information does not dictate an exclusive course of treatment or procedure to be followed and should not be construed as excluding other medical opinions or acceptable methods of practice. Variations taking into account the needs of the individual patient, resources, and limitations unique to the institution or type of practice may be appropriate.

45/4321

Contents

Special Care 307

Preface

There's a lot of information out there about pregnancy—from magazines, newsletters, and books to television shows and Web pages. It's hard for a woman to sift through it all and know what's current and accurate. That's why the American College of Obstetricians and Gynecologists (ACOG)—America's leading authority on women's health—has written this book. *Planning Your Pregnancy and Birth*—the official guide to pregnancy and birth—provides a woman with all she wants to know about her pregnancy. It is written with the collective knowledge of 40,000 experts in the field of obstetrics, but with the pregnant woman's concerns and interests in mind. All of the information and advice contained in this resource have been screened, reviewed, and tested by experts from ACOG. Throughout its almost 50-year history, ACOG's main goal has been to maintain the highest standards of health care for women. To that end, members of ACOG are kept up-to-date on the latest innovations and changing issues facing women's health care. *Planning Your Pregnancy and Birth* features the most current advances and practices in obstetrics and answers the common questions patients ask ob-gyns before, during, and after pregnancy.

With this book, a woman can work with her doctor to become an active participant in one of the most thrilling and fulfilling times of her life. *Planning Your Pregnancy and Birth* starts in the preconception period, a time when a woman can make any needed adjustments to her health and lifestyle before becoming pregnant. It then leads a woman through prenatal care, labor, delivery, and the postpartum period. The information is designed to help a woman become informed about her pregnancy as well as empower her to make certain choices and discuss with her doctor any questions or concerns she may have.

Now in its third edition, *Planning Your Pregnancy and Birth* has become a classic, guiding almost 2 million women through their pregnancies. This edition has been completely updated, expanded, and reorganized. The book has been divided into four sections: "Planning Your Pregnancy," "Pregnancy," "Labor, Delivery, and Postpartum," and "Special Care." All women will relate to the first three sections on normal pregnancy, and those women with special needs or high-risk pregnancies also will be interested in the "Special Care" section. Many women will want to read the book cover-to-cover, regardless of their situation, whereas other women will only want to read the sections about a normal, healthy pregnancy.

To help readers get the most out of this new edition, key features have been added. Special icons alert readers to answers to common questions and warning signs. Checklists and questionnaires allow a woman to use *Planning Your Pregnancy and Birth* as a tool to guide her pregnancy. Throughout the 40 weeks, a woman can check off items to do or remember and fill in information specific to her and her baby. Then, if she likes, she can bring the book with her to doctor's visits to discuss certain points. After the baby is born, the book can serve as a memento of her pregnancy, as well as a reference for the next one.

This edition also covers new areas of emerging interest to prospective parents. Because breastfeeding is something both the newborn and the mother must learn together, an all-new chapter provides detailed how-to advice with illustrations. Also included is valuable new information about second pregnancies, the use of alternative medicines, automobile safety (including airbags), insurance information, and calculating how much having a baby may cost. Hints are offered to help pregnant women relieve physical and emotional discomforts of pregnancy. Popular features of earlier editions have been retained, including the complete subject index, a personal pregnancy diary that can be used to chart the progress of the pregnancy and note key events, and an extensive glossary that defines terms marked in *boldface italic* type at first mention in the text.

Planning Your Pregnancy and Birth equips a woman for one of the most important and exciting events of her life. We hope our book helps women meet their goal—a safe pregnancy and a healthy baby.

Planning YOUR PREGNANCY and BIRTH

Third Edition

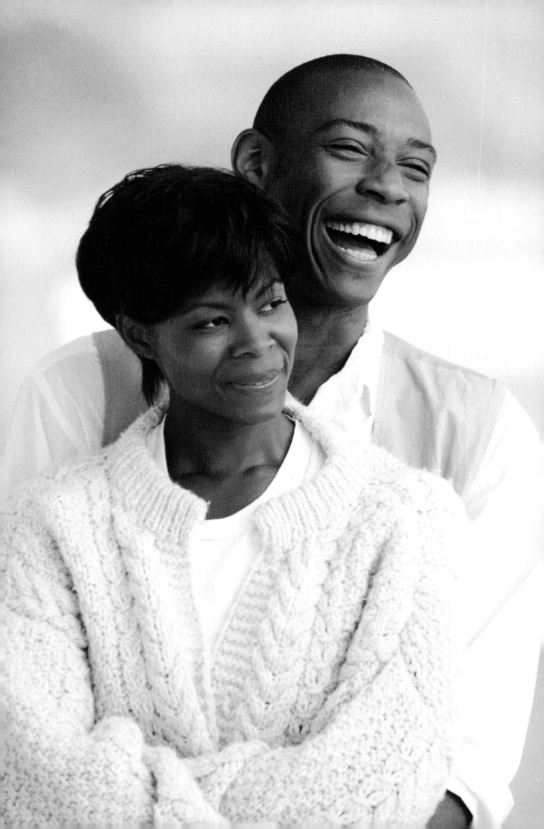

Planning Your Pregnancy

So you're planning to have a baby. Congratulations, and welcome to the first leg of a journey that will transform your life. As great as it is, though, being a parent is a major commitment that's filled with challenges and choices. By planning ahead and making needed changes now—before you become pregnant—you are more likely to be prepared. Certain aspects of pregnancy can't be controlled, but there are some things you can do. Good care and a healthy lifestyle before and during pregnancy increase the odds that you'll end your 40-week journey (and begin a whole new one) with a healthy baby in your arms.

CHAPTER 1

Before You Become Pregnant

If you plan for your pregnancy, you can make choices that are good for your baby. Also, if you are prepared, it will help your body handle the stress of pregnancy, labor, and delivery.

Many women don't know they are pregnant until several weeks after they have *conceived*. These early weeks are key for the baby growing inside you. It's during this time, for instance, that the brain and other organs start to form. Poor health, smoking, drinking alcohol, and using certain drugs can harm normal growth. A healthy body and lifestyle will help promote it. That's why getting proper health care before you even begin trying to get pregnant is so important. It will decrease the chance that either you or your baby will be exposed to harmful things. It also will provide a chance to lower any risks and find and treat any medical problems that you may have.

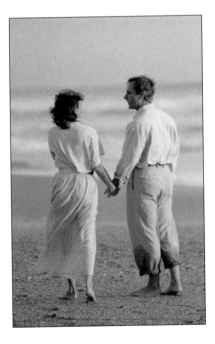

The Pre-Pregnancy Checkup

If you're planning to become pregnant and have already planned a pre-pregnancy checkup, good for you—it's a smart move. If not, do so right away. As a part of this visit, your doctor will ask about your medical and family history, medications you take, any past pregnancies you've had, and your diet and lifestyle. Be open and honest when you respond to these questions. Your answers will help your doctor decide whether you need special care during pregnancy.

This is also a time for you to ask questions. You can seek advice or discuss concerns you might have. There's no such thing as a stupid question, and your health care team is there to inform and guide you.

Your Medical History

Some women have medical conditions—such as *diabetes*, high blood pressure, and seizure disorders—that can cause problems during pregnancy. If you have such a condition, the treatment may vary around the time of pregnancy. Ask your doctor what changes, if any, need to be made to bring your condition under control before you try to get pregnant.

Even if a health problem is well managed, the demands of pregnancy can cause it to worsen. To keep such conditions in check, you may need to make lifestyle changes, see your doctor more often, or get other special care during pregnancy. (The effects of these conditions during pregnancy are discussed in Chapter 14.)

Medications, Herbal Remedies, and Supplements

Many women use medications, remedies, and nutritional supplements to promote their health. Sometimes drugs, herbs, and even vitamins can have the opposite effect during pregnancy. Some medications—including those bought over the counter—can be

Keeping a Menstrual Calendar

When you are thinking of becoming pregnant, you'll want to keep track of your menstrual cycle. By charting your menstrual periods on a calendar for a few months, you'll be able to spot patterns in your cycle (how many days your periods last, for instance, and whether your cycle is typically 25 or 30 days long). You'll also be able to pinpoint the days that you are most fertile—it is most often halfway between the start of one period and the start of the next. To use the calendar, simply circle the days that you menstruate each month. If you can, chart your cycle for a few months and bring the calendar along with you to your checkup.

Jan.	1	2	3	4	5	6	7	8	9	10	11	12	13	14	15	16	17	18	19	20	21	22	23	24	25	26	27	28	29	30	31
Feb.	1	2	3	4	5	6	7	8	9	10	11	12	13	14	15	16	17	18	19	20	21	22	23	24	25	26	27	28	29		
March	1	2	3	4	5	6	7	8	9	10	11	12	13	14	15	16	17	18	19	20	21	22	23	24	25	26	27	28	29	30	31
April	1	2	3	4	5	6	7	8	9	10	11	12	13	14	15	16	17	18	19	20	21	22	23	24	25	26	27	28	29	30	
May	1	2	3	4	5	6	7	8	9	10	11	12	13	14	15	16	17	18	19	20	21	22	23	24	25	26	27	28	29	30	31
June	1	2	3	4	5	6	7	8	9	10	11	12	13	14	15	16	17	18	19	20	21	22	23	24	25	26	27	28	29	30	
July	1	2	3	4	5	6	7	8	9	10	11	12	13	14	15	16	17	18	19	20	21	22	23	24	25	26	27	28	29	30	31
Aug.	1	2	3	4	5	6	7	8	9	10	11	12	13	14	15	16	17	18	19	20	21	22	23	24	25	26	27	28	29	30	31
Sept.	1	2	3	4	5	6	7	8	9	10	11	12	13	14	15	16	17	18	19	20	21	22	23	24	25	26	27	28	29	30	
Oct.	1	2	3	4	5	6	7	8	9	10	11	12	13	14	15	16	17	18	19	20	21	22	23	24	25	26	27	28	29	30	31
Nov.	1	2	3	4	5	6	7	8	9	10	11	12	13	14	15	16	17	18	19	20	21	22	23	24	25	26	27	28	29	30	
Dec.	1	2	3	4	5	6	7	8	9	10	11	12	13	14	15	16	17	18	19	20	21	22	23	24	25	26	27	28	29	30	31

harmful to your baby and shouldn't be taken while you are pregnant. For instance, isotretinoin, a drug to treat acne, can cause *miscarriage* or birth defects. Certain medications used to treat high blood pressure can cause kidney problems in the *fetus*. Herbal remedies (blue cohosh, for instance) may be harmful, too. Just because something is natural doesn't mean it's safe.

Even common nutritional supplements could be harmful. For instance, some multivitamins contain high levels of vitamin A, which has been shown to cause severe birth defects if taken in large doses during pregnancy.

If you take any medications, herbs, or supplements, let your doctor know. Better yet, take the bottles along with you to your

When Should I Stop Birth Control?

Depending on what you use, you may need to switch to another form of birth control a few months before trying to get pregnant. This is because some methods can affect your fertility even after you are no longer using them. When you stop taking *oral contraceptives* ("the Pill"), for instance, it may be a few months before *ovulation* resumes and your menstrual periods become regular. That makes it harder for you to know when you're fertile, so it may take longer to conceive. Periods that aren't regular also make it harder to pinpoint your due date once you become pregnant. If you do conceive while or shortly after using birth control pills, do not worry. It does not cause birth defects as once believed.

There may be a delay in getting pregnant after stopping other forms of hormonal birth control, such as implants and injections. If you're using either method and want to become pregnant, have your doctor remove the implants or stop the injections a few months before you try to conceive. Use a backup method, such as condoms and spermicide, in the meantime.

If you have an *intrauterine device (IUD)*, be sure to have it removed before trying to get pregnant. If you become pregnant with an IUD in place, your doctor will need to remove the device right away so that its presence doesn't lead to infections or pregnancy loss.

pre-pregnancy checkup. You may need to stop using them or switch to others before you try to get pregnant. For more information about harmful agents during pregnancy, see Chapter 5.

Your Family History

Some health conditions occur more often in certain families or ethnic groups. If a close relative has a certain condition, you or your baby could be at greater risk of having it. Your doctor will ask if any family member has diabetes, high blood pressure, seizure disorders, or mental retardation, for instance. Your doctor also will ask if any relatives have a history of twin pregnancies. Ask your closest relatives about their health history before your visit. This way, you'll have the information your doctor needs to detect any risk factors.

Based on your family history or ethnic background, you may be at risk for having a baby with a genetic disorder—a condition that's passed from parent to child. In that case, it's wise to seek genetic counseling before trying to become pregnant. Genetic counselors have been specially trained to assess the risk of inherited disorders. They can help couples understand their chances of having a baby with such a condition. Genetic counseling involves taking a detailed family history and sometimes doing a physical exam and lab tests to pinpoint the risk of inherited disorders. (Even if you show no signs of having a certain disorder yourself, it's possible to be a "carrier" and pass it along to your baby.) For further information about these disorders, see Chapter 13.

Past Pregnancies

Your doctor will review your obstetric history. He or she will ask about any previous pregnancies and any problems you may have had during them.

If you had a problem in a past pregnancy, that doesn't

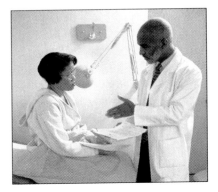

mean it will happen again or that you shouldn't try to get pregnant. Some problems do recur in later pregnancies, but most do not—especially if you receive proper care before and during your pregnancy.

Women who have lost a pregnancy often fear that it will happen again. It's true that 1 in 5 known pregnancies ends in miscarriage and many more occur before a woman even knows she is pregnant. However, most women who miscarry once go on to have normal pregnancies and healthy babies the next time around.

If you have chosen to end a prior pregnancy, you may worry that you'll have trouble getting pregnant again. You may fear you will not be able to carry a baby to term. Most doctors agree that having a single abortion has no effect on future pregnancies. It is possible, though, that having more than one abortion might increase the risk for a low-birth-weight or *preterm* baby. Even in that case, the chance of having a healthy baby is good.

Be sure to let your doctor know if a past pregnancy was complicated by diabetes, high blood pressure, premature labor, preterm birth, or birth defects. If you and your doctor keep a close eye on your health and take steps to reduce your risk, the odds are that problems such as these won't happen again.

Your Lifestyle

Diet

You and your baby will start out with a good supply of the nutrients you both need if you eat right before you become pregnant. A balanced diet is important at all times in your life, but it's vital during pregnancy. The food you eat is the main source of nutrients and energy for your baby. As the baby grows and places new demands on your body, you'll need more calories and nutrients. If you eat a healthy diet before you are pregnant, it's much easier to make minor changes to your diet while you are pregnant.

The nutritional needs of the fetus are small at first, but there's one nutrient that's vital for normal development from the start: folic acid. This B vitamin helps prevent *neural tube defects* (abnormalities of the brain, spine, or their coverings). It's also believed that folic acid helps prevent *cleft lip, congenital heart disease,* and other birth defects. See the box and Chapter 6 to find out more about this important vitamin.

Your doctor will want to know about your diet, so think about these questions before your checkup:

▸ Are you a vegetarian? If so, do you eat dairy products?

▸ Do you have any food allergies?

▸ Do you have trouble digesting milk and other dairy products?

▸ Do you ever fast?

▸ Are you trying to lose weight?

▸ Do you have an eating disorder (*anorexia nervosa* or *bulimia*)?

Folic Acid: The Vital Vitamin

Folic acid, taken before pregnancy and for the first 3 months of pregnancy, can reduce the risk of neural tube defects. The U.S. Public Health Service suggests that all women (even if they are not trying to get pregnant) consume 0.4 mg of folic acid a day. Although folic acid is found in foods such as leafy dark-green vegetables, citrus fruits, and beans, it's hard to eat enough of them to meet the requirement. Breads and cereals are supplemented with folic acid, but they also do not contain enough of the vitamin to meet the requirement. For this reason, doctors advise women to take a daily vitamin with the nutrient.

Women who have had a previous pregnancy that involved a neural tube defect have a higher than average risk of the problem recurring. Such women should take 4 mg daily—10 times the amount normally recommended—for 1 month before conception and during the first 3 months of pregnancy. These women should take folic acid alone rather than as part of a multivitamin. That way, they don't risk overdosing on the other vitamins contained in multivitamin formulas.

Weight

Keeping your weight in a normal range before and during pregnancy is good for your health and your baby's. Excess weight can cause high blood pressure or diabetes. It also puts a strain on the heart. This strain becomes even greater during pregnancy, when your heart works harder to supply blood to you and your baby.

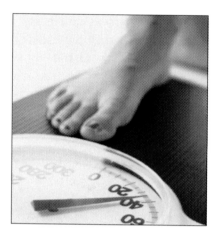

Being too thin, though, can lead to trouble getting pregnant. Being underweight may raise the odds of delivering a low-birth-weight baby. These babies are not easier to deliver and are at risk for problems during labor and after birth.

A woman who's slightly underweight most often can make up the difference by gaining a few extra pounds during pregnancy. But a woman who is overweight should never try to lose weight while she's pregnant. A low-calorie diet could deprive her baby of nutrients needed to grow and develop. In either case, the safest bet is to reach a healthy weight well before you get pregnant. Your doctor can give you advice on the best ways to do that or refer you to a nutritional specialist if needed.

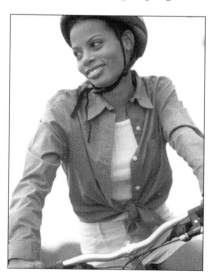

Fitness Level

Good health at any time in your life involves getting plenty of exercise. The type and amount you can do safely during pregnancy depends on your health and how active you are before you are pregnant (see Chapter 5 for specific guidelines).

? Fit or Fat?

Fat is the form in which energy is stored. If you consume too many calories, your body stores the excess as fat. To lose 1 pound, you must use up 3,500 of these stored calories.

Body weight alone isn't a good measure of fat. Exercise burns fat and builds muscle—and muscle is heavier than fat. So a fit woman can have an above-normal body weight, but a below-normal amount of fat. A woman who is not very active, by contrast, may weigh just as much as a fit woman but have more fat and less muscle.

A method for evaluating your weight is "body mass index" (BMI), which compares height to weight. To find out your BMI, find your height on the left-hand column of the chart below. Next, read across the column until you find the weight that's closest to yours. Then look at the bold-faced number at the top of the column. That number is your BMI. Having a BMI above 25 means that you need to shed some pounds. Any amount above 29 is thought to be obese.

Body Mass Index Chart

	19	**20**	**21**	**22**	**23**	**24**	**25**	**26**	**27**	**28**	**29**	**30**	**31**	**32**
Height (inches)						Weight (pounds)								
58	91	96	100	105	110	115	119	124	129	134	138	143	148	153
59	94	99	104	109	114	119	124	128	133	138	143	148	153	158
60	97	102	107	112	118	123	128	133	138	143	148	153	158	163
61	100	106	111	116	122	127	132	137	143	148	153	158	164	169
62	104	109	115	120	126	131	136	142	147	153	158	164	169	175
63	107	113	118	124	130	135	141	146	152	158	163	169	175	180
64	110	116	122	128	134	140	145	151	157	163	169	174	180	186
65	114	120	126	132	138	144	150	156	162	168	174	180	186	192
66	118	124	130	136	142	148	155	161	167	173	179	186	192	198
67	121	127	134	140	146	153	159	166	172	178	185	191	198	204
68	125	131	138	144	151	158	164	171	177	184	190	197	203	210
69	128	135	142	149	155	162	169	176	182	189	196	203	209	216
70	132	139	146	153	160	167	174	181	188	195	202	209	216	222
71	136	143	150	157	165	172	179	186	193	200	208	215	222	229
72	140	147	154	162	169	177	184	191	199	206	213	221	228	235
73	144	151	159	166	174	182	189	197	204	212	219	227	235	242
74	148	155	163	171	179	186	194	202	210	218	225	233	241	249

Adapted from the National Institutes of Health, National Heart, Lung, and Blood Institute. Clinical Guidelines on the Identification, Evaluation, and Treatment of Overweight and Obesity in Adults. Washington, DC: U.S. Government Printing Office, 1998

It is best to exercise regularly before getting pregnant. If you are just starting out, decide on your goals—do you want to improve your heart and lung function, strengthen your muscles, or both? Then choose the exercises that will help you meet your goals. It's best to start with walking, swimming, or bicycling. If you are not used to a lot of exercise, discuss safety guidelines with your doctor ahead of time and take it slow at first. Your target heart rate is a good guide to tell how hard you are working.

Substance Use

Most women know that heavy smoking, drinking, and drug use during pregnancy can have a harmful effect on their baby's health. But what many don't know is that even using these sub-

Target Heart Rate for Nonpregnant Women

To check your heart rate, locate the pulse on the inside of your wrist. Count your pulse for the first 10 seconds after you stop exercising. Multiply this number by 6 to calculate how many times a minute your heart is beating. To find your target heart rate as well as the heart rate it may be unsafe to exceed, find the age category closest to yours on the table below and read across.

Age (years)	Target heart rate (beats per minute)
20	100–150
25	98–146
30	95–142
35	93–138
40	90–135
45	88–131
50	85–127
55	83–123
60	80–120
65	78–116
70	75–113

National Heart, Lung, and Blood Institute, American Heart Association. Exercise and Your Heart. NIH Publication No. 93-1677. Washington, DC: U.S. Government Printing Office, 1993

stances only once in a while, or in small doses, still can do harm. This is also true of medications that are not used as prescribed.

Women who smoke or drink alcohol may have a harder time getting pregnant. What's more, there's growing evidence that if your partner smokes, drinks, or uses drugs, it can lower his fertility, damage his sperm, and have a harmful effect on the fetus. At the very least, living with someone who smokes means that you are likely to breathe in harmful amounts of secondhand smoke. In turn, your developing baby is exposed. This is also a risk for the baby after he or she is born.

If you smoke tobacco, drink alcohol, or take drugs, now is the time to quit. Even if you can't quit, cutting back helps. It takes patience and plenty of support to end a habit—especially if it's long-standing. Don't be afraid or ashamed to ask for help. Your doctor can suggest ways to get through the early stages as well as refer you to support groups. Giving up something that you rely on to relax or to deal with stress may be one of the hardest things you'll ever do, but it also will be one of the most worthwhile.

Your Environment

Some substances found in the home or the workplace may make it harder for a woman to conceive or could harm her fetus. If you are planning to get pregnant, look closely at what's around you. Think about the chemicals you use in your home or garden. Some hobbies, such as stained glass and darkroom work, might expose you to harmful substances. Find out from your employer whether you might be exposed at work to toxic substances such as lead or mercury, chemicals such as pesticides or solvents, or radiation. Then discuss your level of exposure with your doctor as well as your employee health division, personnel office, or union representative. If you do come into regular contact with a substance that may be harmful, take steps to avoid it (see "Harmful Agents" in Chapter 5).

Radiation, a form of energy sent out in invisible waves, is used in certain medical and industrial jobs. It's also used to take X-rays to diagnose disease. Women who are planning a pregnancy and who come into contact with radiation at work should ask for monthly exposure readings. The amount of radiation used to take a chest X-ray or single dental film won't affect fertility or harm a fetus. It's wise, though, to avoid being exposed as much as you can and to wear abdominal shields if you have an X-ray done. However, the level of radiation used to treat diseases such as cancer is much higher and can be harmful during pregnancy.

Infections

Certain infections during pregnancy can cause severe birth defects or illness in a fetus. These infections may be prevented with proper *vaccination*. Before you start trying to get pregnant, ask your doctor if you need to be immunized against measles, mumps, tetanus, polio, hepatitis, chickenpox (varicella), or rubella (German measles). Try to get your childhood vaccination record before your pre-pregnancy checkup. Even if you were vaccinated as a child, though, your immunity to certain diseases may have worn off.

Some vaccines cannot safely be given during pregnancy. If you need vaccines, get them at least 3 months before trying to conceive. During this time, keep using birth control. If you are planning a trip to a country where you might come into contact with diseases that aren't common in the United States, you may need other vaccines. (For more information, see "Travel" in Chapter 5 and "Vaccines" in Chapter 16).

Other infections that can be harmful during pregnancy are those passed on by sexual contact—*sexually transmitted diseases (STDs)*. These diseases can affect your ability to conceive and can infect and harm your baby. The most common STDs are:

▶ *Chlamydia*

▶ *Gonorrhea*

▶ *Genital herpes*

▶ *Genital warts*

▶ *Trichomoniasis*

▶ *Hepatitis B virus*

▶ *Syphilis*

▶ *Human immunodeficiency virus (HIV)*

Using condoms and spermicide regularly will lower your risk of getting an STD. A woman who isn't using these forms of birth control (for instance, if she's trying to conceive) is at a higher risk of getting an STD if she has sex with more than one partner or if her partner has sex with someone else.

If you suspect that you may have been exposed to an STD, see your doctor right away to be tested and treated. Your partner also should be treated. Neither of you should have sex until treatment is finished. STDs such as herpes, HIV, and hepatitis B

? Are Your Immunizations Up-to-Date?

Although some vaccines are safe to receive during pregnancy, it's best to have all needed immunizations before you become pregnant. Women should have the following immunizations:

3 months before pregnancy
Measles–mumps–rubella vaccine (once if not immune)

1 month before pregnancy
Varicella vaccine*

Safe during pregnancy
Tetanus–diphtheria booster (every 10 years)
Hepatitis A vaccine*
Hepatitis B vaccine*
Influenza vaccine (if you will be in the second or third trimester of pregnancy during flu season)
Pneumococcal vaccine*

See Chapter 16 for more information about infections during pregnancy.

*These immunizations are given as needed based on risk factors. If you don't know whether you need one, check with your health care provider.

have no known cures. If your doctor knows that you have one of these conditions, though, he or she can take steps during your pregnancy and delivery to lower the risk of your baby being harmed by the disease or catching it from you.

Keep in mind, too, that many STDs have no symptoms in the early stages. The earlier an STD is found and treated, the lower the long-term risk.

Later Childbearing

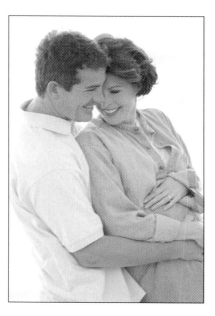

These days, women are becoming mothers later in life than in prior generations. This may be because more women are working and living longer and healthier lives. Women also can use new techniques to promote their fertility. Older moms often worry that their age will affect their fertility and the health of their baby. There's no set age that is unsafe for women to become pregnant. For women older than age 35, the chances of having a normal pregnancy and healthy baby are great—especially if they get good pre-pregnancy and *prenatal care*. Even so, more mature mothers often have concerns about pregnancy that don't apply to younger mothers. Among them:

▸ *Infertility.* A woman's fertility slowly declines starting in her early 30s. After that time, it may take longer to get pregnant.

▸ *Medical and obstetric problems.* As women get older, conditions such as high blood pressure and diabetes tend to occur more often. Because pregnancy puts new demands on a woman's body, the risk of complications may be higher for expectant mothers with these problems. They are more likely to need to visit the doctor more often, need special tests, stay in the hospital before their baby's birth, and require special care during labor and delivery.

▶ *Birth defects.* The risk of some birth defects increases with age, but it remains low well into a woman's 30s. In most cases, women age 35 and older are offered testing for genetic disorders and other medical problems before and during pregnancy. If there's a problem, it often can be spotted early enough to allow time to decide whether to become pregnant or continue a pregnancy. (For more information on birth defects, see Chapter 13.)

▶ *Breast cancer.* Because of changes that occur in women's breasts during pregnancy and after the baby is born, breast cancer screening through self-exams or breast exams by the doctor are less able to detect breast cancer. Thus, if you are planning a pregnancy and are age 40 or older, you may wish to have a *mammogram* (an X-ray of the breasts) before getting pregnant.

Planning Your Pregnancy Care

Aside from you and your partner, the person who will care for you during pregnancy is one of the most important players in your pregnancy. Choosing a caregiver isn't a choice to make lightly.

What's the best way to go about finding the right person? Some women are happy to stick with the health care provider they have been seeing for routine gynecologic care. Other women ask friends or relatives who have become mothers not too long ago. Still others choose the hospital or birthing center where they'd like to deliver their baby and ask the staff there to refer them to someone. (Keep in mind that your health insurance policy may restrict your choices.)

Three types of providers offer medical care for pregnancy and birth: obstetrician–gynecologists (ob-gyns), family practitioners, and certified nurse–midwives (CNMs).

▸ *Obstetrician–gynecologists.* Ob-gyns are doctors who specialize in the reproductive care of women. After graduating from medical school, ob-gyns complete a 4-year course of specialized training in obstetrics and gynecology. To be certified, a physician must pass written and oral tests to show that he or she has obtained the knowledge and skills required for the medical and surgical care of women. A certified ob-gyn can become a Fellow of the American College of Obstetricians and Gynecologists. This group offers continuing educational programs to help physicians stay up-to-date with the latest medical advances.

▸ *Family practitioners.* Doctors in family practice provide general care for most conditions, including pregnancy. After completing medical school, family practitioners receive further training in family practice (including obstetrics) and become certified by passing an exam. They are able to care for normal pregnancies and deliveries.

▸ *Certified nurse–midwives.* CNMs are registered nurses who have been specially trained to care for women and their babies from early pregnancy through labor, delivery, and the weeks after birth. They have completed an accredited nursing program and have a graduate degree in midwifery. To be certified, they must pass a national exam and maintain an active nursing license. They also must have an arrangement with a qualified doctor to provide backup support. They are trained to care for healthy women with normal pregnancies and consult with or refer patients to a doctor if medical problems arise.

Other specialists are part of a team of health professionals that provides care based on an expectant mother's special needs. Some may be employed by the doctor's practice or the teaching hospital where the doctor works. Others are consulted as needed. Their qualifications differ, but each one has an important role in making sure your pregnancy and birth go well. Here's a brief look at who may be members of this team.

Physicians

▸ Residents are physicians who have graduated from medical school but are still in training at a teaching hospital.

▸ Pediatricians are doctors with specialized training in the medical care of infants and children.

▸ Neonatologists are pediatricians with special training in the medical care of newborns.

▸ Anesthesiologists are doctors who provide pain relief during labor and delivery. This also can be done by a nurse anesthetist.

▸ Maternal–fetal medicine specialists are ob-gyns with extra training in handling pregnancies complicated by medical or obstetric problems. Women most often are referred to them by their regular doctor.

Nurses

▸ Nurse practitioners perform duties such as taking medical histories, doing physical exams, and diagnosing and treating common illnesses. They are registered nurses who have completed further training and, in some cases, passed a certification exam.

▸ Registered nurses assist obstetricians in providing care, education, and medical counseling to women. They have graduated from nursing school and passed a number of exams.

▸ Labor and delivery nurses help care for women and their babies during labor, delivery, and right after birth.

▸ Neonatal nurses help care for newborns before they are discharged from the hospital.

▸ Postpartum nurses help care for the mother after birth.

Other

▸ Childbirth educators teach parents-to-be about pregnancy, childbirth, and parenting.

- Dietitians give advice on nutrition during pregnancy and breastfeeding.

- Genetic counselors evaluate a baby's risk of having birth defects and provide counseling to expectant parents.

- Social workers can provide counseling and information about community services for families.

- *Lactation* specialists are breastfeeding experts who can tell you more about such things as methods of breastfeeding and pumping your breast milk.

- Physician assistants work under the guidance of doctors and perform a variety of medical duties.

Another factor to think about is whether a pregnancy-care provider is in a group, collaborative, or solo practice. In a group practice, constant coverage is provided by two or more doctors. You may have a primary doctor but receive care from the other members from time to time. In a collaborative practice, a doctor and a nurse, certified nurse–midwife, or other health professionals work as a team. In a solo practice, one doctor provides complete care for all of his or her patients.

Your Baby's Birthplace

The day your baby enters the world may seem like it's ages away. But the setting for your newborn's delivery can have a big impact on your pregnancy care and your birth experience. Thus, it's wise to weigh your options before you are pregnant.

Your choices will depend on what your area offers, where your caregiver handles deliveries, and what your health insurance provider will cover. The areas for labor and delivery vary from one hospital to another. You will be given information about the choices available. You can tour the hospitals in your community to see which types of settings appeal to you.

Many hospitals offer birthing rooms where the family can stay with you and provide support. Birthing rooms share the staff and services of a more traditional labor and delivery suite, which may

Interviewing the Provider

Before you decide who will care for you during your pregnancy, visit different providers until you find one that you like and trust. Call the practice ahead of time to get basic questions about location, hours, and insurance out of the way before you meet with the doctor. During the interview, feel free to discuss anything that is of concern to you or your partner. Some questions to think about:

How close is the practice to your home or work? _____

Does the practice accept your insurance plan? _____

What are the provider's fees and how is payment handled? _____

_____

Where does the doctor have hospital privileges? _____

How are urgent questions or emergency care handled? _____

_____

What's the provider's belief about pain relief during labor, *fetal monitoring, episiotomy, cesarean birth,* breastfeeding, and other issues that interest you? _____

_____

_____

Is it likely that your doctor will deliver the baby? _____

What is the doctor's cesarean birth rate and how does it compare with the hospital's rate of cesarean births? _____

_____

be needed if a problem occurs. They provide a comfortable setting for labor, delivery, and, in most cases, postpartum recovery. Some allow the entire birth process, including the postpartum stay, to happen in one room. These rooms are called LDRs (labor/delivery/recovery) or LDRPs (labor/delivery/recovery/postpartum).

There are also freestanding birthing centers that are not in a hospital. These centers may not offer all the services you may need if an emergency arises. Because of this, the safest places to give birth are thought to be a hospital or birthing center within the hospital complex.

When selecting your care, you may wish to ask about policies regarding fathers or others in the delivery room. Most hospitals

Evaluating Birth Sites

When you tour a facility, be sure to come with a list of questions about certain policies. For instance:

Who's allowed to be present at the birth? _____

Are there a limited number of birthing rooms (meaning you may be booked into a traditional delivery room if they are full)?

_____

Does the hospital have set rules about the use of medical procedures such as fetal monitoring and intravenous (IV) lines during labor, or does it leave such decisions up to individual caregivers?

_____

Are women in labor allowed to move about freely or are they required to stay in bed? _____

What special care (such as a Neonatal Intensive Care Unit) can the hospital provide if your baby is born with a medical problem?

_____

Will your baby be allowed to room with you after birth, or will he or she need to stay in the newborn nursery? _____

Does the hospital or birthing center employ a lactation consultant or provide other services to help new mothers breastfeed?

_____

Does the hospital have an anesthesiologist on site full time?

_____

permit support people in both labor and delivery rooms. It is wise to know the hospital's policy in advance so you can plan.

If you have health problems during your pregnancy or complications are likely during birth, you may have to deliver at a specific hospital. It is possible that the hospital, which must be equipped to handle complex procedures, may not be near where you live.

Money Matters

The cost of having a baby is high. You should consider in advance how you will pay for it. If you have insurance, it's vital to make sure that you are covered for all that you think you are. Some health plans, for instance, don't include pregnancy care or will pay for only the most routine medical tests and procedures. That could become an issue if you develop problems during pregnancy or birth or have a baby with health problems. Read your policy to make sure you are covered. Also check to see how much of the cost of infertility treatments (if needed), obstetric care, prenatal tests, hospital charges, well-baby care, and postpartum birth control your insurer will cover.

If your coverage doesn't start until a certain date, you may want to think about delaying your pregnancy until then. Also make sure that the provider you'd like to see is part of the plan, as is the hospital where you want to deliver. In many cases, seeing a provider or going to a facility that's out of an insurance company's "network" means that you'll be out, too—that is, out-of-pocket for some or all expenses.

The Health Insurance Portability and Accountability Act, passed in 1996, protects most women who switch health plans during pregnancy or enroll in a plan after she becomes pregnant. This means that if you change jobs and insurance plans during your pregnancy, you cannot be denied insurance coverage for care related to your pregnancy. It does not matter how long you were with your insurance plan before you switched. Also, your newborn cannot be denied coverage as long as you sign him or her up for health insurance within 30 days of birth.

How Much Do Babies Cost?

To get a better idea of the impact a baby can have on your pocketbook, think about these questions:

Will you need to move to a bigger house or apartment to make room for the baby? How much more money will you need to pay for it? _____

How long will you take off work? Are you planning to leave your job? How much income will you lose? _____

_____

Do you have a partner who earns enough to cover costs during your time at home? _____

If not, do you have money in savings you could use? How much?

_____

Will you need to pay for childcare? What can you afford? _____

_____

Can you get baby clothes and supplies from friends or relatives, or will you need to purchase these items?

_____

Does your state or county have programs that can help you? (You may qualify for help even if you are working. Federal assistance programs also are available.) _____

_____

Taking these steps before you even start trying to get pregnant may seem like a lot of work. Making plans ahead of time is well worth the time and effort, though. Starting your pregnancy with a healthy body will give your baby the best start in life. Knowing the issues involved in becoming a parent will make them seem more fun and less scary. You and your partner will be well prepared to deal with all that's in store during the thrilling months ahead.

CHAPTER 2

How Reproduction Occurs

Now that you have taken care of your pre-pregnancy checkup and made some healthy lifestyle changes, you can start trying to make a baby. A finely tuned series of events must take place for conception to occur and for the cells to start growing into a tiny human being.

Knowing how reproduction works will help you figure out when you are most fertile—in other words, when you're most likely to get pregnant. It also will help you understand the rapid changes that take place in your body during early pregnancy.

The Menstrual Cycle

A woman's fertility depends on her menstrual cycle. Changes that occur during each cycle are caused by hormones—substances made by your body to control certain functions. Each month, hormones direct your *uterus* to build up a lining of blood-rich tissue (*endometrium*). These hormones also send a signal for an egg to ripen in a *follicle*—tiny, fluid-filled clusters of cells in your *ovaries*. When the egg is ripe, it's released from the ovary and moves into a fallopian tube, one of a pair of ducts that connects the ovaries to the uterus. This process is called ovulation. Signs that you may be ovulating include a twinge or cramp—called mittelschmerz, for "middle pain"—in your lower abdomen or

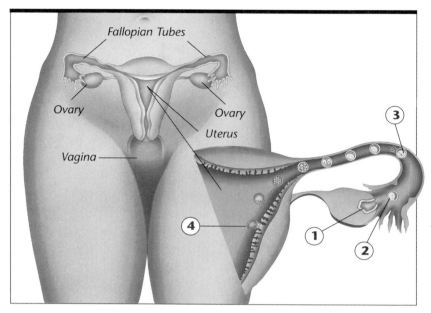

Each month during ovulation an egg is released (*1*) and moves into one of the fallopian tubes (*2*). If a woman has sex around this time, an egg may meet a sperm in the fallopian tube and the two will join (*3*). This is called fertilization. The fertilized egg then moves through the fallopian tube into the uterus and becomes attached there to grow during pregnancy (*4*).

back. You also may notice some breast tenderness, an increase in cervical mucus (vaginal discharge), or an increase in sexual desire around the time an egg is released.

The average menstrual cycle lasts about 28 days, counting from the first day of one period (day 1) to the first day of the next. Cycles ranging from as little as 23 days to as many as 35 days are normal. Your own cycle may vary somewhat from month to month. By keeping a menstrual calendar (see Chapter 1) for a few months, you can get an idea of what's normal for you. When you become pregnant, the calendar will make it easier to figure out your baby's due date.

Ovulation most often occurs halfway through your cycle—on day 14 of 28, for instance. After you have ovulated, the egg moves through one of the fallopian tubes toward your uterus. If it isn't

The Menstrual Cycle

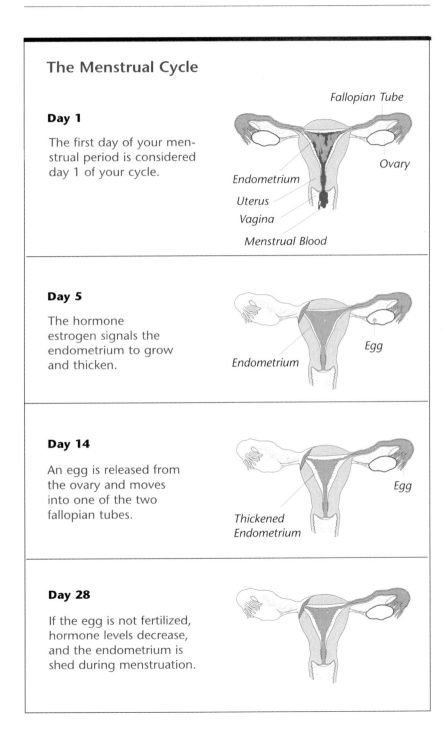

Day 1

The first day of your menstrual period is considered day 1 of your cycle.

Fallopian Tube

Ovary

Endometrium

Uterus

Vagina

Menstrual Blood

Day 5

The hormone estrogen signals the endometrium to grow and thicken.

Egg

Endometrium

Day 14

An egg is released from the ovary and moves into one of the two fallopian tubes.

Egg

Thickened Endometrium

Day 28

If the egg is not fertilized, hormone levels decrease, and the endometrium is shed during menstruation.

fertilized (joined by a sperm) in the fallopian tube, your body absorbs it. Then, the levels of hormones decrease. This signals the lining of the uterus to shed. This shedding is your monthly period.

If the egg is fertilized, it becomes attached to the lining of the uterus. The fertilized egg then starts to grow in the lush uterine lining that will become its home for the next 40 weeks. You may not know it for weeks, but you're pregnant!

Fertilization

Fertilization is the fusion of an egg and a sperm in the fallopian tube. If all goes according to plan during the days and weeks that

Hormones:
Key Players in Menstruation and Pregnancy

Each step in the creation of new life—from *menstruation* to ovulation to implantation—is led by these hormones:

▶ *Estrogen* and *progesterone.* Produced by the ovaries, these hormones trigger the lining of the uterus to thicken during each menstrual cycle and to be shed if pregnancy doesn't occur. After an egg is fertilized, a sharp increase in estrogen and progesterone levels prevents further ovulation.

▶ *Follicle-stimulating hormone (FSH)* and *luteinizing hormone (LH).* These hormones are made by the **pituitary gland,** a small organ at the base of the brain. FSH causes eggs to ripen in the ovaries. LH triggers their release.

▶ *Gonadotropin-releasing hormone* (GnRH). This hormone, also made in the brain, tells the pituitary gland when to produce FSH and LH.

▶ *Human chorionic gonadotropin* (hCG). Made by certain cells from the fertilized and quickly dividing egg, hCG spurs increased estrogen and progesterone production during pregnancy. It's the telltale hormone that pregnancy tests are designed to detect.

follow this union, pregnancy results. Each sperm and egg contains half of a fetus's genetic makeup.

Sperm are tiny cells made by a man's testes in the sac (scrotum) below his penis. When sperm cells mature, they leave the testes through small tubes called the vas deferens. The vas deferens transport the sperm to the seminal vesicles and the prostate gland, small organs located near the bladder. There, the sperm mix with seminal fluid to create semen.

When a man climaxes during sex, this semen spurts (ejaculates) from his penis through a tube called the **urethra**. This deposits millions of sperm in a woman's **vagina**. A man's orgasm, therefore, is vital to conception. A woman, however, doesn't have to climax to get pregnant.

After ejaculation, the sperm "swim" up through the **cervix**, into the uterus, and out into the fallopian tubes. Sperm can live inside a woman's body for 3 days or more. An egg's life span, though, is short—12–24 hours. If an egg is waiting in a fallopian tube when a man ejaculates, or if one is released during the next few days and fuses with a sperm, fertilization occurs.

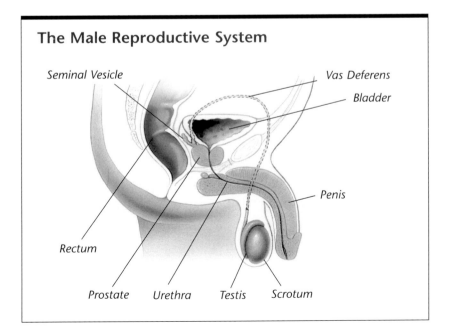

The Male Reproductive System

The fused egg and sperm then move through the fallopian tube to the lining of the uterus. There it implants and starts to grow. This fertilized egg is called an **embryo** for the first 8 weeks. Then it is called a fetus.

Some couples worry that having sex every day will reduce the number of sperm from a man's body and make it harder for him to get his partner pregnant. There's no need for concern—healthy testes produce new sperm all the time, so daily sex shouldn't be a problem as long as a man's sperm count is normal. The sperm count is the number of active sperm in one milliliter (less than a half teaspoon) of semen. A normal sperm count—one of the first things doctors check if a couple is having trouble conceiving—is between 20 million and 250 million per milliliter.

Detecting Ovulation

To raise the odds of getting pregnant, sex has to happen during a small window of time near ovulation. How do you know when you are ovulating? There's no foolproof method to make sure that an ovary has released an egg, but there are a number of methods that are useful. One method is to note changes in your body. Look out for telltale signs of ovulation: cramps, tender breasts, cervical mucus, or an increased desire to have sex. Other methods—especially when they are used in combination—can give you a pretty good idea:

▶ *Chart your cycle.* The simplest way to spot your fertile days is to check the menstrual calendar you have been keeping. First, figure out how long your cycles tend to last and pinpoint the day your next period is due to start. If your periods are regular, count back 14 days. If they are not regular, count back to the first day of your last period and divide the total. Chances are, the result will be the day you will ovulate.

▶ *Know when you are most fertile.* You also can detect ovulation by watching for changes in your cervical mucus. A few days after your period ends, rising estrogen levels trigger the production of cervical mucus. As your body prepares to release an egg,

Ovulation

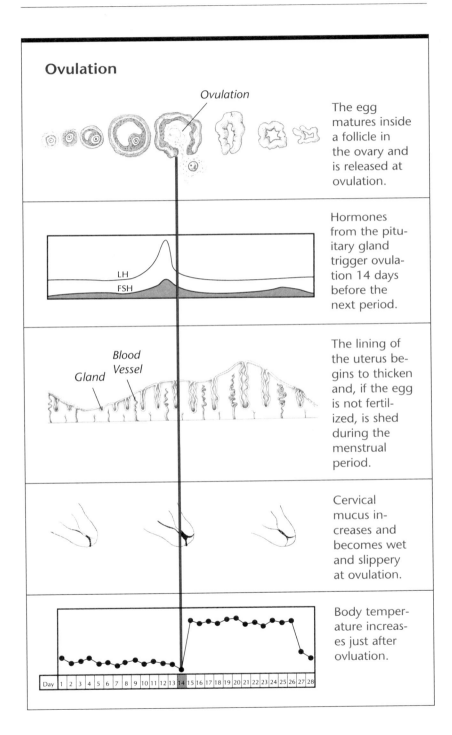

Ovulation

The egg matures inside a follicle in the ovary and is released at ovulation.

LH

FSH

Hormones from the pituitary gland trigger ovulation 14 days before the next period.

Gland

Blood Vessel

The lining of the uterus begins to thicken and, if the egg is not fertilized, is shed during the menstrual period.

Cervical mucus increases and becomes wet and slippery at ovulation.

Body temperature increases just after ovulation.

| Day | 1 | 2 | 3 | 4 | 5 | 6 | 7 | 8 | 9 | 10 | 11 | 12 | 13 | 14 | 15 | 16 | 17 | 18 | 19 | 20 | 21 | 22 | 23 | 24 | 25 | 26 | 27 | 28 |

this mucus increases in volume and becomes thicker. (To get a good look at your cervical mucus, gently wipe your vaginal opening with a clean finger or a piece of toilet tissue before you urinate.) Just before ovulation, you produce more cervical mucus. It becomes clear, slippery, and stretchy—it looks and feels like a raw egg white. This kind of mucus smoothes the way for sperm to enter the uterus and swim up the fallopian tubes. Your fertile period begins with the first signs of slippery mucus and continues through the day you ovulate. After ovulation, an increase in progesterone makes cervical mucus sparse and dense. This makes it harder for sperm to swim through the cervix.

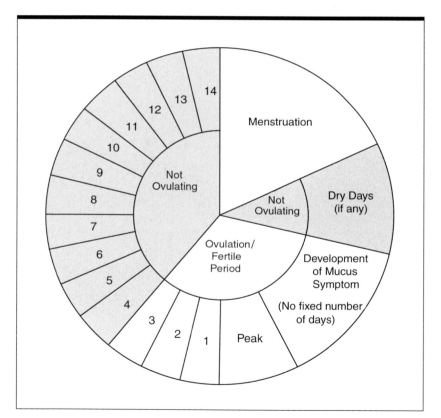

This chart may help you predict the days you will be ovulating. You produce more cervical mucus just before ovulation—about halfway through your menstrual cycle.

▶ *Track your temperature.* Most women's **basal body temperature** increases slightly—about half a degree—after they ovulate. To use this method, take your temperature at the same
time every morning, before you get out of bed. Chart the temperature on a graph that also shows the days you menstruate.
After you have done this for a few months, you'll begin to
spot a pattern that will help you predict when you will ovulate. Your temperature will go up 24–48 hours after you ovulate.

▶ *Use ovulation-predictor kits.* Ovulation-predictor kits are
home tests that you can buy without a prescription. They measure the level of luteinizing hormone (LH) in your urine. When
LH levels increase, it means that one of your ovaries is about to
release an egg.

Fertility

How long will it take before you become pregnant? That
depends on a number of factors—your age, your health, and
how often you have sex, for instance. Most couples are able to
conceive within 6 months of having regular sex without birth
control. Almost all (85 out of 100) are pregnant within a year.
The remaining 15% face fertility problems—they have tried to
get pregnant but cannot.

Couples who have not been able to conceive after 12
months of having regular sex should discuss it with their doctor. Many of these couples will be able to have children with-

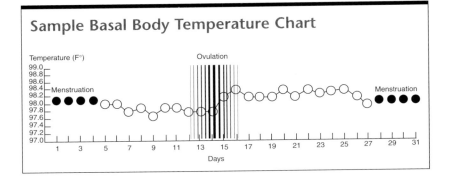

Sample Basal Body Temperature Chart

out medical help—it's just a matter of time. Women older than age 35, whose natural fertility has begun to decline and whose reproductive time is more limited, may want to consult a doctor after 6 months of trying.

A fertility evaluation begins with a medical history and general physical checkup for the woman and the man. The medical history includes questions about past pelvic surgery or illness such as appendicitis or sexually transmitted diseases (STDs), which can harm the reproductive organs. The doctor also asks about the couple's sexual habits to find out if infertility may be tied to the timing or frequency of sex. In that case, they may simply need advice on their sexual practices. Also, possible physical causes of infertility, such as diabetes or being over- or underweight, are ruled out.

If the medical histories and physical exams don't turn up any clues, more in-depth testing will be needed to find the cause of the problem and to find out whether it can be treated. An infertility workup often includes:

▸ *Semen analysis.* A sample of a man's semen is examined under a microscope. This is done to count sperm and to see whether they are formed correctly and move the way they should.

▸ *Hormone screening.* The levels of the hormones that allow ovulation and implantation to take place are measured in a woman's blood and urine.

▸ *Evaluation of reproductive organs.* A doctor examines the uterus, fallopian tubes, or ovaries using an X-ray, **ultrasound** (a device that uses sound waves to examine the fetus), or a laparoscope (a tiny device like a telescope that is inserted into the body to view the pelvic organs or perform surgery). The purpose is to see whether these organs are normal.

In some cases, these tests find nothing and the reason for a couple's infertility remains unknown. If doctors can find the cause of the problem, though, they often can correct it. Treatment options include:

▸ Medications to induce ovulation

▸ Artificial insemination with sperm from the partner or a donor

▸ Assisted reproduction techniques (such as *in vitro fertilization*)

▸ Surgery to open blocked fallopian tubes

Your doctor can tell you more about these methods and help you figure out which of them may be worth trying. Keep in mind that fertility treatment isn't for everyone.

The Months Ahead

Once conception has taken place, a new life begins to grow inside a woman's body. Whether your pregnancy is a long-wished-for goal or a pleasant surprise, the coming months will bring with them drama and suspense, questions and knowledge, and tears and joy.

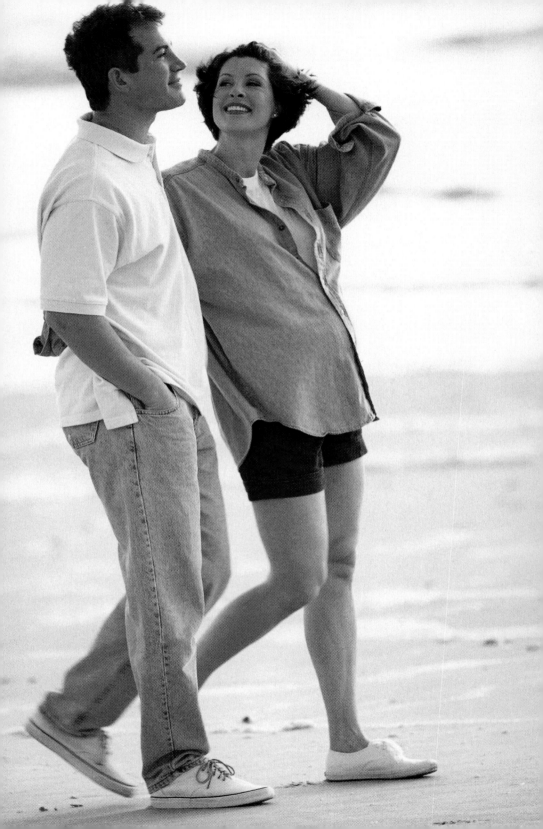

Pregnancy

Pregnancy is a time of major change. From the very start, your baby-to-be alters your body and the way you live your daily life—not to mention your hopes and plans for the future. For 40 weeks, the baby depends on you for all the things it needs to grow and thrive. You'll barely make a move without thinking about how it will affect your small passenger.

It's normal to worry about your baby. Keep in mind that most infants are born healthy. A few women, though, have problems during pregnancy that can affect their baby's health. See your doctor as soon as you suspect you are pregnant, get regular prenatal care, make well-informed decisions, and stick to a healthy lifestyle. If you do, the odds are good that your pregnancy will be as joyful as it should be. It's up to you to take an active role in your pregnancy. This allows you to give your baby a great gift: the chance to start life with a body and mind that are as strong and healthy as possible.

CHAPTER 3

A New Life Begins

After conception, your fetus grows while nestled safely in your uterus. The uterus is a small, pear-shaped organ located in your pelvis between your bladder and rectum. During pregnancy, the lining of this muscular structure thickens and its blood vessels enlarge to nourish a growing fetus. As pregnancy progresses, the uterus expands to make room for the growing baby. By the time your baby is born, your uterus may be nearly a thousand times its normal size.

Once conception has taken place, the changes in your body— and your baby—are rapid. After an egg is fertilized, it splits into identical cells. These cells then split again and again—two cells become four, four cells become eight, and so on.

By the time the cluster of cells reaches your uterus and sinks into its lush lining, it's shaped like a tiny sphere. Half of this budding ball of life (called a blastocyst) will develop into an organ called the *placenta*. The placenta functions as a life-support system during pregnancy, taking substances from the mother's blood and delivering them to her baby. The other half of the sphere will become your baby.

As the placenta begins to take shape, small fingerlike projections grow out of it. In these projections, called *chorionic villi*, blood vessels form. The tips of the vessels burrow into the uterine wall and tap the mother's blood supply. The blood systems of the mother and fetus are in close contact during pregnancy.

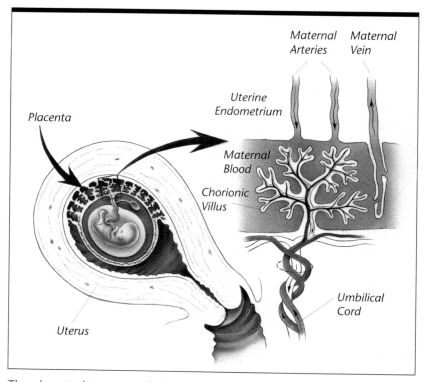

The placenta is composed of many lobes of chorionic villi. Chorionic villi contain fetal cells. One of these lobes is shown on a larger scale at right.

The placenta delivers oxygen, nutrients, and hormones from mother to fetus. It also can transfer more harmful agents, such as drugs, viruses, and other products. The exchange goes both ways. The placenta filters waste products from the fetus's blood and deposits them in the mother's blood. This waste then is disposed of by her kidneys. Once the baby is born and the placenta has finished serving its purpose, it's delivered as the afterbirth.

On the side of the placenta nearest the fetus, the *umbilical cord* forms. This tube-like structure is attached to your baby in the center of his or her belly. Once the cord is cut after delivery, it becomes the baby's navel. Inside the cord are three blood vessels. One delivers blood enriched with oxygen and nutrients to the fetus. The other two transport blood filled with waste products from the baby back to the placenta.

The fetus grows very quickly. It starts as a single cell that carries the genetic blueprint for the baby's entire physical makeup. Just 40 weeks later, it's a fully formed human being that's able to cry, feed, and kick.

Are You Pregnant?

The first sign that you are pregnant often is a missed menstrual period. A late period doesn't always mean that a baby's on the way, though. Not all women start their periods at the same time each month. Even if you usually have regular periods, stress, illness, or a change in your exercise or eating habits can delay menstruation. Thus, also be on the lookout for these other symptoms of early pregnancy:

▶ Spotting or a very light menstrual period

▶ Tender breasts

▶ Feeling very tired

Warning Signs

Get medical help right away if you suspect you are pregnant or are in early pregnancy and have any of these symptoms:

▶ Cramps or severe abdominal pain

▶ Spotting that lasts more than 1 day

▶ Bleeding that's as heavy as a menstrual period or soaks a sanitary pad each hour

▶ Blood clots, bright red blood, or flesh-like tissue from your vagina

▶ Heavy, foul-smelling vaginal discharge

▶ Faintness or dizziness

▶ Painful urination

▶ Vomiting so severe that you can't keep any food or liquid down

- Upset stomach or nausea

- Feeling bloated

- Frequent urination

- Being moody

If you have missed your period and have one or more of these signs, you could be pregnant. This is true even if you have been using birth control. The next step: buy a home pregnancy test or visit your doctor's office or clinic.

Pregnancy Tests

Thanks to advances in testing, pregnancy can be confirmed as early as the first day of a missed period. How? Soon after conception, the developing placenta produces human chorionic gonadotropin (hCG). This hormone is released into the mother's urine and blood, where it is picked up by a pregnancy test.

Home pregnancy tests are simple to use and can be bought over the counter. Most tests involve urinating on a chemically treated stick or dipping it in a cup of your urine. If hCG is present, the chemicals in the stick will react to the hormone and produce a signal in the test's result window—a blue line, a pink dot, or a red "plus" sign, for instance.

The tests are accurate as long as you use them correctly. Still, they can give an incorrect (false-positive or false-negative) result if you are taking certain medications, if you don't follow the directions, or if you take the test too early. A false-positive result tells you that you are pregnant when you really aren't. A false-negative result tells you that you aren't pregnant when you really are.

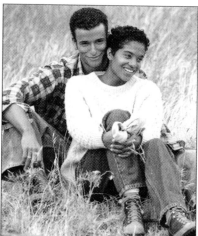

If a home test result is negative but your period doesn't start in a couple of days or you develop other pregnancy symptoms, repeat the test or ask your doctor to give you a test. (See the doctor right away if you have heavy vaginal bleeding or stomach pain, no matter what the test results are.) If a home test is positive, visit your doctor as soon as possible. The sooner you start your prenatal care, the better off you and your baby will be. If you're not already taking prenatal vitamins, ask your doctor for a prescription.

Counting Down

The first day of my last menstrual period was: _____

I think I ovulated on: _____

My pregnancy test result was positive on: _____

The type of test I used was: _____

My symptoms are: _____

_____

_____

_____

My first prenatal check-up is on: _____

Questions for my doctor: _____

_____

_____

_____

_____

_____

_____

_____

_____

The Countdown Begins

At times in the coming months, you may feel like you have been pregnant forever. A "typical" pregnancy lasts for 280 days, counting from the first day of your last menstrual period. That's roughly 40 weeks. A normal range, however, is from as few as 259 days to as many as 294 days (37–42 weeks). The 40 weeks of pregnancy are divided into three *trimesters*. These last about 12–13 weeks each (or about 3 months):

▸ 1st trimester: 0–13 weeks

▸ 2nd trimester: 14–28 weeks

▸ 3rd trimester: 29–40 weeks

Many changes begin taking place inside your body as your baby grows. You won't see most of these changes at first. There's no doubt you'll feel them, however. Although the basics of carrying a baby are the same for almost every woman, no two pregnancies are alike. Even for the same woman, pregnancy is often very different the second or third time around. (For more details on the physical changes you are likely to experience and on how each pregnancy can differ, see Chapter 7.) Knowing what's taking place in your body and with your developing baby will help you prepare for the weeks ahead.

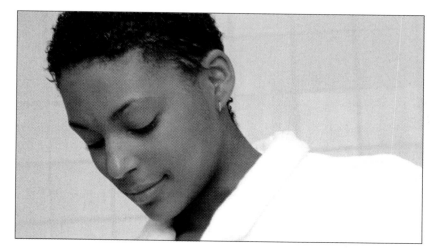

Growth and Changes During Pregnancy

The First Trimester: 0–13 Weeks

Mother

▶ Your period stops or menstruation is very light.

▶ Your breasts may become larger and more tender.

▶ Your nipples may stick out more.

▶ You may need to urinate more often.

▶ You may feel very tired.

▶ You may feel nauseous and even vomit.

▶ You may crave certain foods or lose your appetite.

▶ You may have heartburn or indigestion.

▶ You may be constipated.

▶ You may gain or lose a few pounds.

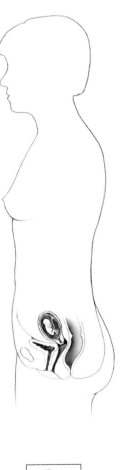

Fetus

▶ The placenta develops.

▶ The major organs and nervous system form.

▶ The heart starts beating.

▶ The lungs begin to develop.

▶ Bones appear.

▶ The head, face, eyes, ears, arms, fingers, legs, and toes form.

▶ The genitals develop.

▶ Hair starts to grow.

▶ 20 buds for future teeth appear.

Fetus in week 4 (actual size)

Growth and Changes During Pregnancy
(continued)

The Second Trimester: 14–28 Weeks

Mother

▶ Your appetite increases.

▶ Your abdomen begins to expand. By the end of this trimester, the top of your uterus will be near your rib cage.

▶ The skin on your abdomen and breasts stretches and may feel tight and itchy. You may see stretch marks.

▶ Between weeks 16 and 20, you start to feel the fetus move.

▶ Your abdomen may ache on one side or the other, as the ligaments that support your uterus are stretched.

▶ A dark line, the **linea nigra**, may appear down the middle of your stomach from your navel to your pubic hair.

▶ You may get brown patches (**chloasma**, or the "mask of pregnancy") on your face.

▶ Your **areolas**, the darker skin around your nipples, may darken.

▶ Your feet and ankles may swell.

Fetus

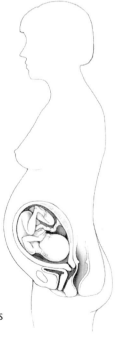

▶ The fetus grows quickly from now until birth.

▶ The organs develop further and begin to function.

▶ Eyebrows, eyelashes, and fingernails form.

▶ The skin is wrinkled and covered with a waxy coating (**vernix**) and fine hair (**lanugo**).

▶ The fetus moves, kicks, sleeps, and wakes. It can swallow, hear, pass urine, and even suck his or her thumb.

Growth and Changes During Pregnancy
(continued)

The Third Trimester: 29–40 Weeks

Mother

▶ You can feel the baby's movements strongly.

▶ You are short of breath as the uterus pushes up against the diaphragm, a muscle that aids in breathing. (Toward the end of this trimester, the baby may "drop" into a lower position. This will make it easier for you to catch your breath.)

▶ You need to urinate more often after the baby drops and puts extra pressure on your bladder.

▶ *Colostrum*—a yellow, watery pre-milk—may leak from your nipples.

▶ Your navel may stick out.

▶ You may have *contractions*—abdominal tightening or pain. These can signal false or real labor.

▶ Your cervix may begin to *efface* (thin out) and *dilate* (open).

Fetus

▶ The fetus kicks and stretches. (This activity may slow down as the fetus grows and its uterine home becomes more cramped.)

▶ Lanugo disappears.

▶ With its major development finished, the fetus gains weight very quickly.

▶ Bones harden, but the skull remains soft and flexible for delivery.

▶ The fetus usually turns into a head-down position for birth.

Growth of the Fetus

Week 12:
2 1/2 inches

Week 16:
6–7 inches,
5 ounces

Week 20:
10 inches,
1/2–1 pound

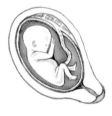
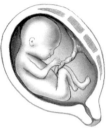
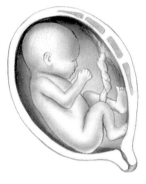

Week 24:
12 inches
1–1 1/2 pounds

Week 28:
14 inches,
2–2 1/2 pounds

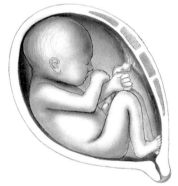
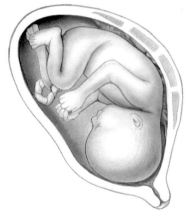

Growth of the Fetus (continued)

Week 32:
15 inches, 3 pounds

Week 36:
18 inches, 5 pounds

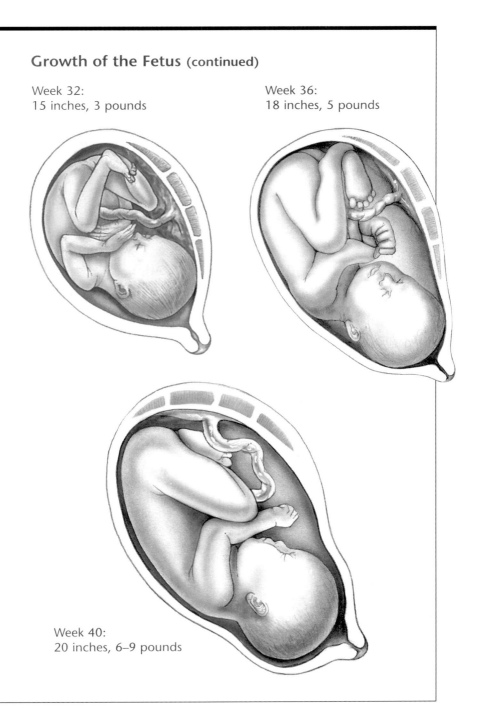

Week 40:
20 inches, 6–9 pounds

CHAPTER 4

Prenatal Care

During prenatal visits, you'll learn about what's going on in your body. You can ask for advice on coping with common changes during pregnancy and gather the information you need to make important choices.

These visits also allow your doctor to keep close tabs on your health and your baby's progress. Pregnancy and birth are a natural part of life, but there can be some risks. That's why it's important to get prenatal care as soon as you know a baby's on the way.

What if you're a veteran mom and had a normal pregnancy in the past? Regular prenatal care is still important. No two pregnancies are alike, and problems can come up without warning.

During your pregnancy, each member of your health care team—your doctor, midwife, nurse practitioner, and others—will keep an eye on your health and well-being. A series of tests will give clues to how your baby is doing.

Keep in mind that prenatal care isn't just medical care. It also helps you learn good health habits, get counseling or support if needed, find out about local family services, and prepare for childbirth and being a parent.

Informed Care

The more you know about your health care, the better equipped you are to make choices. During prenatal visits, your doctor will explain what's happening and why. Before you give your OK for a test or a treatment, be sure you know what it is and why it's needed. You also should be told about the risks, benefits, and options. This is called "informed consent."

If you don't understand something you have heard, ask your doctor to explain it more clearly. The doctor will make a note on your chart that something has been explained to you. He or she also will note what you have chosen to do. In some cases, you may be asked to sign a form saying that you have been informed of something or that you have agreed to have a certain procedure done.

Prenatal Visits

One of your early prenatal checkups will be longer and more involved than later visits. At this visit, your doctor will take a detailed health history, do a physical exam, order lab tests, figure your due date, and set up a schedule for your prenatal care. Throughout your pregnancy you will see your doctor on a regular basis. These visits provide a good chance to discuss any questions or concerns and learn more about your pregnancy.

History

Will you need special care during your pregnancy? There's no way to tell for sure, but your health and obstetric history will give your doctor clues. You may want to fill out the checklist "Your Health History" and take it with you to your doctor's visit. Be honest, and answer these questions as completely as you can.

Physical Exam

After your health history is taken, your height, weight, and blood pressure will be measured. Next comes a physical exam, which may involve the following:

- Ears, eyes, nose, throat, and teeth
- Thyroid gland

Your Health History

Fill this list out and take it with you to your first doctor's visit.

Medications you are taking_____

Allergies you have (including latex) _____

Medical conditions you have _____

_____

Immunizations you have had, and when you had them _____

_____

Childhood diseases you have had _____

_____

Your age when you got your first period _____

How long your menstrual cycles tend to last _____

When your last period started _____

What birth control you have used_____

Whether you smoke, drink alcohol, or use drugs _____

Whether you are exposed to anything that could put your baby at risk _____

If you have been pregnant before, the doctor will ask:

If you have had a miscarriage, *induced abortion, ectopic pregnancy, stillbirth,* or *multiple pregnancy* _____

If you had problems such as preterm labor or high blood pressure during pregnancy_____

How long your labor lasted _____

If you delivered vaginally or by cesarean birth _____

How much your children weighed at birth _____

If you have had a child with a birth defect _____

What kind of pain relief, if any, you used_____

Partners in Health Care

Both you and your health care providers have rights and responsibilities.

You have the right to:

▶ Get quality care without discrimination

▶ Be given privacy

▶ Know the professional status of your health care providers and their fees

▶ Know your diagnosis, treatment options, and expected outcome

▶ Be involved in decisions about your care

▶ Refuse treatment

▶ Agree or decline to be involved in research that affects your care

You have the responsibility to:

▶ Provide correct and complete health information

▶ Let your providers know that you understand what's being done to you and what you are expected to do

▶ Accept responsibility if you refuse treatment or don't follow the doctor's plan

Your health care provider has the right to:

▶ Stop treating you as long as you have time to find other care

He or she has the responsibility to:

▶ Give you quality medical treatment while you are in his or her care

‣ Breasts

‣ Heart, lungs, back, abdomen, arms, and legs

‣ *Lymph nodes*

‣ Skin

Next, a **pelvic exam** may be done to check the health of your reproductive organs: cervix, vagina, ovaries, fallopian tubes, and uterus. Using a device called a **speculum**, the doctor will look at your vagina and cervix and gently remove cells for testing.

Then the doctor will insert one or two gloved fingers into your vagina while pressing down on your abdomen with the other

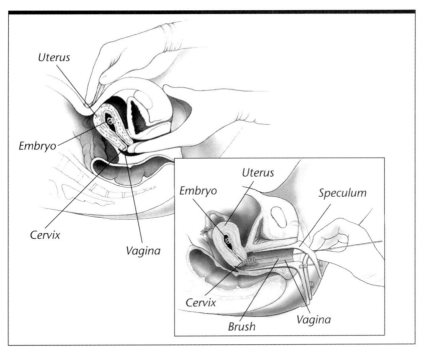

During your visit, your doctor may check your pelvic organs for any changes (*left*). Your doctor also may do a Pap test (*right*). For the Pap test, a speculum is inserted into the vagina. A small sample of cells is collected with a small brush or swab and scraper. The brush or swab is inserted into the cervical canal to reach the higher cells.

hand. This allows him or her to check the size of your pelvis. The doctor also may feel your uterus and ovaries and check their size, shape, and position. Lastly, the doctor will try to get an idea of the size of the inside of your pelvis.

Lab Tests

To double-check the findings of a home pregnancy test, your blood or urine may be tested for the hormone human chorionic gonadotropin (hCG). Also, the doctor will order a series of lab tests to make sure you don't have a disease or a condition that could harm your baby. These tests may include:

▸ *Urine tests.* Urine is collected and checked for sugar, protein, and bacteria. Their presence can signal diabetes or a bladder or kidney problem.

▸ *Blood tests.* Blood is drawn and checked for **anemia** (low red blood cell count) and infection. All women are offered testing for human immunodeficiency virus (HIV) infection. Most women also are tested for syphilis and antibodies to hepatitis B virus surface antigen. Your blood also may be checked for other sexually transmitted diseases (STDs) and signs that you are immune to rubella (German measles) and chickenpox (varicella). Any of these infections could harm your baby. Your blood type and Rh factor also are noted. (See Chapter 15 for more information about the Rh factor.)

▸ *Pap test.* The cells from the cervix collected during your pelvic exam may be checked for infection, cancer, or conditions that could lead to cancer. A swab may be used to check for infections, such as chlamydia or gonorrhea.

Due Date

The day your baby is due is called the "estimated date of delivery," or EDD. Although only about one in 20 women deliver on their exact due date, your EDD is useful for a number of reasons. It is used as a guide for checking the baby's growth and your pregnancy's progress. Your due date also affects the timing of prenatal tests. In some cases, the test results depend on the stage of pregnancy. Finally, the EDD gives a rough idea of when your baby will be born. Most women go into labor within about 2 weeks before or after their due date. Keep in mind that if your doctor says you are 6 weeks pregnant, for instance, that means you have been pregnant for a full 6 weeks. You are in week 7 of your pregnancy.

There are a number of methods to figure your due date. They often are used together to help predict when your baby will arrive:

▶ *The date of ovulation.* This is the best way to figure the age of a fetus (and thus your due date). However, it is rarely known. See Chapter 2.

▶ *The date of menstruation.* Your due date is most often pinpointed based on the first day of your last period. This method isn't exact, though. The length of your menstrual cycle affects your due date. These cycles differ from one woman to another and from one month to the next. Unless you made a note of it, it's easy to forget when your last period started. This is why keeping a menstrual calendar comes in handy (see Chapter 1). To get an idea of your due date by using your menstrual calendar, take the date that your last period started. Add 7 days. Then count back 3 months. Say the first day of your last period was January 1, for instance. Add 7 days to get January 8. Then count back 3 months. Your due date is October 8.

▶ *The size of your uterus.* At about 12 weeks, the top of the uterus (fundus) grows up and out of the pelvic cavity and can be felt just above your pubic bone. At 20 weeks, it reaches your navel. At term, when your baby is fully grown, it will be under your rib cage.

▶ *The fetal heartbeat.* No sound is sweeter to a pregnant woman than the rapid "whoosh" of her baby's tiny heart. It also can tell the doctor how far along you are in your preg-

What's Your Due Date?

There's no way to know for sure your delivery date. Here's how to get an idea: simply find the first day of your last menstrual period (LMP) on this chart. Then look at the estimated date of delivery (EDD) directly below it.

LMP: Jan.	1	2	3	4	5	6	7	8	9	10	11	12	13	14	15	16	17	18	19	20	21	22	23	24	25	26	27	28	29	30	31
EDD: Oct./Nov.	8	9	10	11	12	13	14	15	16	17	18	19	20	21	22	23	24	25	26	27	28	29	30	31	1	2	3	4	5	6	7

LMP: Feb.	1	2	3	4	5	6	7	8	9	10	11	12	13	14	15	16	17	18	19	20	21	22	23	24	25	26	27	28
EDD: Nov./Dec.	8	9	10	11	12	13	14	15	16	17	18	19	20	21	22	23	24	25	26	27	28	29	30	1	2	3	4	5

LMP: Mar.	1	2	3	4	5	6	7	8	9	10	11	12	13	14	15	16	17	18	19	20	21	22	23	24	25	26	27	28	29	30	31
EDD: Dec./Jan.	8	9	10	11	12	13	14	15	16	17	18	19	20	21	22	23	24	25	26	27	28	29	30	31	1	2	3	4	5	6	7

LMP: April	1	2	3	4	5	6	7	8	9	10	11	12	13	14	15	16	17	18	19	20	21	22	23	24	25	26	27	28	29	30
EDD: Jan./Feb.	8	9	10	11	12	13	14	15	16	17	18	19	20	21	22	23	24	25	26	27	28	29	30	31	1	2	3	4	5	6

LMP: May	1	2	3	4	5	6	7	8	9	10	11	12	13	14	15	16	17	18	19	20	21	22	23	24	25	26	27	28	29	30	31
EDD: Feb./Mar.	8	9	10	11	12	13	14	15	16	17	18	19	20	21	22	23	24	25	26	27	28	1	2	3	4	5	6	7	8	9	10

LMP: June	1	2	3	4	5	6	7	8	9	10	11	12	13	14	15	16	17	18	19	20	21	22	23	24	25	26	27	28	29	30
EDD: Mar./April	8	9	10	11	12	13	14	15	16	17	18	19	20	21	22	23	24	25	26	27	28	29	30	31	1	2	3	4	5	6

LMP: July	1	2	3	4	5	6	7	8	9	10	11	12	13	14	15	16	17	18	19	20	21	22	23	24	25	26	27	28	29	30	31
EDD: April/May	8	9	10	11	12	13	14	15	16	17	18	19	20	21	22	23	24	25	26	27	28	29	30	1	2	3	4	5	6	7	8

LMP: Aug.	1	2	3	4	5	6	7	8	9	10	11	12	13	14	15	16	17	18	19	20	21	22	23	24	25	26	27	28	29	30	31
EDD: May/June	8	9	10	11	12	13	14	15	16	17	18	19	20	21	22	23	24	25	26	27	28	29	30	31	1	2	3	4	5	6	7

LMP: Sept.	1	2	3	4	5	6	7	8	9	10	11	12	13	14	15	16	17	18	19	20	21	22	23	24	25	26	27	28	29	30
EDD: June/July	8	9	10	11	12	13	14	15	16	17	18	19	20	21	22	23	24	25	26	27	28	29	30	1	2	3	4	5	6	7

LMP: Oct.	1	2	3	4	5	6	7	8	9	10	11	12	13	14	15	16	17	18	19	20	21	22	23	24	25	26	27	28	29	30	31
EDD: July/Aug.	8	9	10	11	12	13	14	15	16	17	18	19	20	21	22	23	24	25	26	27	28	29	30	31	1	2	3	4	5	6	7

LMP: Nov.	1	2	3	4	5	6	7	8	9	10	11	12	13	14	15	16	17	18	19	20	21	22	23	24	25	26	27	28	29	30
EDD: Aug./Sept.	8	9	10	11	12	13	14	15	16	17	18	19	20	21	22	23	24	25	26	27	28	29	30	31	1	2	3	4	5	6

LMP: Dec.	1	2	3	4	5	6	7	8	9	10	11	12	13	14	15	16	17	18	19	20	21	22	23	24	25	26	27	28	29	30	31
EDD: Sept./Oct.	8	9	10	11	12	13	14	15	16	17	18	19	20	21	22	23	24	25	26	27	28	29	30	31	1	2	3	4	5	6	7	8

nancy. By about 12 weeks, your doctor can hear your baby's heart by using a special device. This device uses a form of ultrasound to convert sound waves into signals you can hear.

▸ *Ultrasound.* Ultrasound uses sound waves to create a picture of your uterus and the baby growing inside it. A technician measures the size of the fetus to figure its age. During the first half of pregnancy, ultrasound can be used to set the age of the fetus within a week or so. Later on, this method is less reliable.

Future Visits

The timing of prenatal visits depends on two things: your health and the amount of risk present. Women with medical or obstet-

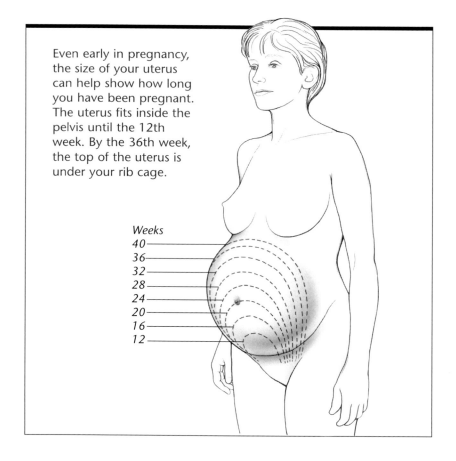

Even early in pregnancy, the size of your uterus can help show how long you have been pregnant. The uterus fits inside the pelvis until the 12th week. By the 36th week, the top of the uterus is under your rib cage.

Weeks
40
36
32
28
24
20
16
12

ric problems need special care. Healthy women with no known risk factors often need less care. If you develop a problem during your pregnancy, you'll need to see the doctor more often. As long as mother and baby are both doing well, though, your checkups will more than likely follow a schedule like this one:

From the first visit to 28 weeks	Every 4 weeks
From 28 to 36 weeks	Every 2–3 weeks
From 36 weeks to delivery	Weekly

During each prenatal visit, you will be examined to check how your pregnancy is coming along. Your health also will be monitored closely to make sure no new problems occur. During a checkup:

▸ Your weight may be measured and written on your chart.

▸ Your blood pressure may be taken.

▸ Your urine may be checked for protein and sugar.

▸ The height of your fundus may be measured to gauge the baby's growth.

▸ Your face, ankles, hands, and feet may be examined for swelling.

▸ After about the 12th week, the fetal heartbeat may be checked.

▸ Later in the pregnancy, your abdomen may be felt to note the position of the fetus.

▸ If needed, lab tests and pelvic exams will be done.

Finally, you will be asked if you have any questions or concerns. It never fails: you may be bursting with questions between visits, but draw a blank once you are in the exam room. It's a good idea to jot down your questions ahead of time and bring them with you. Also make a note of any symptoms you have between visits and mention them to the doctor. (Using the Personal Pregnancy Diary at the back of this book is a handy way to chart the course of your pregnancy.)

Risks Factors That May Need Special Care in Pregnancy

Medical

- High blood pressure
- Heart, kidney, lung, or liver disease
- STDs, urinary tract infections, or other infections caused by a virus or bacteria
- Diabetes
- Severe anemia
- Epilepsy or other seizure disorders
- Mental health problems

Obstetric

- Problems in past pregnancies
- Being younger than age 15 or older than age 35 during pregnancy
- Previous birth defects
- Multiple pregnancy (carrying more than one baby)
- Bleeding, especially during the second or third trimester
- Pregnancy-induced high blood pressure (*preeclampsia*)
- Abnormal fetal heartbeat
- Intrauterine growth restriction (the fetus doesn't grow at the rate it should)

Lifestyle

- Smoking cigarettes
- Drinking alcohol
- Taking drugs that aren't prescribed by a doctor
- Eating poorly
- Not gaining enough weight
- Having more than one sexual partner

If your questions are pressing or your symptoms alarm you, don't wait until your next visit. Talk to your doctor or nurse right away.

Prenatal Tests

Tests can be done to help your doctor spot possible health problems. They also will give clues to how your baby is growing and developing. The results of these tests will be noted on your chart. The tests you have depend on your medical history, family background, ethnic background, or exam results. (See the box "Tests During Pregnancy.") There are new tests being evaluated to detect other genetic disorders. Chapter 13 has more information about how and why these tests are done.

Fetal Movements

In mid-pregnancy, the nausea you may have been feeling is replaced by a new sensation in your belly: the gentle flutter of your baby moving inside you. The first time you feel the baby move is called *quickening,* and it's likely to be one of the most thrilling moments of your pregnancy.

Quickening usually occurs between 16 and 20 weeks. It can happen sooner for thin women and second-time moms. The feeling varies from woman to woman. Many compare it to the flapping of butterfly wings.

During the second half of pregnancy, your baby's soft movements will become stronger and more lively. Such fetal movement is a good sign of well-being, so your doctor will ask at each visit if you have noticed any change in the way your baby moves. He or she also may ask you to perform daily *kick counts.* See Chapter 17 for details on how to perform kick counts.

Other Tests

Even if you passed your earlier tests with no problems, your doctor may want to run a few more later in pregnancy. These tests will reassure you that your baby is doing well and that your preg-

Tests During Pregnancy

Alpha-fetoprotein (AFP) and *multiple marker screening* are *screening tests* routinely offered to pregnant women. Other tests are done for certain women based on their history or risk factors. Those tests are best done at a certain time in pregnancy:

Weeks	Test	Reason
10–12	*Chorionic villus sampling (CVS)*	Tests placental tissue for chromosomal disorders (such as *Down syndrome*) and genetic conditions (such as sickle cell anemia)
15–18	*Amniocentesis*	Tests cells for genetic and chromosomal disorders
16–18	Alpha-fetoprotein screening	Checks blood for risks of neural tube defects or Down syndrome
16–18	Multiple marker screening	Measures hormone and AFP levels to check for risk of Down syndrome
18–20	Ultrasound	Detects some congenital malformations and multiple pregnancy, tracks baby's growth, and checks position of fetus and placenta
24–28	*Glucose* screening	Tests for *gestational diabetes*
35–37	Group B streptococci (GBS) screening	Checks for GBS in the mother, which can be passed to the baby during delivery

nancy is coming along the way it should. Among the tests and checks you may need:

▸ *Nonstress test.* During a nonstress test, an ultrasound device is strapped to your abdomen to measure changes in your baby's heart rate. If the heart rate goes up when the fetus moves, it's a sign of good health.

▶ *Contraction stress test.* This involves tracking the baby's heart rate in response to mild uterine contractions. These contractions are brought on with a drug called *oxytocin*. The test gives clues to how well a baby can handle the stress of labor and delivery.

▶ *Biophysical profile.* A biophysical profile often is done at the same time as a nonstress or contraction stress test. A technician looks at the fetus on an ultrasound monitor and notes its movements, muscle tone, and breathing patterns. The level of *amniotic fluid* also is measured.

During the last weeks of pregnancy, your doctor also may check your cervix for changes that can signal the onset of labor. Before delivery, the cervix often begins to move forward in the vagina, thin out, soften, and open slightly as it gets ready for the baby's passage. All of these things may happen weeks before labor begins. Many women have none of these signs, yet go into labor within hours.

Choices

If you haven't done so yet, now is the time to make choices about your baby's birth and after-delivery care. Even the best-laid plans may not work out, but it's vital to think about your options and resolve as much as you can well before delivery day.

Among the issues to think about ahead of time:

▶ What kind of birth do you hope for?

▶ Do you want pain relief during labor, or will you try for a natural childbirth?

▶ Who will be at your side during labor and delivery?

You'll also need to think about breastfeeding, circumcision (if you have a boy), and what to do about birth control after the baby's born. (Work and travel plans, which also may need advance planning, are covered in Chapter 5.)

Childbirth Preparation

Your baby won't arrive for a few months yet. Still, your doctor will want to talk about childbirth now. He or she will talk to you about what to expect in the delivery room.

The doctor also can direct you to a childbirth education class that's a good match for you and for the kind of birth you hope to have. These classes often meet over the course of a few weeks or months, so start looking into them as soon as you can. The class will inform you about the labor and delivery process and teach you how to help it go smoothly. You can't know how your labor will play out ahead of time. However, childbirth preparation will help ease your fears, teach you methods for coping with labor pain, and help you feel more in control.

The most common methods of preparation—Lamaze, Bradley, and Read—vary greatly, but each is based on the idea that pain is made worse by fear and tension. Classes aim to relieve labor pain through education, emotional support, relaxation techniques, and touch.

Some childbirth education classes will help you draft a birth plan. This is a written outline of what you'd like to happen during labor and delivery. It might include the setting you want to deliver in, the people you want to have with you, and the pain medications you want, if any. It also allows you to let your health care team know about the things you feel strongly about (such as episiotomy and circumcision). It is useful to make sure you and your doctor have the same ideas. Be sure to check your plan with the hospital in which you'll be delivering your baby, in case parts of it do not fit the hospital's policy.

Once you have drawn up your plan, go over it with your doctor. He or she will help you amend the plan based on your situation. The doctor also will let you know if your wishes conflict with hospital policies. Be sure to keep your birth plan both realistic and flexible. Each birth is unique, after all, and you won't know exactly what yours will be like until it happens.

Your Childbirth Partner

Another choice to make well ahead of time is your childbirth partner. The constant support of a spouse, partner, relative, or friend will help ease the many stresses of pregnancy. It also will help labor and delivery go more smoothly.

If possible, your partner should come with you to prenatal visits and tests. Your partner also needs to attend childbirth classes with you. They have almost as much to learn as you do, after all. This person will help you practice breathing or relaxation exercises. On delivery day, your partner will coach you through each contraction and help you carry out what you learned in class.

Most mothers-to-be are happy to have their baby's father, a friend, or a family member with them in the delivery room. But a growing number are also hiring professional labor assistants, or doulas. Doulas provide emotional support and hands-on comfort during labor and delivery. Although the childbirth partner still plays a vital role, a doula can take some of the pressure off during a long or intense labor.

Breastfeeding

Will you nurse your baby or give him or her formula? This is yet another issue to think about before delivery. Only you can decide what's right for your family. Still, there's plenty of proof that breastfeeding is the healthier choice. Chapter 10 has details about breastfeeding.

Circumcision

Whether to circumcise a baby boy is another important issue for parents-to-be. Circumcision means cutting away the *foreskin*. This is the layer of skin that covers the *glans*, the sensitive end of the penis. Circumcision is most often done by an ob-gyn soon after birth, before the baby leaves the hospital.

Circumcision is a matter of choice. More than half of newborn boys in the United States are circumcised. That number is on the

Circumcision

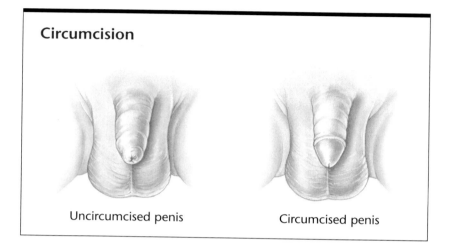

Uncircumcised penis   Circumcised penis

decline, though. Personal and emotional factors need to be considered. Some parents have their sons circumcised for religious or cultural reasons. Muslims and Jews, for instance, have circumcised their sons for centuries.

In most cases, there's no medical reason to circumcise. It's not required by law or hospital policy. Parents who want their sons circumcised must request it.

No matter which way you and your partner are leaning on this issue, talk to your doctor about circumcision long before your due date. That way, you'll have time to make an informed decision.

Ask for details about the procedure. Find out about the care needed for both a circumcised and uncircumcised penis. If you choose to circumcise your son, be sure to ask about options for pain relief. Not all doctors routinely use pain relief, and some question its value.

Birth Control and Sterilization

Your doctor will tell you when you can resume having sex. It likely will be a month or so after delivery. You might not feel ready then, though. After your baby is born, sex may be the last thing on your mind. Believe it or not, though, desire will return. It'll happen before you know it—and, chances are, before you're ready for another baby. That's why it's vital to think about post-delivery birth control now. Chapter 12 gives you more details about birth control options and sterilization.

Banking Cord Blood

The blood in a baby's umbilical cord contains stem cells. These cells can be transplanted into genetically matched persons to treat diseases such as leukemia and other forms of cancer. For this reason, private companies have been set up to collect and store cord blood samples for possible future use. There is a cost involved, and the value of this process has been questioned. This is a new area. There are many unknowns and some concerns. Ask your doctor if you have questions. Decisions about donating cord blood need to be made early in pregnancy.

Teamwork

In the coming months, you and your doctor will become partners. By working together, you'll know that you're doing all you can to have a normal pregnancy and healthy baby.

CHAPTER 5

A Healthy Lifestyle

Many of the choices you make in your daily life affect your baby. This is true of the things you do—exercise, rest, and eat well, for instance. It's also true of the things you don't do, such as drink, smoke, or use drugs.

It's best to cut out bad health habits before you get pregnant. Because so many pregnancies come as a surprise, though, you can't always do that. Some women may need to make a few lifestyle changes after they become pregnant. In some cases, that may simply mean being sure to get extra rest and eat healthy foods. (Chapter 6 has information about healthy eating during pregnancy.) In other cases, it might mean kicking a drinking or drug habit or changing an abusive relationship. In any case, keeping healthy is the best thing you can do for you and your baby.

Exercise

If you are active now, pregnancy need not get in the way of your fitness routine. If you have not been active, now is a great time to start. Keeping fit is good for you in many ways. It builds bones and muscles, gives you energy, and keeps you healthy. Exercise is just as vital when you are pregnant. Prenatal exercise will:

▸ Help you look and feel better

▸ Reduce constipation, leg cramps, bloating, and swelling

71

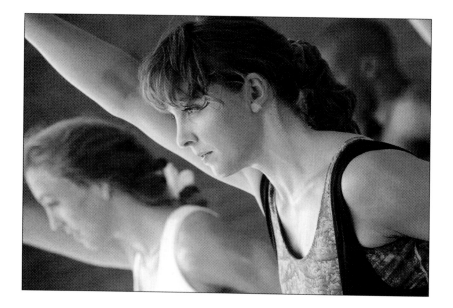

- ▶ Lift your spirits

- ▶ Help you relax

- ▶ Improve your posture

- ▶ Promote strength and stamina

- ▶ Help you sleep better

- ▶ Help your body prepare for the hard work of labor and delivery

- ▶ Give you a head start in getting back in shape after the baby is born

Some exercise routines also will help you ward off pregnancy-related aches and pains. For instance, the extra weight you are carrying—along with posture changes—can be hard on your back. Certain moves can lessen back pain by stretching muscles and making them stronger (see the "A Healthy Back" box).

Fitness is good, but think about safety, too. The many changes that come along with pregnancy affect the sort of exercise you can do safely. These changes affect your:

▶ *Joints.* Some pregnancy hormones cause the ligaments that support your joints to stretch. This makes them more prone to injury.

▶ *Balance.* The weight you are gaining and the fact that it's pooled in your middle shifts your center of gravity. This puts stress on your joints and muscles—mostly those in the lower back and pelvis. It also can make you less stable and more likely to fall.

▶ *Heart rate.* Extra weight also makes your body work harder than it did before you were pregnant. This is true even if you are working out at a slower pace. Intense exercise boosts oxygen and blood flow to the muscles and away from other parts of your body—such as your uterus. If you can't talk at a normal level during exercise, then you are working too hard. Slow down.

Before you start your exercise program, talk with your doctor to make sure you do not have any health conditions that may limit your activity. Ask about any specific exercises or sports that you like to do. Almost any form of exercise is safe if it is done with caution and if you don't do too much of it. Follow these tips for a safe and healthy exercise program that's geared to the special needs of pregnancy:

▶ Exercise to reach or keep a safe fitness level during pregnancy—not to shed excess pounds. Exercise often—at least 3 times a week, but every day is best. Spurts of heavy exercise followed by long periods of no activity put strain on your body and offer few benefits.

▶ If you didn't exercise much before getting pregnant, start your workout routine with slow, low-impact activities such as walking or cycling. As you become more fit, you can move to higher levels bit by bit.

▶ Don't do brisk exercise when it's hot and humid outside. Wear comfortable clothes that will help you stay cool. Also, don't exercise if you are running a fever.

▶ Be sure you have all the equipment you need for a safe workout. Wear the right shoes for your sport. There are shoes made just for walking, running, aerobics, and tennis, for instance. Also, be sure the shoes have plenty of padding and give your feet good support. Be sure to wear a sports bra that fits well and gives plenty of support. Your breasts are growing and may be very tender.

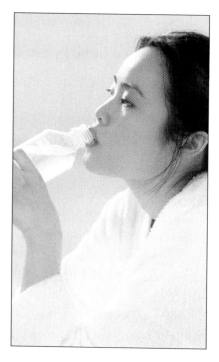

▶ Drink enough fluid. Take a bottle of water with you for a drink before, during, and after your workout. If you're getting hot or feeling thirsty, take a break and drink more water.

▶ Your workout should begin with warming up for 5 minutes to prevent muscle strain. Slow walking or riding a stationary bike are good warm ups.

▶ Avoid jerky, bouncy, or high-impact motions. Jumping, jarring motions, or quick direction changes can strain your joints and cause pain. Low-impact exercise such as walking or swimming is best.

▶ Work out on a wooden floor or a tightly carpeted surface. This cuts down impact and gives you better footing. Avoid deep knee bends, full sit-ups, double leg lifts (raising and lowering both legs at once), and straight-leg toe touches.

▶ Get up slowly after lying or sitting on the floor. This will prevent feeling dizzy or fainting. Once you're standing, walk in place briefly. After 20 weeks of pregnancy, don't do any exercises on your back. This can cut down the blood flow to your baby.

- Be sure to take a break if you need one. If you have trouble talking at a normal level during your workout, ease up. Never exercise until you are exhausted.

- Follow intense exercise with cooling down for 5–10 minutes. Slow your pace little by little and end your workout by gently stretching. Don't stretch too far, though. This can injure the tissue that connects your joints.

- Reduce your workout levels in late pregnancy. Exercise that may have been easy earlier in pregnancy becomes harder as your belly expands.

The type of exercise you can safely do depends on your health and fitness level. Pregnancy is not the time to take up a new sport. If you were active before getting pregnant, though, you should be able to keep it up, within reason.

Certain sports are safe even for beginners. Others are OK for those who have done them for a while. Still others are off-limits during pregnancy. With any type of exercise you'd like to try, be

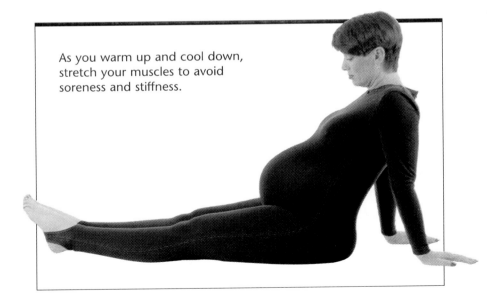

As you warm up and cool down, stretch your muscles to avoid soreness and stiffness.

A Healthy Back

The following exercises strengthen and stretch the muscles of the back, abdomen, hips, and upper body. These muscles support the back and legs and promote good posture. The exercises will help ease back pain as well as help prepare you for labor and delivery.

Upper Body Bends

This exercise strengthens the muscles of your back and torso.

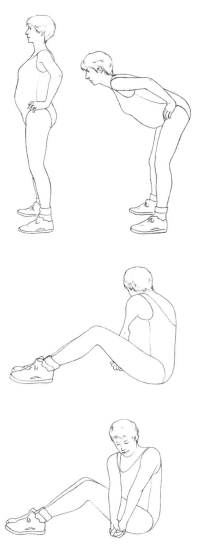

▶ Stand with your legs apart, knees bent slightly, with your hands on your hips.

▶ Bend forward slowly, keeping your upper back straight. You should feel a slight pull along your upper thigh.

▶ Repeat 10 times.

Diagonal Curl

This exercise strengthens the muscles of your back, hips, and abdomen. If you have not already been exercising regularly, skip this exercise.

▶ Sit on the floor with your knees bent, feet on the floor, and hands clasped in front of you.

▶ Twist your upper torso to the left until your hands touch the floor.

▶ Do the same movement to the right.

▶ Repeat on both sides 5 times.

A Healthy Back (continued)

Forward Bend

This exercise stretches and strengthens the muscles of your back.

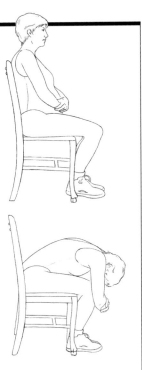

- Sit in a chair in a comfortable position. Keep your arms relaxed.

- Bend forward slowly, with your arms in front and hanging down.

- If you feel any discomfort or pressure on your abdomen, do not push any further.

- Hold this position for a count of 5, then get up slowly without arching your back.

- Repeat 5 times.

Trunk Twist

This exercise stretches the muscles of your back, spine, and upper torso.

- Sit on the floor with your legs crossed, with your left hand holding your left foot and your right hand on the floor at your side for support.

- Slowly twist your upper torso to the right.

- Do the same movement to the left after switching your hands (right hand holding right foot and left hand supporting you).

- Repeat on both sides 5–10 times.

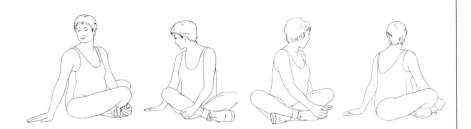

A Healthy Back (continued)

Backward Stretch

This exercise stretches and strengthens the muscles of your back, pelvis, and thighs.

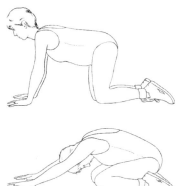

- Kneel on hands and knees, with your knees 8–10 inches apart and your arms straight (hands under your shoulders).

- Curl backward slowly, tucking your head toward your knees and keeping your arms extended.

- Hold this position for a count of 5, then come back up to all fours slowly.

- Repeat 5 times.

Leg Lift Crawl

This exercise strengthens the muscles of your back and abdomen.

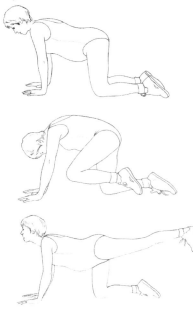

- Kneel on hands and knees, with your weight distributed evenly and your arms straight (hands under your shoulders).

- Lift your left knee and bring it toward your elbow.

- Straighten your leg without locking your knee.

- Extend your leg up and back.

- Do this exercise to a count of 5. Move slowly—don't fling your leg back or arch your back.

- Repeat on both sides 5–10 times.

A Healthy Back
(continued)

Rocking Back Arch

This exercise stretches and streng-thens the muscles of your back, hips, and abdomen.

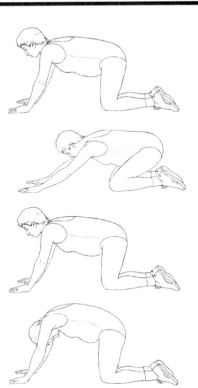

- Kneel on hands and knees, with your weight distributed evenly and your back straight.

- Rock back and forth, to a count of 5.

- Return to the original position and curl your back upward as much as you can.

- Repeat 5–10 times.

Back Press

This exercise strengthens the muscles of your back, torso, and upper body and promotes good posture.

- Stand with your back against a wall and your feet 10–12 inches away from the wall.

- Press the lower part of your back against the wall.

- Hold this position for a count of 10, then release.

- Repeat 10 times.

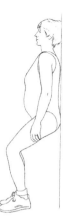

> **!**
>
> ## Signs of a Problem
>
> If you have any of these symptoms when you exercise, stop your workout and call the doctor:
>
> ‣ Dizziness or faintness
>
> ‣ Increased shortness of breath
>
> ‣ Irregular or rapid heartbeat
>
> ‣ Chest pain
>
> ‣ Trouble walking
>
> ‣ Pain
>
> ‣ Vaginal bleeding
>
> ‣ Uterine contractions that continue after rest
>
> ‣ Fluid gushing or leaking from your vagina

sure to discuss it with your doctor ahead of time. Here are some options:

‣ *Walking.* If you were not active before getting pregnant, walking is the ideal way to start an exercise program. Try to walk briskly for 30 minutes at least 3 times a week.

‣ *Swimming.* This is great for your body because it works many different muscles. The water supports your weight so you avoid injury and muscle strain. Stay off the diving board, though. Hitting the water with great force can be harmful.

‣ *Cycling.* This provides a good aerobic workout. Your growing belly can affect your balance and make you more prone to falls, though. As your belly grows, stick to stationary cycling.

‣ *Jogging.* If you were a runner before you became pregnant, you can keep hitting the road now. Be careful, though. Avoid getting too hot. Stop if you feel tired or any pain. Drink plenty of water to replace the fluid you lose in sweat.

‣ *Aerobics.* Low-impact aerobics is a safe and good way to keep your heart and lungs strong. There are aerobics classes designed just for pregnant women. Water aerobics also is a good class to try. It combines the benefits of swimming and aerobics.

▸ *Tennis.* Tennis likely is safe during pregnancy. You should be aware of how your changing balance affects rapid movements, though.

▸ *Body building or strength training.* Your muscles will become stronger with strength training. The workouts also help prevent some of the aches and pains so common in pregnancy. To avoid harming your muscles and joints, do strength training only under the watchful eye of an expert. Use slow, controlled movements and do short sets (10 or fewer repetitions). Don't hold your breath while bearing down.

▸ *Golf and bowling.* These may be fun, but they don't do much to tone your body, heart, and lungs. With either sport, you may have to adjust to your change in balance.

▸ *Snow skiing.* This may be OK if you are skilled and careful. Keep in mind that some hazards are beyond your control. One hazard is altitude. The air is thinner on slopes at very high altitudes. This makes it harder for you to breathe and may cut down on the oxygen your baby gets. Downhill skiing also poses a risk of severe injuries and hard falls. Stick to safe slopes—you can tackle harder ones after the baby arrives. Lastly, your changing center of gravity can cause balance problems. Cross-country runs are safer than downhill slopes for pregnant skiers. They also give your heart a better workout. The ski machines at many gyms are fine.

▸ *In-line skating.* Again, if you are very skilled and very careful, you may be able to keep rolling during your pregnancy. Keep in mind that your balance is affected and there's a risk of crashes and falls.

▸ *Water skiing, surfing, and scuba diving.* It's best to sit out water skiing and surfing when you're pregnant. That's because you can hit the water with great force. Taking a fall at such fast speeds could harm you or your baby. Little is known about how water pressure affects a growing fetus.

Rest

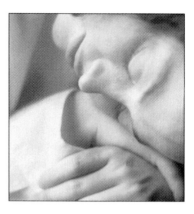

It's little wonder that pregnant women are so tired. After all, even when you are sleeping, your body is hard at work building a whole new human being from scratch. Fatigue will be a fact of daily life during the coming months. Although feeling tired is normal, there are some ways you can get some needed rest.

Take short breaks during the day to relax. At work, try to find a couch or a quiet room where you can close your eyes and put your feet up for a few minutes. Take a catnap if you can and if it doesn't prevent you from sleeping well at night.

A brisk walk or other exercises will increase your energy level. This will release tension (which is tiring on its own) and help you feel more refreshed.

Keeping house and caring for kids can leave you feeling even more tired and stressed. Try to get some help. Do the things that need to be done, and let the other things go. Build in time to relax.

?

Are Hot Tubs, Baths, and Saunas Safe?

A warm bath can be a safe—and relaxing—treat during pregnancy. But, just as it is not safe to exercise until you are overheated during pregnancy, it also is not a good idea to become overheated in a hot tub, very hot bath, or sauna. During pregnancy, your core body temperature should not rise above 102.2°F (39°C) for more than 10 minutes. You can check the water temperature by dipping a thermometer into the water. One sign of being overheated is that you feel uncomfortable or you stop sweating.

If you soaked in a hot tub before you knew you were pregnant, most likely your baby will be fine. Most women get out of the hot tub before the temperature reaches a harmful level because they start to feel too hot.

If your rest time involves a nap, try to lie on your side (your left side is best). After about 20 weeks of pregnancy, the weight of your growing uterus puts pressure on the vena cava. This is a major vein that returns blood from your lower body to your heart. Spending a long time on your back can restrict the flow of blood to your baby. It also can leave you feeling faint and dizzy. Don't panic if you wake up on your back, though. Just turn onto your side.

Stress

Stress—on the body and mind—is a fact of most women's lives these days. Too much stress, though, may cause problems. Problems caused by stress can be serious at any time. They may be even harder to cope with during pregnancy. The box suggests ways to manage and avoid stress.

Work

Today two thirds of American women of childbearing age work outside the home. More than 1 million of them become pregnant each year. Many work right up until delivery and return to their job within weeks or months of the baby's birth.

This trend—along with a growing concern about on-the-job health and safety—has prompted a number of questions: How safe is it for a pregnant woman to work? How long, under what conditions, and with what effects can she work? These questions have no easy answers. As long as you and your baby are healthy and your job presents no special hazards, though, you should be able to work as long as you want. No matter what type of work you do, discuss it with your doctor early in pregnancy.

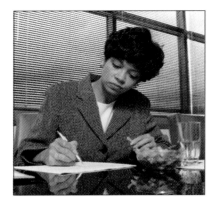

De-Stressing Tips

You can't avoid stress. But you can take steps to cut down on the stress in your life:

- Ask for help. Let your partner or a friend help with household and childcare duties. Ask friends and relatives to run some errands for you.

- Do first things first. Every day, make a list of the things you hope to get done. Then go through your list and circle the things that you must get done. Focus on these, and tackle the less pressing tasks only if you have the time and energy. In fact, this is good training for the kind of scaling back you'll need to do after the baby arrives.

- Exercise. Staying fit helps you blow off steam and leaves you better able to cope when things get stressful.

- Relax. Use meditation, deep breathing, visualization, or muscle relaxation exercises when you need a break. Call a friend. Take a walk at lunch. Listen to soothing music.

- Find support. If you are feeling stressed, talk to your partner, a relative, or a friend. Sometimes just talking about the problem will help you feel better. Also, let your doctor know if you are really stressed out. He or she can offer advice or direct you to support groups and other resources.

Jobs That May Cause Concern

Pregnant women often can keep doing their normal jobs. But strenuous jobs—those that involve a lot of heavy lifting, climbing, carrying, or standing—may not be safe during pregnancy. That's because the dizziness, nausea, and fatigue common in early pregnancy can increase the chance of injury. Later on, extra weight and a growing belly throw off balance and can lead to falls.

If your job is heavy duty, discuss safety with your doctor. You may need to cut back on the hours you work, give up certain tasks, transfer to another position, or stop working until after the baby is born.

Being exposed on the job to harmful substances is fairly rare. Still, agents found in some workplaces pose a risk. It makes sense, then, to think about the things you come into contact with during the course of your workday. You also may come in contact with these agents through a hobby.

Pesticides, chemicals, cleaning solvents, and heavy metals such as lead can cause serious problems during pregnancy. Women who work in farming, factories, dry cleaners, printing, or crafts businesses such as painting or pottery glazing may be exposed to harmful agents.

Health care workers also are at risk. Viruses such as hepatitis B, rubella, and chickenpox can cause miscarriage or birth defects if a woman is infected during pregnancy. Breathing or absorbing medical gases and toxic drugs is another danger. Ionizing radiation is used to take X-rays and treat certain diseases, such as cancer. In high doses, it can harm a fetus. Most women who work around radiation are protected from exposure, though.

If you think your job may bring you into contact with something harmful, find out for sure by asking your employee health office, personnel office, or union. Then let your doctor know right away. Workplace safety hazards and tips can be found at the Web sites of the Occupational Safety and Health Administration (www.osha.gov) and the National Institute for Occupational Safety and Health (www.cdc.gov/niosh). Keep in mind that just because a toxic agent is present doesn't mean you are exposed to harmful levels of it. In some cases, proper clothing and safety measures can greatly reduce or prevent exposure.

If a problem can't be easily fixed, your employer may be able to relieve you of certain duties or move you to another job. If not, your doctor may advise you to stop working.

Pregnancy-Related Disability

Having a disability means that health problems keep you from doing your normal duties. Most pregnancies are not disabling. For some women, pregnancy could become a disability if problems arise. Your pregnancy may be partly or totally disabling— only you and your doctor can decide. There are three types of pregnancy-related disability:

1. *Disability caused by the pregnancy itself.* Some pregnant women suffer from nausea, vomiting, extreme fatigue, dizziness, or swollen legs and ankles. These symptoms may cause short-term or partial disability. (Most often, though, they are minor.) Giving birth also causes short-term disability.

2. *Disability due to pregnancy complications.* More severe problems such as infection, bleeding, preterm labor, or early rupture of the *amniotic sac* (which surrounds the fetus) may cause disability. Also, conditions you had before getting preg-

Your Workplace Rights

Three major federal laws protect the health, safety, and employment rights of pregnant working women. If you are denied your rights, contact the agencies listed.

Pregnancy Discrimination Act

The Pregnancy Discrimination Act (PDA) requires employers to treat pregnancy as they would any other medical condition. That means they must offer the same disability leave and pay. The PDA also makes it illegal to hire, fire, or refuse to promote a woman because she's pregnant. If you think you are the victim of pregnancy discrimination, contact the Equal Employment Opportunity Commission at 1-800-669-EEOC or the Woman's Bureau of the Department of Labor at 1-800-827-5335.

Occupational Safety and Health Act

The Occupational Safety and Health Administration (OSHA) requires employers to provide a workplace free from known hazards that cause, or are likely to cause, death or serious physical harm. It also requires employers to give workers facts about harmful agents. If you think your employer may be breaking these rules, contact OSHA at 1-202-576-6339

The National Institute for Occupational Safety and Health (NIOSH) finds workplace hazards, figures out how to control them, and sug-

nant—such as heart disease, diabetes, or high blood pressure—may become disabling in pregnancy.

3. *Disability due to job exposures.* Being exposed at work to agents that could harm the fetus may cause disability. This type of pregnancy-related disability is rare, though.

If your doctor decides that your pregnancy is disabling, ask for a letter from him or her that says you qualify for disability. Likewise, if your employer wants you to stop working but your doctor says you can continue, get a letter from the doctor to give to your boss.

Your Workplace Rights (continued)

gests ways to limit the dangers. If you, your union, or your doctor asks it to, this group will inspect your workplace for hazards. Contact NIOSH at 1-800-356-4674.

Certain state and city laws also give workers and unions the right to ask for the names of chemicals and other substances used in the workplace. If you have questions or concerns, ask your employer or call the numbers listed.

Family and Medical Leave Act

The Family and Medical Leave Act (FMLA) requires employers with 50 or more employees to allow up to 12 weeks of unpaid leave during any 12-month period:

1. On the birth, adoption, or foster care of a child

2. When needed to care for a spouse, a child, or a parent with a serious health condition

3. When a worker isn't able to do her job because of her own serious health condition, including a pregnancy- or birth-related disability

To find out more about family and medical leave, contact the U.S. Department of Labor at 1-800-959-3652. A few states have better leave laws than the federal FMLA. For details, contact your state department of labor.

Leave

Maternity- and disability-leave policies vary from company to company and state to state. Only about 4 in 10 working women in the United States get paid leave after giving birth. Others must use sick leave and vacation time or take time off without pay.

The Family and Medical Leave Act protects a woman's right to take off up to 12 weeks, without pay during any 12-month period, for pregnancy-related problems or after giving birth. To take family leave, a woman must:

▶ Work for a company at a location where there are at least 50 employees of the same employer within a 75-mile area (at a branch office, for instance)

▶ Have worked there for at least 12 months

▶ Have worked at least 1,250 hours during the past year

An employee may have to use stored-up vacation, personal, or sick leave for some or all of her time off. If an employer provides health care benefits, this coverage must be kept at the same level during the leave period. When she returns to work, an employee must be given the same or equal job and the same benefits she had when she left. If an employee uses some of the 12 weeks for a difficult pregnancy, it may be counted as part of the 12-week FMLA leave entitlement.

The Pregnancy Discrimination Act requires employers that have at least 15 workers to treat workers disabled by pregnancy or childbirth the same as workers disabled by illness or accident. If you're partly disabled by pregnancy and your company gives lighter duty to other partly disabled workers, it must do the same for you. Because many employers don't offer their workers any disability benefits, though, they don't have to provide paid leave. If you are not covered by a disability plan at work, you may be able to get state unemployment or disability benefits. For details, contact your local unemployment office. Many states also have maternity/family leave laws.

Travel

You don't need to cancel your travel plans because you are pregnant. As long as you get your doctor's OK and follow a few simple guidelines, in most cases you can travel safely until close to your due date.

The best time to hit the road is mid-pregnancy (14–28 weeks of pregnancy). By that time many women are past the morning sickness phase. During late pregnancy, it's often harder to move around or sit for a long time. During mid-pregnancy, though, your energy has returned, morning sickness is a fading memory, and you are still mobile.

The best travel rule is to follow your body's signals. Paying heed to the way you feel is the best guide for your well-being and safety—whether you are on the road or at home. When choosing your mode of travel, think about how long it will take to get where you are going. The fastest way is often the best. Whether you go by train, plane, car, bus, or boat (motorcycles are not a good idea), take steps to ensure your comfort and safety. Here are some healthy travel tips:

▸ Think about having a prenatal checkup before you leave.

▸ If you'll be far from home, take a copy of your health record with you.

▸ In case of emergency, ask your doctor for the name and phone number of a doctor where you're visiting.

▸ Check with your doctor before you plan to travel late in pregnancy. After all, you don't want to go into labor far from home.

▸ Keep your travel plans easy to change. Pregnancy problems can come up at any time and ground you before you leave home. Buy travel insurance to cover tickets and deposits that can't be refunded.

▸ While you are en route, walk around about every hour. Stretching your legs will lessen the risk of blood clots and make you more comfortable. It also will decrease the amount of fluid that pools in your ankles and feet.

▸ Wear comfortable shoes, support stockings, and clothing that doesn't bind. Choose natural fabrics like cotton or wool that absorb sweat.

▸ Carry some crackers or other light snacks with you to help prevent nausea.

▸ Take time to eat regular meals. A balanced and healthy diet during your trip will boost your energy and keep you feeling good. Be sure to get plenty of fiber to ease constipation, a common travel problem.

▸ Drink extra fluids. Take some juice or a bottle of water with you.

▸ Don't take any medication not prescribed for you. Traveling can upset your stomach and disrupt your sleep. Don't take any medicine—including motion-sickness pills, laxatives, diarrhea remedies, or sleeping pills—before checking with your doctor.

▸ Get plenty of sleep, and rest often so you won't feel tired.

▸ Don't do too much. It's tempting to squeeze in as many sights as you can, but it's vital to slow your pace when you are pregnant. After all, you can't conquer Rome (or most other places) in a day.

By Land

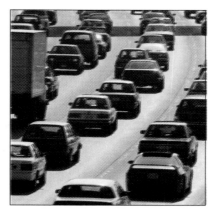

For short trips, a car can be a good way to travel. Make each day's drive brief, though. Spending hours on the road is tiring even when you're not pregnant. Try to limit driving to no more than 5 or 6 hours each day.

Be sure to wear your seat belt every time you ride in a car or truck, even if your car has an air bag. If you get in a crash—even a minor fender-bender—see your doctor to make sure you and your baby are OK.

Many new cars have air bags to protect the driver and the passenger riding in the front seat. Air bags are inside the steering wheel and dashboard in front of the passenger seat. In a crash, air bags inflate very fast. The force of an airbag can hurt people who are close to it—especially if they are small. To prevent injury, buckle up with both the lap and shoulder belts on every trip. Keep your seat as far back from the dashboard as you can.

Buckling Up During Pregnancy

For the best protection in a vehicle, wear a lap–shoulder belt every time you travel. The safety belt will not hurt your baby. You and your baby are far more likely to survive a car crash if you are buckled in.

When wearing your safety belt:

- Always wear both the lap and shoulder belt.
- Buckle the lap belt low on your hipbones, below your belly.
- Never put the lap belt across your belly.
- Place the shoulder belt across the center of the chest (between your breasts)—never under your arm.
- Make sure the belts fit snugly.

The upper part of the belt should cross your shoulder without chafing your neck. Never slip the upper part of the belt off your shoulder. Safety belts worn too loosely or too high on the belly can cause broken ribs or injuries to your belly. More damage is caused when they aren't used at all.

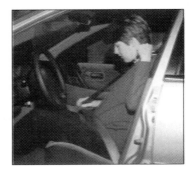

If you plan to travel by bus or train, there are a few things to keep in mind. Buses have narrow aisles and small bathrooms. Trains have more space for walking, but the bathrooms are often just as small. With both modes of transport, the ride may not always be smooth. Be sure to have a good hold on railings or seat backs when you are 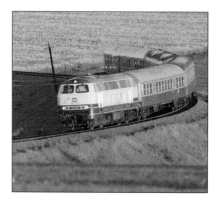 up and about. Don't worry that a bumpy ride could bring on labor—it won't.

By Air

Flying in an airplane is almost always safe during pregnancy. Most airlines allow pregnant women to fly until about 36 weeks of pregnancy.

Commercial planes are pressurized. That means the air in the cabin has more oxygen than the air outside. Many private planes are not pressurized. It's best to avoid altitudes higher than about 7,000 feet in unpressurized planes.

Don't worry about walking through the metal detector at the airport security check. These machines give off very low levels of radiation, but not nearly enough to harm you or your baby. Some tips for your flight:

▸ Book an aisle seat. This will make it easier for you to get up and walk around every hour or so. What's more, you won't have to climb over your fellow fliers to get to the bathroom. Also try to get a seat near the front of the plane. The ride often is smoother there. Avoid sitting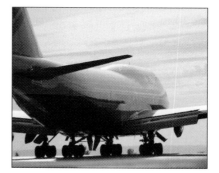

near an exit, where you are asked to help out in an emergency. A seat just behind the wall that divides first class and coach has extra room to stretch your legs.

▶ Wear a few layers of light clothing. Dressing in layers allows you to add clothes or peel them off as the cabin cools down or heats up. If you are cold, ask for a blanket.

▶ Get some pillows and prop them behind your back and neck to make your seat more comfortable.

▶ Bring crackers or other snacks to help ward off sickness. Having a few snacks also comes in handy while you are waiting for the meal cart. If you need a special meal, be sure to order it ahead of time.

▶ The air in the cabin is very dry. Make sure to drink plenty of fluids.

▶ Rest after a long flight. This will help your body get over jet lag.

By Sea

A cruise or sailing trip can be a treat. Sea travel can upset your stomach, though. If you have never been on a ship before, now is not the time for your maiden voyage. If you have done this before and you think your stomach can stand it, check on cruise rules for pregnant women. Make sure the ship has a doctor or a nurse on board and that it docks in areas 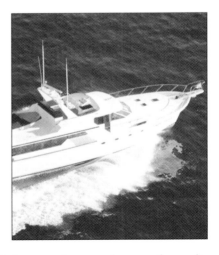 with modern medical facilities. Ask your doctor about safe medicines for calming seasickness. Or try a pair of the seasickness bands for sale at many drug stores. These bands use acupressure to help ward off nausea.

Foreign Travel: Let the Traveler Beware

If you are planning a trip out of the country, discuss it with your doctor before calling the travel agent. He or she can help you decide if foreign travel is safe for you. Your doctor also can help you figure out what steps to take before your trip. Allow plenty of time to get any shots you may need. Also be sure to get a copy of your health record to take with you.

When you are planning your trip, call the International Travelers Hotline at the Centers for Disease Control and Prevention (CDC). This service has safety tips and up-to-date vaccination facts for many countries. The number is 1-404-332-4559. The CDC Web site (www.cdc.gov) also has world travel health facts.

Unsafe Food and Water

Traveling to other countries means you may be exposed to other kinds of germs. The locals are used to the organisms in the food and water, but those same organisms can make you very ill. This is true whether you're staying in a city or a rural area.

Traveler's diarrhea may be a minor problem to someone who's not pregnant. It's a greater concern for you, though. That's because severe dehydration can rob your baby of needed fluid and nutrients. Talk with your doctor about using medicine to prevent diarrhea.

If you do get diarrhea, drink plenty of fluids to combat dehydration. Before taking a diarrhea remedy, check with a doctor to make sure it's safe. The best way to prevent illness is to avoid unsafe food and water. Be sure to:

▶ Drink only pure bottled water, bottled or canned juices and soft drinks, pasteurized dairy products, hot tea, or broth. Iodine used to purify water may not be safe for pregnant women.

▶ Don't put ice in your drinks. Don't drink out of glasses that may have been washed in impure water. Drink straight from the bottle or use paper cups.

▶ Avoid fresh fruits and vegetables unless they have been cooked or peeled.

▶ Don't eat raw or undercooked meat or fish.

Foreign Travel: Let the Traveler Beware (continued)

Malaria

Malaria is a tropical infection passed on by mosquito bites. It causes anemia and flu-like symptoms. Malaria can result in miscarriage, stillbirth, and small babies. To avoid mosquito bites, wear long-sleeved shirts and use mosquito netting. Ask your doctor about the safety of insect sprays or lotions during pregnancy.

No drug fully protects against malaria. A medicine called chloroquine can help prevent and treat the disease, though. Chloroquine is safe to use during pregnancy. You must start taking it before you travel and keep taking it for a few weeks after you return. In certain areas, though, mosquitoes carry strains of malaria that don't respond to chloroquine.

Immunizations

A disease that's rare in the United States may be common in other areas. As a result, some countries require visitors to get vaccinations before they travel there. Immunization rules vary, so find out before your trip which shots you may need.

It's best to get vaccines before you get pregnant. You can't always plan that far ahead, though. The good news: some vaccines are safe during pregnancy. Discuss the shots you need with your doctor. Together, you can decide which is the greater risk—the disease or the vaccine. The bad news: if neither option—getting the vaccine or risking the disease—is safe, you should delay your trip.

Medical Care

Even if you are in perfect health before going on a trip, you never know when an emergency will come up. Before leaving home, locate the nearest hospital or medical clinic in the place you are visiting. To find a doctor there, call the International Association for Medical Assistance to Travelers at 1-716-754-4883 or International SOS Assistance at 1-800-523-8930 (this group requires you to be a member). If you need to see a doctor who doesn't speak English, it's a good idea to have a foreign language dictionary with you. After you arrive, register with an American embassy or consulate. This will help if you need to leave the country because of an emergency.

Sex

Pregnancy affects just about every aspect of your life, including sex. In some cases, body changes make you or your partner want sex or enjoy sex less (see "Changes for Your Partner and Family" in Chapter 7).

You also may worry that having sex will harm your baby. The fetus is safe in the uterus. Don't worry that a penis will poke or jab it. Also, the amniotic sac and the thick mucus plugging your cervix shield the baby from germs.

Unless your doctor has told you not to, you can keep having sex right up until you go into labor. As your belly grows, though, you'll need to try some new positions:

▸ *The side-lying position.* You and your partner each lie on your side. You can either face each other or have your partner enter you from behind.

▸ *The woman-on-top position.* This takes the pressure off your belly.

▸ *The man-behind position.* This way, your growing belly won't come between you.

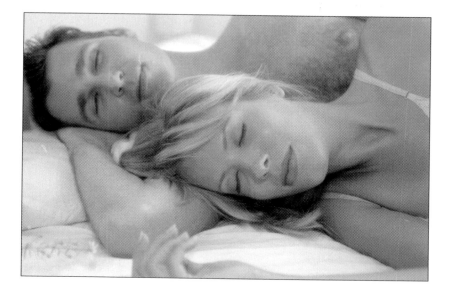

You may be advised to limit or avoid sex if you have had:

▸ Preterm labor or birth

▸ More than one miscarriage

▸ *Placenta previa* (the placenta covers part or all of the cervix)

▸ Infection

▸ Bleeding

▸ Breaking of the amniotic sac or leaking amniotic fluid

If sex is off-limits, there are other ways to express your sexuality and love. Cuddling, kissing, "petting," mutual masturbation, and oral sex can feel just as nice and close. If you have a condition that limits sex, ask your doctor what is safe for you.

Harmful Agents

Almost all that goes into your body—food, drink, medicine, even viruses—is shared with your baby. If you put good things in your body, it will be good for your baby. If you put something harmful in your body, you may put your baby at risk.

Teratogens are agents that can cause birth defects when a woman is exposed to them during pregnancy. They include certain medications, chemicals, and infections (Chapter 16 has details on infections during pregnancy). These agents can prevent the fetus from growing normally and cause defects of the brain or body. Their effect depends on the level of exposure and when in pregnancy it occurs. Other substances, such as tobacco, alcohol, and illegal drugs, also are harmful during pregnancy.

Some substances once were thought to be harmful, but now they are thought to be safe during pregnancy. For instance, many women worry that using hair dye during pregnancy

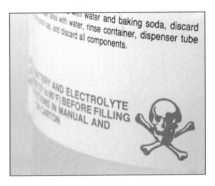

Agents to Avoid During Pregnancy

Certain medications (including prescription medication) and drugs are known to be harmful to your baby if you are exposed to them during pregnancy. Some agents may be more harmful than others—it often depends on the amount taken or when in pregnancy the fetus was exposed. If you are prescribed or exposed to any of the following substances, be sure to talk to your doctor:

- Alcohol
- Androgens and testosterone by-products (for instance, danazol)
- Angiotensin-converting enzyme (ACE) inhibitors (for instance, enalapril or captopril)
- Coumarin by-products (for instance, warfarin)
- Carbamazepine
- Anti-folic acid drugs (for instance, methotrexate or aminopterin)
- Cocaine
- Diethylstilbestrol (DES)
- Lead
- Lithium
- Organic mercury
- Phenytoin
- Streptomycin and kanamycin
- Tetracycline
- Thalidomide
- Trimethadione and paramethadione
- Valproic acid
- Vitamin A and its by-products (for instance, isotretinoin, etretinate, or retinoids)

might be harmful to their baby. It is believed that hair dyes are most likely safe to use during pregnancy. One thing you should know: because pregnancy causes a change in hormone levels, the hair color may not come out as expected. Also, there's no proof that small amounts of caffeine (for instance, 1 or 2 cups of coffee) cause problems during pregnancy. Caffeine is a stimulant and a diuretic (it increases urine production). It is found in coffee, cola and some other soft drinks, some teas, and chocolate.

If you are addicted to harmful substances, it may be hard to stop. Try to quit for your sake and your baby's. After all, carrying a new life inside you is one of the best reasons there is to break the cycle.

If you need help, talk to your doctor right away. He or she can get you the treatment you need to make a new start in your life—and to help your baby get the best start in his or hers.

Medications

Medications cross the placenta and enter the baby's bloodstream. In some cases, a medication could cause birth defects, addiction, or other problems in the baby. That doesn't mean you need to trash the contents of your medicine cabinet once you become pregnant. It means that you need to be careful.

Some medicines are safe to take during pregnancy. Also, the risks of some medicines may be outweighed by the effects of not taking them. Certain diseases are more harmful to a fetus than the drugs used to treat them, for instance. Don't stop taking a medication prescribed for you. Ask your doctor about them.

Tell anyone who prescribes medications for you that you are pregnant. That includes the

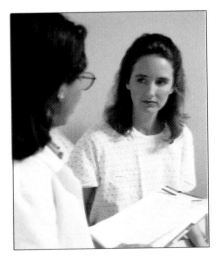

doctor you see for nonpregnancy problems, your dentist, or a mental health provider. Be sure that the doctor who cares for you during your pregnancy knows about any medical problems you may have. Tell him or her about the medications you take. Also tell the doctor if you have any drug allergies. If a medication you are taking poses a risk, your doctor may advise cutting down the amount or switching to a safer drug while you are pregnant.

Prescription medications also can be harmful if they are abused. A woman who abuses prescription drugs risks overdose and addiction as well.

Medicines sold over the counter can cause problems during pregnancy, too. Pain relief such as aspirin, acetaminophen, and ibuprofen may be harmful to a fetus. Check with your doctor before taking any over-the-counter drug. This includes pain-relief medications, laxatives, cold or allergy remedies, and skin treatments. You don't have to suffer through headaches or colds without relief, though. Your doctor can give you a list of medications that are safe for pregnant women.

Smoking

If you smoke when you're pregnant, every puff you take exposes your baby to harmful chemicals. These chemicals include tar, nicotine, and carbon monoxide. Nicotine causes blood vessels to constrict, so less oxygen and nutrients reach the fetus. Carbon monoxide travels to the baby's blood and lowers the amount of oxygen the baby and mother receive.

What's more, women who smoke during pregnancy are more likely to have:

▸ An *ectopic pregnancy*

▸ A miscarriage

▸ Vaginal bleeding

▸ Problems with the way the placenta attaches to the uterus

▸ A stillbirth

> A preterm baby

> A low-birth-weight baby (weighing less than 5 ½ pounds)

> A baby with deformed limbs or mental defects

Smoking isn't just harmful during pregnancy. If you or your partner light up after the baby is born, he or she may breathe in harmful amounts of smoke from your cigarettes (secondhand smoke). This raises the odds of asthma and *sudden infant death syndrome (SIDS).*

The sooner you quit, the better off both you and your baby will be. If you stop smoking early in your pregnancy, the chance of having a low-birth-weight baby is the same as that of a woman who didn't smoke at all. If you can kick the habit now, you may be able to kick it for a lifetime. You and your family will be healthier as a result.

If you can't quit, at least cut down on the number of cigarettes you smoke. The less you smoke, the less harm it will do. Cutting down or stopping smoking at any time in your pregnancy is better than not stopping at all.

If you have tried to quit on your own but failed, tell your doctor that you need help. If you are a heavy smoker, chewing nicotine gum or wearing a nicotine patch may help. Using these during pregnancy has some risks so they should be used only if, in your case, the benefits of quitting smoking outweigh the risks of nicotine replacement or smoking.

You may want to ask your partner and other family members to quit, too. This will help support you in your efforts to give up smoking. Even if you don't smoke but people around you do, secondhand smoke can harm your baby.

Alcohol

Many women—about 6 in 10—drink alcohol. Some of them use alcohol. Some abuse it. Having a glass of wine with dinner or a cocktail once in awhile is using alcohol. Having several drinks each day or binge drinking (having several drinks in one sitting) is abusing it. There's a fine line between the two. It's often hard to

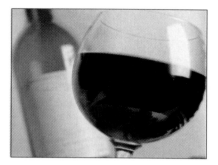

tell what is alcohol use and what is abuse. Because it is unclear how much alcohol is too much during pregnancy, the best course is not to drink at all.

When a pregnant woman drinks alcohol, it quickly reaches her fetus. The same amount of alcohol that's in her blood is in her baby's blood. Alcohol is much more harmful to a fetus than it is to an adult. The more a pregnant woman drinks, the greater the danger to her baby. Drinking at any time during pregnancy can cause problems.

Alcohol raises the odds of having a miscarriage or a preterm baby. One of the worst effects of drinking in pregnancy is *fetal alcohol syndrome.* This is a pattern of major physical, mental, and behavioral problems in babies exposed to alcohol during pregnancy.

Babies with fetal alcohol syndrome may have:

- Small bodies (even with special care, their growth doesn't catch up)

- Problems with joints and limbs

- Heart defects

- Abnormal facial features

- Behavioral problems, including hyperactivity, anxiety, and poor attention span

Some babies with fetal alcohol syndrome are born with all of these problems. Others have only some of them. Smoking, drug use, poor diet, and stress also may play a role in this condition.

Because so much is yet to be known, the wisest choice is to not drink alcohol when you are pregnant. It's best to stop drinking before you get pregnant. Find other ways to relax. Soak in a warm bath. Take a long walk. Listen to soothing music. Talk with a friend. Replace a wind-down drink with a steaming mug of herbal

? Do You Have a Drinking Problem?

Do you use alcohol or abuse it? Sometimes it's hard to tell. If you're not sure, asking a few simple questions can help you figure out if your drinking is a problem.

T   How many drinks does it take to make you feel high? (TOLERANCE)

A   Have people ANNOYED you by criticizing your drinking?

C   Have you felt you ought to CUT DOWN on your drinking?

E   Have you ever had a drink first thing in the morning to steady your nerves or get rid of a hangover? (EYE OPENER)

If your answer to the first question is more than two drinks, give yourself 2 points. Give yourself 1 point for every "yes" response to the other questions. If your total score is 2 or more, you may have an alcohol problem.

   Talk to your doctor about your drinking habits. He or she can help you decide if you have a problem. The doctor will refer you for counseling or treatment if needed. You also may want to think about contacting a substance abuse program. These groups can help you find someone to talk to about your problem and give you needed support when you are trying to quit. Check your local yellow page listings.

Modified from Sokol RJ, Martier SS, Ager JW. The T-ACE questions: practical prenatal detection of risk drinking. Am J Obstet Gynecol 1989;160:865

tea, a soothing cup of hot cocoa, or a cool glass of fruit-juice spritzer.

Drugs

Drug use during pregnancy can harm the health of the mother and the fetus. It can lead to long-term problems.

   There's no safe time to use drugs. Using them early in pregnancy, when the body systems form, can do severe damage. Using them in mid- to late pregnancy can affect brain growth. During late pregnancy, drug use can stunt fetal growth and bring on preterm labor. After birth, some drugs can be passed to the baby through breast milk.

It's safest to quit taking drugs well before getting pregnant. Still, giving them up or cutting back at any time is better than nothing. Here's a look at the effects of certain drugs during pregnancy.

Marijuana

Marijuana can be smoked or eaten. It affects a user's mood and sense of reality. The active compound in marijuana (THC) stays in the body for weeks, leading to higher levels of fetal exposure. Like cigarettes, smoking marijuana releases carbon monoxide. This can prevent the fetus from getting enough oxygen.

Cocaine

Cocaine can be snorted, injected, or smoked. No matter what its form, cocaine is very addictive. During pregnancy, cocaine can cause the placenta to tear away from the uterus—a condition called **abruptio placentae** (placental abruption). This can cause bleeding, preterm birth, or fetal death. Pregnant women who use cocaine also are at high risk of preterm labor. Babies exposed to cocaine may:

▸ Have withdrawal symptoms

▸ Grow more slowly

▸ Have brain injury

▸ Be very fussy

▸ Have long-lasting behavioral, emotional, and learning problems

Methamphetamine

Methamphetamine ("meth") is snorted, swallowed, smoked, or injected. It's highly addictive. Methamphetamine can cause placental abruption or even fetal death. A user's lifestyle can be just as harmful as the drug itself. That's because users often go on binges and may not sleep or eat for days.

Babies exposed to methamphetamine may:

▸ Have intrauterine growth restriction, or IUGR (grow too slowly in the womb)

▸ Have trouble bonding with others

▸ Have tremors

▸ Be very fussy

Heroin and Other Narcotics

Heroin is smoked, snorted, or injected. If heroin is used during pregnancy, it can cause:

▸ Fetal death

▸ Addiction in the fetus

▸ IUGR

▸ Preterm birth

▸ Low birth weight

▸ Delays in development

▸ Behavioral problems

A woman who uses heroin can quickly become addicted to it. If she tries to kick the habit, sudden withdrawal can harm her and her baby.

Drug treatment programs often replace heroin with methadone, a prescription drug. Women in methadone treatment programs may be able to stick to a healthier lifestyle than women who are addicted to heroin. Still, the drug itself is not good for a growing fetus. It also may be just as addictive. Because of this, methadone should be used only under a doctor's care.

"T's and blues" is the street name for a mix of a prescription drug and an over-the-counter allergy medication. It's often used as a cheap standby for heroin. Babies whose mothers use T's and blues are more likely to have IUGR. They also may suffer withdrawal symptoms after birth.

PCP and LSD

PCP often is smoked. It also can be eaten, snorted, or injected. It may cause a user to lose touch with what's real. They may become violent. A woman who uses PCP can have flashbacks, seizures, heart attacks, or lung failure. Babies exposed to PCP during pregnancy may have withdrawal symptoms after birth, be smaller than normal, and have poor control of their movements.

LSD ("acid") is swallowed. It can cause someone who has used it to hear and see things that aren't there, have flashbacks, and become violent. LSD use during pregnancy can cause birth defects.

Glues and Solvents

Inhalant use makes a user feel light-headed and dizzy. It also can damage the liver, kidneys, bone marrow, and brain. It can even cause sudden death. During pregnancy, glue and solvent abuse can lead to miscarriage, IUGR, and preterm birth. The birth defects linked with glue sniffing during pregnancy are much like those caused by alcohol.

The Abused Woman

Physical, sexual, and emotional abuse of women is one of America's worst health problems. Millions of women are abused each year. Pregnancy often offers no break from an abuser's blows. In fact, nearly 1 in 6 pregnant women is abused by her partner. Also, 1 in 5 women visiting an emergency room is there for injuries received by her partner. More than 1 in 3 female murder victims is killed by her husband or boyfriend. Domestic abuse crosses all racial, class, economic, and religious lines.

This abuse often starts or gets worse during pregnancy. It puts both a mother and her baby at risk. An abuser is likely to aim his blows at a pregnant woman's breasts and belly. The dangers of this violence include miscarriage, vaginal bleeding, low birth weight, and fetal injury.

Sometimes abuse lessens during pregnancy. A woman may feel safe from her partner only when she's carrying a child. As a result, she may get pregnant to escape her partner's rage. All too often, though, his rage returns and may worsen after the baby's born. Then, there are two victims.

If you are in a violent relationship, it's vital to take steps to protect yourself and your baby. First, know that you are not at fault for your partner's actions. Abusers often blame their wives or girlfriends. Women may stay with violent men because they feel they deserve the treatment they get. No matter what he says, though, it's not your fault. He alone is to blame for his actions.

Second, tell someone you trust—a close friend, a family member, your doctor, a counselor, or a clergy member—about the abuse. Talking about a problem you have kept bottled up can be a huge relief. What's more, the person you confide in can put you in touch with crisis hotlines, domestic violence programs, legal-aid services, and shelters for abused women. These services offer counseling that can help you get out of a bad situation.

Next, learn to spot violence before it happens. Danger signs include:

- Yelling, taunting, or name-calling

- Threatening to use a weapon

- Threatening or harming children or other family members

- Forcing you to have sex

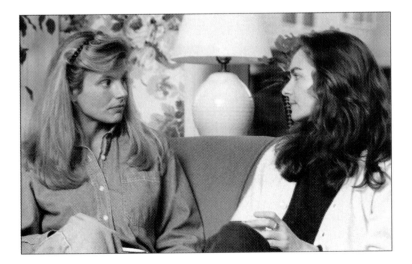

For your safety, come up with a fast-exit plan. That way, you can leave quickly when you see these signs. Key moves to make:

▸ Pack a suitcase. Include toilet items, a change of clothes for you and your children, and an extra set of car and house keys. Store the bag with a friend or neighbor you trust.

▸ Hide some cash. Each week, put aside as much money as you can spare. Having a stash of money may help you work up the nerve to leave.

▸ Keep needed items in a safe place. Have them handy so you can take them with you on short notice. Include:

—Prescription medicines
—Birth certificates
—Social Security cards
—Health insurance cards
—Driver's license
—Extra cash and change for phone calls
—Checkbook
—Savings account book
—Credit cards
—Medical and financial records
—A special toy for each child

▸ Have a safe place. Know a friend or relative's home or shelter where you can go, no matter what time of day or night. Keep the address and phone number in your purse.

▸ Know what to do after you are hurt. Call your doctor or head to an emergency room if you don't get out in time and your partner harms you. Tell the doctor how you were hurt. Be sure to ask for a copy of your medical record in case you want to file charges.

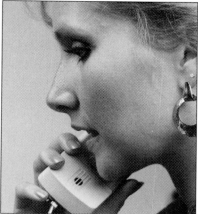

? Is Your Relationship Abusive?

Fights, even heated ones, are a normal part of relationships. Physical violence and other abuse are not. How do you know if your relationship has crossed the line? Ask yourself these questions:

- Does your partner make jokes at your expense or put you down?
- Has he forced or pressured you to perform a sexual act?
- Does he threaten you or throw things when he's angry?
- Has he physically hurt you in the past year?
- Does he say it's your fault if he hits you?
- Does he promise it won't happen again, but it does?

If your answer to any of these is "yes," your relationship is not healthy. Get help right away.

- Call the police. Physical abuse is a crime, even if you are living with or married to your abuser. Tell the police what happened to you. Get the officer's badge number and a copy of the report in case you want to press charges at any time.

It's hard to break the cycle of violence. If you do nothing, though, chances are the abuse will happen more often and become more severe. With help, some violent men can learn to stop hurting their wives or girlfriends. The only way for your partner to get help is for you to get help first.

No one deserves to be abused: not you, not your fetus, and not your children. Leaving your partner or having him arrested during your pregnancy takes great courage. But you owe your baby a safe and loving home, and you owe yourself an end to the violence.

For more information or to get help, check the section of your phone book for domestic violence services or hotlines. You also can call the National Domestic Violence Hotline at 1-800-799-SAFE (7233).

Healthy Lifestyle, Healthy Baby

Few things are more vital to your baby's health than your lifestyle choices during pregnancy. If you led an active, healthy lifestyle before pregnancy, keep it up. If you do want to make a few changes, make them now to give your baby the best start you can. You'll also make a change for the better in your own life. Years from now, you'll still be reaping the rewards.

CHAPTER 6

Nutrition

A well-balanced diet is key to good health. It is even more important during pregnancy, when there are added demands on your body to meet the needs of the growing fetus. A good diet can help ensure the health of your body and the growth of your baby.

Eating right during pregnancy may take a little effort, but it will be a major benefit for you and your baby. If you already have a balanced diet, all you have to do is add a few extra calories and nutrients. (Breastfeeding mothers need to pay careful attention to their diet as well. See Chapter 10 for details.)

A variety of foods can be used to create a healthy diet for you and your baby. Women all over the world with vastly varied diets have healthy babies. To nourish your growing baby, make sure you are getting the nutrients both of you need.

A Healthy Diet

The Food Guide Pyramid

One way to be sure you're eating a balanced diet is to follow the Food Guide Pyramid. This pyramid was devised by the U.S. Department of Agriculture. It offers guidelines to help you get the nutrients you need. It stresses a diet that's low in fat, sugar, and *cholesterol* (a substance that carries fat through the bloodstream) and high in vegetables, fruits, and grains. If you don't want to

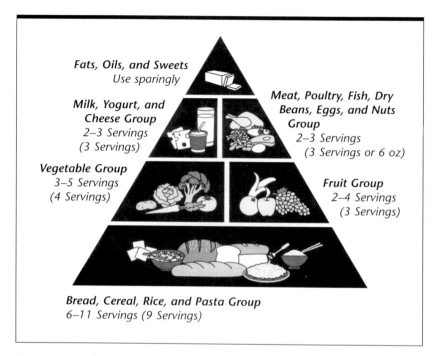

Fats, Oils, and Sweets
Use sparingly

Milk, Yogurt, and
Cheese Group
2–3 Servings
(3 Servings)

Meat, Poultry, Fish, Dry
Beans, Eggs, and Nuts
Group
2–3 Servings
(3 Servings or 6 oz)

Vegetable Group
3–5 Servings
(4 Servings)

Fruit Group
2–4 Servings
(3 Servings)

Bread, Cereal, Rice, and Pasta Group
6–11 Servings (9 Servings)

The food guide pyramid is a guide to help men and nonpregnant women choose foods that will give them the nutrients they need. Because a pregnant woman needs extra calories and nutrients, she should get at least the number of servings shown in parentheses after the standard servings.

Modified from the U.S. Department of Agriculture and U.S. Department of Health and Human Services.

measure out each serving to see if you're getting the right amount, follow this rule: one serving size of a food item is about the size of the palm of your hand. The pyramid has six food groups:

1. *Bread, cereal, rice, and pasta.* This group provides complex carbohdrates (starches). These are a good source of energy, vitamins, minerals, and fiber. Choose whole-grain products, such as whole-wheat bread, as often as you can. Also look for foods made with little fat or sugar. A serving equals: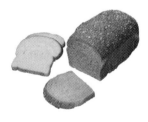

▸ 1 slice of bread

▸ 1 ounce of cold cereal

▸ ¹/₂ cup of cooked cereal, rice, or pasta

2. *Vegetables.* This group provides vitamins such as A and C and folic acid, and minerals such as iron and magnesium. Vegetables are low in fat and high in fiber. When you're planning your meals, choose a wide array of vegetables. This will help ensure that you get a variety of nutrients. Women who are worried about pesticides might want to think about buying vegetables and fruit that are grown without chemicals (organic). Pesticides also can be removed from fruit and vegetables by washing them with warm water and a small amount of soap and rinsing them. Eat a mixture of:

▸ Dark-green leafy vegetables (spinach, romaine lettuce, broccoli)

▸ Deep-yellow or orange vegetables (carrots, sweet potatoes)

▸ Starchy vegetables (potatoes, corn, peas)

▸ Legumes (chick peas and navy, pinto, and kidney beans)

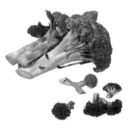

A serving equals:

▸ 1 cup of salad greens

▸ ¹/₂ cup of other cooked or raw vegetables

▸ ³/₄ cup of vegetable juice

3. *Fruits.* This group provides vitamins A and C, potassium, and fiber. Choose fresh fruits, fruit juices, and frozen, canned, or dried fruit. Eat plenty of citrus fruits, melons, and berries. Choose fruit juices instead of fruit drinks, which are mostly sugar. A serving equals:

▸ 1 medium apple, banana, or orange

▸ ¹/₂ cup of chopped, cooked, or canned fruit

▸ $1/2$ cup of fruit juice

▸ $1/4$ cup of raisins or other dried fruit

4. *Milk, yogurt, and cheese.* Dairy products are a major source of protein, calcium, phosphorus, and vitamins. Calcium is a key nutrient in pregnancy and during breastfeeding. If you don't like the taste of milk, eat dairy products such as yogurt, cottage cheese, or sliced cheese. Choose low-fat, skim, or part-skim items as often as you can. A serving equals:

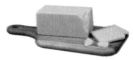

▸ 1 cup of milk or yogurt

▸ 1 $1/2$ ounces of cheese

5. *Meat, poultry, fish, beans, eggs, and nuts.*
   This group provides B vitamins, protein, iron, and zinc. A fetus needs plenty of protein and iron to develop. Choose lean meats and trim off the fat and skin before cooking. One serving equals:

▸ 2–3 ounces of cooked lean meat, poultry, or fish

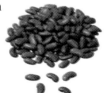

▸ 1 cup of cooked dry beans

▸ 1 egg

▸ 2 tablespoons of peanut butter

6. *Fats, oils, and sweets.* These foods are full of calories and have few vitamins or minerals. You should get no more than 30% of your daily calories from fat. Choose low-fat foods as often as you can. Go easy on butter, margarine, salad dressing, and gravy, too. Save high-sugar foods such as candy, sweet desserts, and soft drinks for a special treat. Also keep in mind that sugar-free sodas and punches, gums, gelatins, and desserts often contain an artificial sweetener called saccharin. There are questions about saccharin's safety during pregnancy. But, another artificial sweetener called aspartame is believed to be safe during pregnancy.

Getting the Nutrients You Need

Every diet should include proteins, carbohydrates, vitamins, minerals, and fat. These fuel your body and help your baby grow. You often can get enough of the nutrients if you eat a healthy diet, but your doctor may suggest you take a supplement or prenatal vitamin to ensure you are getting the right amount. Do not take a supplement without speaking to your doctor about it. Too much of a vitamin can be harmful to you and your baby.

To get the right amount of nutrients, you need to know which foods are good sources. Follow these steps to ensure your diet is healthy:

Step 1: Get in the habit of looking at the labels on food boxes, cans, and bottles. This will teach you a lot about what's going

Reading Food Labels

All packaged foods must be clearly labeled with nutrition information. Reading all food labels can help you make smart food choices. The label will tell you how many grams of fat and how many calories are in each serving.

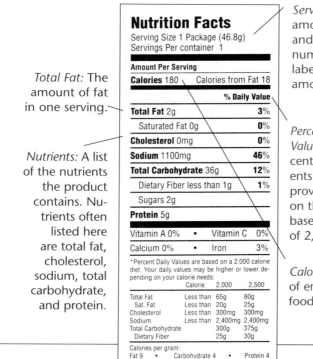

Serving Size: The amount served and eaten. The numbers on the label refer to this amount of food.

Total Fat: The amount of fat in one serving.

Nutrients: A list of the nutrients the product contains. Nutrients often listed here are total fat, cholesterol, sodium, total carbohydrate, and protein.

Percent Daily Value: The percentage of nutrients this product provides based on the RDA. It is based on a diet of 2,000 calories.

Calories: Amount of energy the food supplies.

Nutrition Facts
Serving Size 1 Package (46.8g)
Servings Per container 1

Amount Per Serving

Calories 180   Calories from Fat 18

% Daily Value

Total Fat 2g	3%
Saturated Fat 0g	0%
Cholesterol 0mg	0%
Sodium 1100mg	46%
Total Carbohydrate 36g	12%
Dietary Fiber less than 1g	1%
Sugars 2g	
Protein 5g	

Vitamin A 0%	•	Vitamin C	0%
Calcium 0%	•	Iron	3%

*Percent Daily Values are based on a 2,000 calorie diet. Your daily values may be higher or lower depending on your calorie needs:

		Calorie 2,000	2,500
Total Fat	Less than	65g	80g
Sat. Fat	Less than	20g	25g
Cholesterol	Less than	300mg	300mg
Sodium	Less than	2,400mg	2,400mg
Total Carbohydrate		300g	375g
Dietary Fiber		25g	30g

Calories per gram:
Fat 9   •   Carbohydrate 4   •   Protein 4

TABLE 1. Recommended Dietary Allowances for Nonpregnant, Pregnant, and Breastfeeding Women

Nutrient (unit)	Nonpregnant			Pregnant	Breastfeeding
	15–18 years	19–24 years	25–50 years		
Protein (g)	44	46	50	60	65
Calcium (mg)	1,300	1,000	1,000	1,000	1,000
Phosphorus (mg)	1,250	700	700	700	700
Magnesium (mg)	360	310	320	360	320
Iron (mg)	15	15	15	30	15
Zinc (mg)	12	12	12	15	19
Iodine (µg)	150	150	150	175	200
Selenium (µg)	50	55	55	65	75
Vitamin A (µg)	800	800	800	800	1,300
Vitamin D (µg)	5	5	5	5	5
Vitamin E (mg)	8	8	8	10	12
Vitamin C (mg)	60	60	60	70	95
Vitamin K (µg)	55	60	65	65	65
Thiamin (mg)	1.1	1.1	1.1	1.5	1.6
Riboflavin (mg)	1.3	1.3	1.3	1.6	1.8
Niacin (mg)	15	15	15	17	20
Vitamin B_6 (mg)	1.5	1.6	1.6	2.2	2.1
Folic acid (µg)	180	180	180	400	280
Vitamin B_{12} (µg)	2.0	2.0	2.0	2.2	2.6

Adapted from Recommended Dietary Allowances. 10th ed. © 1989 by the National Academy of Sciences. Courtesy of the National Academy Press, Washington, DC; Committee on Dietary Reference Intakes for Calcium, Phosphorus, Magnesium, Vitamin D, and Fluoride (Washington, DC; National Academy Press, 1997)

into your body. These labels list serving sizes, calories, calories from fat, and the amounts of certain nutrients.

You'll also see the words Daily Value (DV) on most food labels. The daily value is the amount of a nutrient that an average person should eat every day. Keep in mind, though, that pregnant women often need more. Table 1 shows the Recommended Dietary Allowances (RDAs) for key nutrients during pregnancy. Daily values are derived, in part, from RDAs.

Step 2: Keep tabs on the nutrients you are getting. The numbers listed below the daily value are the levels of nutrients in one serving of the product. For instance, if the daily value for fat in a granola bar is listed as 10%, that means the bar contains one tenth of the fat you need that day. Reading labels will help you boost your intake of certain nutrients and limit your intake of others.

Step 3: Don't worry about eating the exact amount of every nutrient. Just try to eat a variety of foods and eat enough servings from the Food Guide Pyramid. If you do, chances are good that your diet is healthy and that your baby is getting the right amount of nutrients. Certain nutrients are key to growth during pregnancy (Table 2). During pregnancy, you need more:

▸ Calories to help nourish your growing fetus

▸ Iron and folic acid to help make the extra blood needed in pregnancy

▸ Protein to help make blood and build your baby's tissues and muscles

▸ Calcium to help build your baby's bones and teeth

Protein

Protein provides the nutrients your body needs to grow, maintain, and repair muscles and other tissues. During pregnancy, protein is the building block for your baby's cells.

Most women should eat 45 grams of protein a day. Pregnant women need 60 grams. Protein comes from animals—meat, fish, poultry, and dairy products. Animal foods rich in protein include:

TABLE 2. Key Nutrients in Pregnancy

Nutrient	Function	Sources
Protein	Builds cells, helps make blood, provides energy stores	Meat, eggs, beans, dairy products
Carbohydrates	Gives energy	Bread, cereal, rice, potatoes, pasta
Fat	Provides energy for growth	Meat, eggs, nuts, peanut butter, margarine, oils
Vitamins		
A	Prevents eye disease, aids vision, helps bone and teeth growth	Green leafy vegetables, deep yellow or orange vegetables (carrots and sweet potatoes), milk, liver
Thiamin (B_1)	Aids in carbohydrate digestion, helps nervous system function	Whole-grain or enriched breads and cereals, fish, pork, poultry, lean meat, milk
Riboflavin (B_2)	Helps body release energy to cells, promotes healthy skin and eyes	Milk, whole-grain or enriched breads and cereals, liver, green leafy vegetables
B_6	Helps form red blood cells; helps body use protein, fat, and carbohydrates	Beef liver, pork, ham, whole-grain cereals, bananas
B_{12}	Aids nervous system, helps form red blood cells	Animal foods: liver, milk, poultry (vegetarians should take a supplement)
C	Promotes healthy gums, teeth, and bones; helps body absorb iron; helps body resist infection; helps form collagen, a flexible tissue that supports the body	Citrus fruit, strawberries, broccoli, tomatoes
D	Helps body use calcium and phosphorus, promotes strong bones and teeth	Fortified milk, fish liver oils, sunshine

TABLE 2. Key Nutrients in Pregnancy (continued)

Nutrient	Function	Sources
E	Helps body use vitamin A, helps body form and use red blood cells and muscles	Vegetable oils, whole-grain cereals, wheat germ, green leafy vegetables
Folic acid	Helps make blood, helps some enzymes function, helps prevent neural tube defects and other problems	Green leafy vegetables; dark yellow or orange fruits and vegetables; liver; legumes and nuts; fortified breads, cereals, rice, and pastas
Niacin	Promotes healthy skin, nerves, and digestion; helps body use carbo-hydrates	Meat, liver, poultry, fish, whole-grain or enriched cereals
Minerals		
Calcium	Builds strong bones and teeth, helps blood clot, helps muscles and nerves function	Milk and dairy products; sardines and salmon with bones; collard, kale, mustard, spinach, and turnip greens; fortified orange juice
Iodine	Helps produce hormones that control energy use	Seafood, iodized salt
Iron	Helps form red blood cells that carry oxygen to the fetus, prevents anemia and fatigue, helps body resist infection	Lean red meat, liver, dried beans, whole-grain or enriched breads and cereals, prune juice, spinach, tofu
Magnesium	Helps nerves and muscles function, helps body use carbohydrates	Legumes, whole-grain cereals, milk, meat, green vegetables
Phosphorus	Builds strong bones and teeth	Milk and dairy products, meat, poultry, fish, whole-grain cereals, legumes
Zinc	Helps produce insulin and certain enzymes	Meat, liver, seafood, milk, whole-grain cereals

▶ Beef, pork, ham, or canned tuna (a 3-ounce serving has 27 grams of protein)

▶ Chicken (a 3-ounce serving has 22 grams of protein)

▶ Low-fat milk (1 cup has 11 grams of protein)

Plant products such as grains and legumes also are good sources of protein. For strict vegetarians (called "vegans"), though, getting enough protein can be a problem. If you don't eat any meat, dairy products, or eggs, talk to your doctor about ways to get more protein. He or she may refer you to a nutritionist or a dietitian to help you plan a high-protein vegetarian diet. The food guide pyramid designed for vegetarians also is helpful.

Carbohydrates

Food sugar—carbohydrates—is the body's main source of energy. There are two types of sugar: simple sugars and starches.

Simple sugars, such as glucose, provide a quick energy boost. That's because they are ready to be used by the body right away. Simple sugars are found in table sugar, honey, syrup, fruit juices, hard candies, and many processed foods.

Starches are a more complex form of sugar. It takes your body longer to process them, so starches provide longer lasting energy than simple sugars do. Starches are found in bread, rice, pasta, fruits, and starchy vegetables such as potatoes or corn.

Starchy foods also contain fiber. Your body doesn't use fiber the same way it uses other nutrients. Still, you can't live without it. Fiber helps flush out your digestive system and keep you "regular." It also helps rid your body of excess fat and cholesterol. Try to eat 20–30 grams (about 1 ounce) of fiber a day. Good sources of fiber include:

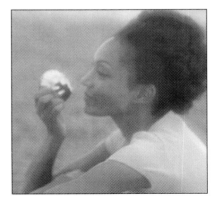

▶ Fruits (such as raisins, prunes, or apples)

‣ Vegetables

‣ Whole-grain products (such as whole-wheat bread or brown rice)

Carbohydrates should make up more than half of the food you eat. It's important to have a balance of fruits, vegetables, and grains. Not all starches offer the same benefits, so variety is the key. Because they have other nutrients, fruits and vegetables are better sources of carbohydrates than bread and grains are.

Try to limit simple sugars. They have more calories than nutrients, and the energy they provide is used up quickly. Eating a candy bar might give you a brief "sugar high." It doesn't offer much nutrition, though, and you'll soon feel tired again. But starches have lots of nutrients and fiber. They give you longer-lasting energy, too.

Fats

Many people have come to think of fat as "bad." It's true that too much fat isn't good for you. You need some fat to function, though.

Fats help your body use vitamins A, D, E, and K, as well as proteins and carbohydrates. Fat that your body doesn't need right away is stored as fat tissue. This tissue is converted back into energy when your body needs more calories than you eat. Those fat stores also will be called on when you start making breast milk for your newborn.

Dietary fat comes in two forms—saturated and unsaturated:

‣ Saturated fats come from meat and dairy products and some vegetables. They tend to be sold chilled—as butter and lard, for instance. Shortening, palm oil, and coconut oil are also saturated fats.

‣ Unsaturated fats tend to be liquid and come mostly from plants and vegetables. Olive oil, canola oil, peanut oil, sunflower oil, and fish oil are all unsaturated fats.

Too much saturated fat can raise your cholesterol level and lead to heart disease. It should make up less than one third of the total fat in your diet, or no more than 10% of the calories you eat each day. The other two thirds of the fat in your diet, or about 20% of your daily calories, should come from unsaturated fat.

Fat is very high in calories. A gram of protein or carbohydrate has just 4 calories, for instance. A gram of fat has 9.

Fat is found in many foods—from meat and baked goods to nondairy coffee creamer. You can reduce the fat in your diet by changing the way you prepare foods:

▸ Broil, bake, poach, or steam your food instead of frying or sautéing it

▸ Skim liquid fat from soups

▸ Trim all fat from meats

▸ Remove skin from poultry

▸ Cut back on butter, margarine, cream, oil, and mayonnaise

▸ Choose unsaturated fats over saturated fats as often as you can

Water

Most people don't think of water as a nutrient. Still, we can't live without it. Water is used to:

▸ Build new tissue

▸ Carry nutrients and waste products within the body

▸ Aid digestion

▸ Help chemical reactions

▸ Form amniotic fluid around the fetus and help prevent the uterus from contracting before it should

Nearly three fourths of your body's weight is water. Water is lost through sweat, urine, and even breathing. To replace what's lost, be sure to drink eight glasses of water a day. One tip to increase your fluid intake: keep a bottle of water on your desk or in your purse. Drink from it often. Other liquids, such as fruit juice and tea, can stand in for some of the water you need each day.

Iron

Iron is used to make hemoglobin. This protein in red blood cells carries oxygen to your organs, tissues, and fetus. Just like the other cells in your body, blood cells die and are replaced in a constant process. The iron from blood cells is used to make more hemoglobin.

Every time you menstruate, you lose blood and thus iron. This means that after you become pregnant, you may not have enough iron stored in your body to make the extra blood you and your baby need. This condition is called anemia. Women need more iron in their diet during pregnancy to support the growth of the fetus and to produce extra blood. Getting plenty of iron when you are pregnant is a must.

Eating certain foods will help provide the extra iron you need. Dried fruits and beans, whole grains, dark leafy greens, and organ meats are all high in iron.

Vitamin C helps your body absorb the iron in food. Calcium, though, can block absorption. Thus, don't take iron and calcium at the same time. It's a good idea to take iron in the morning with orange juice and take calcium before you go to bed.

Talk with your doctor about whether you need extra iron. An iron supplement or a prenatal vitamin with iron will help boost your intake. Be aware, though, that iron pills can cause constipation, bloating, and black stools. If you are taking an iron supplement, keep it away from children (as with all medication).

Folic Acid

Like iron, folic acid is used to make blood. Folic acid is used to make the extra blood your body needs during pregnancy.

Not getting enough folic acid in your diet before conception and in the early weeks of pregnancy increases the risk of birth defects such as neural tube defects (defects of the spine and skull). Lack of folic acid also may increase the risk of congenital (exists from birth) heart defects, oral and facial defects, preterm delivery, and low birth weight.

Pregnant women should take a supplement of 0.4 milligrams of folic acid each day. The best sources of folic acid in foods include:

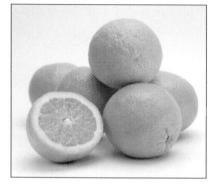

▶ Dark, leafy greens

▶ Whole-grain breads and cereals

▶ Citrus fruit

Women who have had a child with a neural tube defect or certain other birth defects need 10 times the amount of this vitamin—4 milligrams daily. They should take folic acid 1 month before they become pregnant and during the first 3 months of pregnancy. Taking this amount before becoming pregnant and in early pregnancy may prevent a repeat of the problem.

The U.S. government asks food companies to add folic acid to certain products to help lower the rate of neural tube defects. Almost all breads, cereal, pasta, rice, and flour have folic acid added. Still, it can be hard to get all of the folic acid you need from food alone. To be on the safe side, ask your doctor about taking a supplement. Most prescription prenatal vitamins have at least 1 milligram of folic acid. Over-the-counter prenatal vitamins have 0.8 milligrams of folic acid. Keep in mind that you should take folic acid alone to get 4 milligrams daily. It should not be taken as part of a multivitamin. Otherwise, you would get too many of the other vitamins.

Calcium

Calcium is used to build your baby's bones and teeth. If you don't get enough of this mineral from food, your baby will take the calcium it needs from your bones. That can lead to *osteoporosis* (fragile bones) later in your life. It also may cause you to lose a tooth.

To prevent this, pregnant women should get 1,000 milligrams of calcium each day (1,300 for those under age 19). Drinking about 3 cups of milk a day will fill this quota. Milk and other dairy products such as cheese and yogurt are the best sources of calcium. You also can get calcium from:

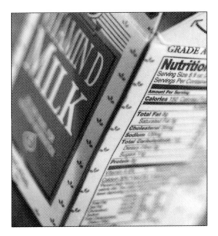

▶ Fortified orange juice

▶ Nuts and seeds

▶ Sardines

▶ Salmon with bones

▶ Collard, kale, mustard, spinach, and turnip greens

If you have *lactose intolerance* (trouble digesting milk products), ask your doctor how you can get enough calcium. He or she may suggest you try pills or drops with an enzyme that helps your body break down milk sugar. Taking a daily antacid made with calcium is another simple way to boost your calcium intake that your doctor may suggest you try. Also, many stores carry low-lactose milk and cheese. Keep in mind that iron prevents calcium from being absorbed, so do not take calcium with iron.

Prenatal Vitamins

Except for iron, folic acid, and maybe calcium, a well-rounded diet should supply all of the nutrients you need during pregnancy. If your doctor thinks your diet is lacking certain nutrients, though, he or she may advise taking a prenatal multivitamin and mineral supplement. You should not take a prenatal vitamin or any other supplement without talking with your doctor.

Take prenatal vitamins only as directed. Large doses of anything—even a good thing—can be harmful. Don't take more than the RDA for any vitamin or mineral—most of all vitamins A and D—without getting your doctor's OK.

Some prenatal tablets have high levels of other vitamins and minerals, or they may skimp on nutrients like calcium. Very high levels of vitamin A have been linked with severe birth defects. Some single-dose supplements have up to 25,000 IUs of vitamin A.

Some prenatal vitamins have as many as 8,000 IUs. Your prenatal multivitamin should contain no more than 5,000 IUs of vitamin A.

Some women take daily herbal supplements or drink medicinal teas to enhance their health. These include herbs such as echinacea, golden seal, ginseng, and gingko biloba. Little is known about the effect of herbs during pregnancy. The safest bet is to avoid taking anything you don't need when you're pregnant. Let your doctor know about any herbal or "natural" supplements you use.

Special Concerns

For most women, careful meal planning and a daily prenatal vitamin will cover all the nutritional bases. Some mothers-to-be need more nutrients than a normal diet provides, though. If you fit into any of these groups, talk to your doctor about your nutrition needs.

Women With Severe Morning Sickness

Early in pregnancy, many women feel sick to their stomach. Some can't bear the thought of eating. Others can eat only certain foods. Still others find that they lose their lunch almost as soon as they have eaten it. (Despite its name, morning sickness doesn't just happen in the morning. For some women, "morning, noon, and night sickness" is more like it.)

Don't panic if you can't eat (or keep down) much during these early weeks. As long as you are keeping something down and taking a daily prenatal vitamin, your baby should be fine.

If your nausea and vomiting are severe, though, you may need medical treatment. You could have a condition called *hyperemesis gravidarum.* It can lead to loss of weight and fluids (dehydration), which puts the fetus at risk. If your doctor suspects that you have hyperemesis gravidarum, you may need to stay in the hospital for a while.

Your doctor may give you fluids through an intravenous (IV) line. You also may be treated with anti-nausea medications. In most cases, you will not be allowed to eat any food until the vomiting stops. Your doctor may suggest that you rest in a dimly lit room where it is quiet and private. This type of treatment in the hospital often relieves symptoms. Call your doctor if you:

▸ Can't keep any food or liquid down

▸ Lose weight quickly

▸ Have dark, scant urine

▸ Vomit blood

Women With Poor Nutrient Stores

Pregnancy demands a lot from your body. Having more than one pregnancy in a short time can wipe out some of the nutrients your body needs to help nourish you and your baby. Iron and calcium, for instance, are minerals that may be low in a woman who has back-to-back babies.

If you have been pregnant more than twice in 2 years (including pregnancies that ended in abortion or miscarriage), you may not have had a chance to replace the nutrients your body has lost. Your stores also may be low if you had complications in a pregnancy, if you had a low-birth-weight baby, or if you are very thin. In that case, your doctor can tell you how to get the extra nutrients you need.

Women With Unusual Cravings

Pregnant women are known for their weird food cravings. Most often, giving in to these cravings does no harm. Cravings can cause problems, though, if you eat only a few types of food for long periods. They also can be less than healthy if you indulge your cravings for french fries and potato chips and neglect the rest of your diet.

Most harmful is a condition called *pica*. During pregnancy, some women feel strong urges to eat nonfood items such as laundry starch, clay, ice, or chalk. If you feel these urges, discuss them with your doctor.

Women Who Don't Gain Enough Weight

More than 7 million American women suffer from eating disorders. These disorders can be deadly. They starve a woman's body—and her baby—of key nutrients. If you have an eating disorder, get help for your baby's sake and your own. Eating disorders include:

▶ *Anorexia nervosa.* Women with anorexia starve themselves because they think they are too fat. In fact, they are far too thin. Women with anorexia have trouble getting pregnant because they often stop menstruating. If they do manage to conceive, these women are more likely to miscarry or to have a cesarean birth. They also are at risk of having a baby that's too small or born too early.

▶ *Bulimia.* Women with bulimia binge on huge amounts of food and then purge (vomit or take laxatives) to rid their body of excess calories. Women with bulimia may have a higher rate of miscarriage. They also risk delivering low-birth-weight babies and babies with certain birth defects.

Pregnancy raises body-image issues for just about every woman. But for a pregnant woman with anorexia or bulimia, anxiety about food and weight gain can cause the disorder to worsen.

Eating disorders may recur during pregnancy. If a woman with the disorder feels bad about her growing body, it may trigger the disorder's return. She may stop taking medication often used to treat eating disorders in an effort to protect the baby.

Counseling and medication help control the emotional aspects of the disorder. If anything is getting in the way of eating a healthy diet or gaining weight, a doctor can offer advice.

Women Who Weigh Too Much

A woman with a body mass index (BMI) of more than 29 is thought to be obese. (See Chapter 1 to learn how to calculate your BMI.) Women who are overweight or obese may have problems during pregnancy, such as gestational diabetes or having an overly large baby (macrosomia).

Women With Certain Diseases

Aside from the health problems they cause, some diseases can lead to nutrition problems as well. Certain medications that are used to keep an ailment under control, for instance, can affect how your body absorbs food. What's more, conditions such as kidney disease, diabetes, and phenylketonuria (in which a woman lacks an enzyme needed to process certain foods) call for special diets. If a lot of foods are off-limits, it can be hard to eat a balanced diet.

Again, tell your doctor about any health problems you have and any medications you take for them. He or she may change your medication, advise another diet, or take other steps to help you get the nutrients you need.

Calories and Weight Gain

Some women worry about adding pounds when they are pregnant. Pregnancy is not the time to fret about putting on weight. It's also not an excuse to eat too much, though. Most women need between 1,800 and 2,200 calories a day when they are not pregnant. Pregnant women need about 300 calories more.

Keep in mind that those calories add up fast—a glass of skim milk and a half-sandwich should do it. "Eating for two" doesn't mean eating twice as much.

How many pounds should you gain? That depends on how much you weighed before getting pregnant. Most women are advised to gain 25–35 pounds. Overweight women can gain less. Underweight women should gain more.

TABLE 3. Weight Gain in Pregnancy

Condition Before Getting Pregnant	Weight Gain (pounds)
Underweight	28–40
Normal Weight	25–35
Overweight	15–25
Obese	15
Carrying Twins	35–45

The amount of weight you need to put on is based on your body mass index, which compares your weight to your height (see Chapter 1). Ask your doctor about the right amount of pregnancy weight gain for you.

A woman who gains too few pounds is more likely to have a small baby (less than 5 1/2 pounds). These babies often have health problems after birth. Women who gain too much weight also are at risk for health problems. These

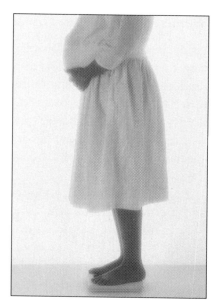

? Where Does the Weight Go?

The average newborn weighs in at about 7 1/2 pounds. Yet most mothers-to-be are advised to gain 25–35 pounds when they are pregnant. Where do the other pounds go? Here's a look at what a normal-weight woman who gains 30 pounds does with the extra weight.

Baby	7 1/2 pounds
Amniotic Fluid	2 pounds
Placenta	1 1/2 pounds
Uterus	2 pounds
Breasts	2 pounds
Body Fluids	4 pounds
Blood	4 pounds
Maternal Stores of Fat, Protein, and Other Nutrients	7 pounds

problems include diabetes, high blood pressure, and a baby that's too large (see Chapter 15).

Women often put on 3–5 pounds in their first trimester, and a pound or two each week after that. This weight isn't all fat. Far from it, in fact. Most of it is from the baby, amniotic fluid, placenta, breasts, and extra fluid and blood your body make during pregnancy.

Eating for Two

Eating well is one of the great pleasures of pregnancy—and of life. If healthy eating is an old habit for you, keep it up now. If it's not, having a baby is a great excuse to improve your diet. In fact, many women discover a bounty of tasty and healthy new foods when they are pregnant. What's more, they often stick with better eating habits long after the baby's born. Try to follow a healthy, balanced, and varied diet as often as you can. If you do, your baby—and your body—will thank you.

CHAPTER 7

Changes During Pregnancy

During pregnancy, your uterus grows from the size of your fist to a size able to hold a baby up to 10 pounds. In fact, your uterus grows to about 1,000 times its normal size.

Other parts of your body are also changing. Many of these changes are triggered by pregnancy hormones. These hormones nurture your fetus and prepare your body for childbirth and breastfeeding. They also can cause physical woes and emotional ups-and-downs.

If you have concerns or questions about what your body is going through, talk with your doctor. He or she can offer tips for dealing with pregnancy changes and also assure you that what you are feeling is normal.

Physical Changes

Backache

Backache is one of a pregnant woman's most common problems. Back pain during pregnancy has many causes. The strain from carrying 30 pounds of extra weight on your back muscles is one cause. The swayback posture you use to offset it is another. Stretched and weakened muscles in your abdomen (which support the spine) are yet one more reason.

Don't think that severe back pain is a normal part of pregnancy, though. It could be a sign of kidney infection or preterm labor. If you have pain in your back that doesn't go away or gets worse, call your doctor.

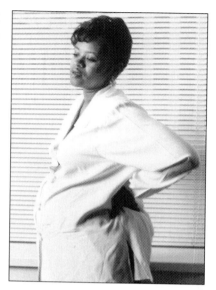

Here are some tips to help lessen back pain:

» Wear low-heeled (but not flat) shoes with good arch support. High heels tilt your body forward and strain your lower-back muscles.

» Avoid lifting heavy objects. Heavy lifting puts even more strain on your back.

» Don't bend at the waist to pick something up. If you must lift something (like a bag of groceries or a small child) here's how to do it: squat down, bend your knees, and keep your back straight.

» Get off your feet. If you have to stand for a long time (to do your job, wash dishes, or prepare meals, for instance), rest one foot on a stool or a box to take the strain off your back.

» Sit in chairs with good back support, or tuck a small pillow behind your lower back.

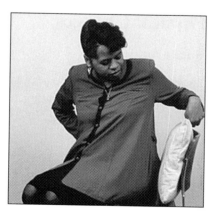

» Keep things within reach. Put objects that you use often in close reach. This way, you won't have to bend or stretch to grab them.

» Sleep on a firm mattress. If your bed is too soft, have

someone put a board between the mattress and box spring to make it firm.

‣ Sleep on your side rather than on your back. Tucking a pillow between your legs will give your back added support.

‣ Exercise to stretch your aching muscles, keep your back and abdominal muscles strong, and promote good posture (see "A Healthy Back" in Chapter 5).

‣ Buy an abdominal support garment (for sale in maternity stores and catalogs). They look like girdles and help take the weight of your belly off your back muscles. Also, some maternity pants come with a wide elastic band that's worn under the curve of your belly to help support its growing weight.

‣ Apply a heating pad, warm-water bottle, or cold compress to ease the pain. Be sure to use a towel to avoid burns.

Breast Changes

For many women, tingling, tender, swollen breasts are the first clue that they are pregnant. By 6 weeks of pregnancy, in fact, breasts may grow a whole cup size. Soon after conception, your breasts ready themselves for feeding the baby. Here's what's going on:

‣ Fat builds up in the breasts, making your normal bra too tight.

‣ Blood flow increases, causing a bluish web of veins to appear just under the skin.

‣ Milk glands increase as your body gears up for making milk.

‣ The nipples and areolas (the pink or brownish skin around your nipples) darken.

‣ Your nipples may begin to stick out more, and the areolas will grow larger.

‣ Small glands on the surface of the areolas called Montgomery's tubercles become raised and bumpy. These glands produce an oily substance that keeps the nipples and areolas soft and supple.

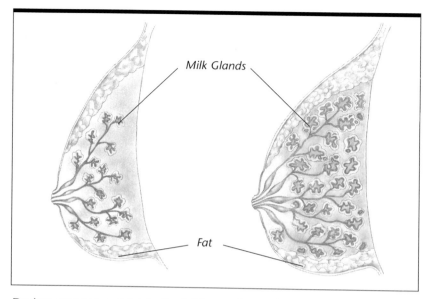

Milk Glands

Fat

During pregnancy (*right*), the fat layer of your breasts thickens and the number of milk glands increases. This makes them larger than before pregnancy (*left*).

Your breasts may keep growing in size and weight during the first 3 months of pregnancy. If they are very tender, wearing a good bra that fits well will help.

What sort of bra to choose? A maternity bra is a good choice. These bras have wide straps to support the weight of your bosom, more coverage in the cups to protect tender breasts, and extra rows of hooks so you can adjust the band size as you baby grows and your ribs expand. You also might want to pick up a special sleep bra to give your breasts nighttime support.

Most women's nipples stick out—even more so when they are pregnant. But some women have nipples that are flat or even recessed (***inverted nipples***). When you press the tissue just behind the nipples, they stay flat or are drawn in rather than sticking out. This can make it hard for your baby to nurse.

If you have flat or inverted nipples and want to breastfeed, you can take steps ahead of time to correct the problem. Talk to your doctor or a lactation consultant (breastfeeding specialist) as early in pregnancy as you can.

By the end of your first trimester, your breasts may start leaking. This fluid, called colostrum, is nothing to worry about—it shows that your breasts are getting ready to do the work they are made to do. Colostrum nourishes your newborn until your breasts start making milk a few days after birth. It is rich in fat and calories and contains water, proteins, minerals, and antibodies that protect against disease.

Early in pregnancy, colostrum is thick and yellow. As birth draws near, it becomes pale and has almost no color. Colostrum may leak on its own or dribble out when your breasts are massaged. It also can leak when you are sexually aroused.

Don't worry if your breasts don't leak during pregnancy, though. It doesn't happen to all women, and it doesn't mean that you won't be able to breastfeed later.

Congestion and Nosebleeds

During pregnancy, your hormone levels increase and your body makes extra blood. Both of these changes cause the mucus membranes inside your nose to swell up, dry out, and bleed easily. This may cause you to have a stuffy or runny nose that seems to last 40 long weeks. You also may get nosebleeds from time to time. To deal with the problem:

▶ Try saline drops to relieve congestion. (Never use other types of nose drops, nasal sprays, or decongestants without your doctor's approval.)

▶ Drink fluids to keep your nasal passages moist.

▶ Use a humidifier to moisten the air in your home.

▶ Dab petroleum jelly around the edges of your nostrils to keep the skin moist.

Constipation and Gas

Most pregnant women get a little backed up at some point. When that happens, gas can build up in your belly and cause bloating and pain.

Constipation occurs when you have infrequent bowel movements with stools that are firm or hard to pass. Constipation (and the gas that results) can occur for many reasons. Hormonal changes may slow digestion. Iron supplements can block you up. Toward the end of pregnancy, the weight of the uterus puts pressure on your rectum, adding to the problem.

If you are constipated and have gas, these tips may help:

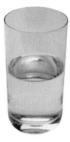

- Drink plenty of liquids. Drinking eight glasses of liquid a day will help to flush out your digestive tract. Drinking prune or other fruit juice also can help make you more regular.

- Eat high-fiber foods. Raw fruits, vegetables, beans, whole-grain bread, and bran cereal are good choices.

- Exercise. Walking or doing another safe activity a few times a week aids your digestive system.

- Ask your doctor about taking a bulk-forming agent. These products absorb water and expand inside your body. That adds to the moisture in stool and makes it easier to pass. Don't take laxatives during pregnancy.

Fatigue

Most women feel very tired when they are pregnant—mostly during early and late pregnancy. Your body is working hard to create a new life (and, later on, to carry, feed, and support that life). The pregnancy hormone progesterone also may make you feel tired.

There's not much you can do about fatigue, other than try to get as much rest as you can. Chapter 5 contains some good tips to help fight fatigue. Exercise and a healthy diet also may help boost your energy.

Frequent Urination

Why is it that the bathroom becomes like a second home for many pregnant women? There are a number of reasons:

▶ During pregnancy, the kidneys work harder than ever to flush waste products out of your body. Hence, frequent trips to the bathroom.

▶ The amount of fluid in your body goes up when you're pregnant. As a result, so does the amount of urine you make.

▶ As your uterus grows, it puts pressure on the bladder. Your bladder may be nearly empty, but may still feel like it's about to burst. In mid-pregnancy some of the pressure should be relieved when your uterus no longer presses down on your bladder.

▶ In the last weeks of pregnancy (later for second-timers), the fetus "drops" into your pelvis. When that happens, the baby's head moves down in the uterus and presses against your cervix and bladder. This is called *lightening*. During this time, you may visit the bathroom more than you ever thought possible. Your need to urinate may wake you up in the middle of the night, too.

There's not much you can do for relief except cut down on coffee, tea, and cola. (Caffeine makes you urinate more.) Don't cut back on liquids, though. Drinking less in an effort to curtail those bathroom trips will rob your body of vital fluids.

The weight of your uterus on your bladder may even cause you to leak a little urine when you sneeze or cough. You can wear san-

---

!

Warnings Signs of a Urinary Tract Infection

Call your doctor if you have any of these warning signs of a urinary tract infection (UTI):

▶ Pain when you urinate

▶ Feeling like you must urinate right away

▶ Urinating blood

▶ Running a fever

itary pads or panty shields for protection. Doing *Kegel exercises* (see box) will help you improve your bladder control.

Headache

Headaches are common during pregnancy. Pregnancy hormones are one cause. Hunger and stress also can be factors. Also, some women cut back on caffeine during pregnancy. This may cause caffeine withdrawal headaches.

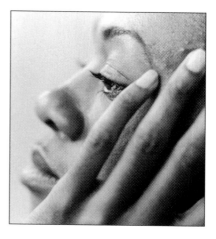

For some women, pregnancy headaches are a minor bother. For others, very painful headaches (called migraine headaches) can affect their daily life.

If you get headaches, ask your doctor what pain relief is safe to use when you're pregnant. Also, place a cold washcloth on your forehead for relief. Gently massage your temples. Rest in a dark, quiet room.

Call your doctor if headaches are a constant problem. Also call if a headache doesn't go away, is very severe, causes blurred vision

Kegel Exercises

Kegel exercises strengthen the muscles that surround the openings of the vagina, anus, and urethra (the tube that carries urine out of the body). If they are done often enough, Kegel exercises will help stop urine leaks. They may even lower the chance that you'll need an episiotomy (a cut to widen the opening of the birth canal) when you give birth.

Here's how to do Kegel exercises: squeeze the muscles that you use to stop the flow of urine. Hold for 10 seconds, then release. Do this 10–20 times in a row at least 3 times a day. You can do Kegel exercises anywhere.

or spots in front of your eyes, or makes you feel sick to your stomach.

Heartburn and Indigestion

Heartburn doesn't mean that something is wrong with your heart. It refers to a burning feeling in the throat and chest. Heartburn is a common problem among pregnant women.

Pregnancy hormones, which relax the muscle valve between your stomach and esophagus (the tube leading from the throat to the stomach), are a main cause. This places stomach acids where they don't belong. As your uterus grows, it adds to the problem by pressing up against your stomach.

The words "heartburn" and "indigestion" often are thought to mean the same thing. They are not. Indigestion is what happens when a sluggish stomach takes hours to empty. Women with indigestion feel very full, bloated, and gassy.

Follow these tips to help relieve (or prevent) indigestion and heartburn:

▸ Eat six small meals a day instead of three big ones.

▸ Eat slowly and chew your food well.

▸ Don't have a lot of liquid with your meals. Drink fluids between meals instead.

▸ Stay away from fried, greasy, and fatty foods.

▸ Avoid foods that bother your stomach. If heartburn is a problem, avoid fizzy drinks, citrus fruits or juices, and spicy or fatty foods.

▸ Don't eat or drink within a few hours of bedtime. Don't lie down right after meals, either.

▸ Try raising the head of your bed. Prop a few extra pillows under your shoulders or stick a couple of books under the legs of your bed.

▸ Talk to your doctor about using antacids.

Hemorrhoids

Pregnant women who are constipated often suffer from hemorrhoids. These are painful and itchy *varicose veins* in the rectal area. (When they occur in the vagina or *vulva*, they are called vulvar varicosities.) The extra blood in the pelvic area along with the pressure the growing uterus puts on veins in the lower body are the main causes.

Constipation can make these swollen, itchy veins worse. That's because straining during bowel movements traps more blood in the veins. It can even cause them to stick out of the rectum. Talk to your doctor about using certain over-the-counter creams and suppositories to make hemorrhoids easier to bear.

Hemorrhoids may be something you have to live with for awhile. Even if they improve during pregnancy, straining during delivery can bring them back. Hemorrhoids often go away for good after the baby's born. In the meantime, try these tips for a little relief (or to avoid the problem in the first place):

▸ Eat a high-fiber diet and drink plenty of liquids. This will help ward off constipation.

▸ Don't gain too much weight. Extra pounds can worsen hemorrhoids. Keep your weight gain within the limits your doctor suggests.

▸ Get moving. Standing or sitting for a long time puts pressure on the veins in your pelvic area. Get up and move around to shift the weight of your uterus off these veins.

▸ If you get hemorrhoids, apply ice packs or witch hazel pads to the area to relieve pain and reduce swelling. Your pharmacist can help you find an over-the-counter witch hazel product.

▸ Try soaking them in water a few times a day.

Insomnia

After the first few months, you may find it hard to sleep at night. As your abdomen grows larger, it may be hard to find a comfortable position. To get the rest you need:

▶ Take a shower or warm bath at bedtime (but be careful not to slip—the changes in your body can make it hard to keep your balance in a wet tub).

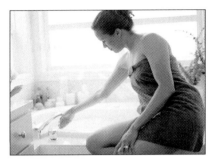

▶ Try the relaxation tips you learned in childbirth classes.

▶ Lie on your side with a pillow under your abdomen and another between your legs.

▶ Limit your daytime rest.

Leg Cramps

During late pregnancy, painful leg cramps may be a bother at night. Although cramps were once thought to be caused by a problem with the amount of calcium in a woman's diet, this is no longer thought to be true. It is not clear what causes leg cramps. Stretching your legs before going to bed can help relieve them. Also, avoid pointing your toes when stretching or exercising.

Lower-Abdominal Pain

As the uterus grows, the round ligaments (bands of tissue that support the uterus on both sides) are pulled and stretched. You may feel this stretching as either a dull ache or a sharp pain on one side of your belly. The pains are most common between 18 and 24 weeks of pregnancy.

If abdominal pain doesn't go away or gets worse, call your doctor. It could be a sign of a problem. To prevent or relieve these pains:

▶ Avoid quick changes of position.

▶ Don't turn sharply at the waist.

▶ When you do feel a pain, bend toward it to help relieve it.

▶ Rest or change your position.

Mouth and Tooth Changes

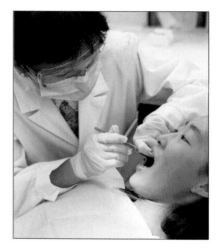

Pregnancy hormones can make your gums swell and bleed. Keep up the brushing and flossing, though. Switching to a softer brush may help.

You also may notice that your mouth waters more during pregnancy. No one knows why this occurs.

Don't cancel your regular dental visit just because you are pregnant. A dental checkup early in pregnancy will help ensure that your mouth stays healthy. Putting off dental work can lead to further problems.

When you go to the dentist, be sure to let him or her know that you are pregnant. Don't worry if you need local anesthesia or dental X-rays. Neither of these poses a risk as long as they are done with your baby's safety in mind. If your dentist has concerns, ask him or her to contact your doctor.

Nausea and Vomiting

Once the first 3 months have passed, you may find that food has never smelled so good or been quite so tasty. Still, the early months of your pregnancy may be spent fighting against nausea triggered by certain food odors. You also may have trouble keeping down the food you have just eaten.

Nausea and vomiting are common during pregnancy, especially during the first part of pregnancy. This is often called "morning sickness," although it can occur at any time of the day. Although no one is certain what causes the nausea and vomiting, rising levels of hormones during pregnancy may play a role. Nausea and vomiting should lessen by about 14 weeks of pregnancy.

Most mild cases of nausea and vomiting do not harm you or your baby's health. Morning sickness does not mean your baby is sick. In most women, symptoms of nausea and vomiting are mild and go away after the middle of pregnancy.

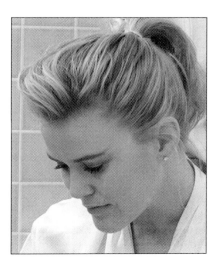

Morning sickness can become more of a problem if you can't keep any foods or fluids down and begin to lose weight. If your nausea and vomiting are severe, call your doctor. You may have a condition called hyperemesis gravidarum. It can lead to loss of weight and body fluids.

If your nausea and vomiting are severe, you may need medical treatment. If your doctor suspects that you have hyperemesis gravidarum, you may need to stay in the hospital for a while.

You may be given fluids through an intravenous (IV) line. You also may be treated with anti-nausea medications. In most cases, you will not be allowed to eat any food until the vomiting stops. Your doctor may suggest that you rest in a dimly lit room where it is quiet and private. This type of treatment in the hospital often relieves symptoms. Don't take any medication to treat nausea or vomiting unless your doctor tells you it's safe. (For more details on hyperemesis gravidarum, see "Women With Severe Morning Sickness" in Chapter 6.)

Until the nausea and vomiting go away, there are some things you can do that might help you feel better:

- Get up slowly in the morning and sit on the side of the bed for a few minutes.

- Eat dry toast or crackers before you get out of bed in the morning.

- Get plenty of fresh air. Take a short walk or try sleeping with a window open.

- Drink fluids often during the day. Cold drinks that are bubbly or sweet may help.

> **!**
>
> ## When To Call Your Doctor
>
> ▶ If you have a small amount of urine and it is dark in color
>
> ▶ If you can't keep down liquids
>
> ▶ If you are dizzy or faint on standing up
>
> ▶ If you have a racing or pounding heart
>
> ▶ If you vomit blood

▶ Eat five or six small meals each day. Try not to let your stomach get empty, and sit upright after meals.

▶ Avoid smells that bother you.

▶ Eat foods that are low fat and easy to digest. The BRATT diet (bananas, rice, applesauce, toast, and tea) may help. This diet will provide vital nutrients that will replace what you have lost.

Prenatal vitamins and iron may cause nausea. A children's chewable vitamin with folate (folic acid) taken at the end of the day may help. Acupressure, ginger, motion sickness bands, or hypnosis also may help relieve symptoms. Talk with your doctor before taking any medication or trying any treatment.

Numbness and Tingling

As your uterus grows, it rests on some of the nerves connecting your legs to your spinal cord. This may cause chronic pain in the hip or thigh (sciatica). Nerves also may get pressed if your legs swell during pregnancy (see "Swelling"). This pressure can cause your legs or toes to tingle or feel numb. Most often, these symptoms are minor and go away after the baby is born.

Your arms or hands may tingle as a result of tissue swelling, too. For instance, a condition called *carpal tunnel syndrome* is common in pregnant women. It causes a burning, tingling feeling in one or both hands and may make your fingers numb. Wearing a special wrist splint can help.

Some women get numbness and tingling that's caused by hyperventilating (overbreathing). Anxiety, or simply pregnancy, can make you feel short of breath. This causes you to breathe deeper and faster in an effort to get some air. When you hyperventilate, you may feel sweaty and dizzy and your heart may pound. If you get these symptoms, breathe into a paper bag for a few minutes. This restores the balance of oxygen and carbon dioxide in your body.

Shortness of Breath

Early in pregnancy, you may feel short of breath because of the increase of progesterone in your body. This may be relieved when you become used to the progesterone. Later in pregnancy, a new cause of shortness of breath occurs. Your uterus is starting to take up more and more room in your abdomen. By about 31–34 weeks of pregnancy, the uterus is so large that it presses the stomach and the diaphragm (a flat, strong muscle that aids in breathing) up toward the lungs. Although you may feel short of breath, this does not affect the amount of oxygen your baby gets.

Some tips to help you breathe easier:

▶ Slow down. When you move more slowly, your heart and lungs don't have to work so hard.

▶ Sit (or stand) up straight. This gives your lungs more room to expand.

▶ Sleep propped up. This stops the stomach and other organs from taking up space for your lungs.

Skin and Hair Changes

Sun block is always a good idea, and it may be even more important in pregnancy. Also, changes in hormone levels can cause not-so-pretty (but harmless) skin problems:

▶ *Acne.* Some mothers-to-be find that their face breaks out more during pregnancy. To treat breakouts, wash your face a few times a day with a mild cleanser. You may want to buy a good,

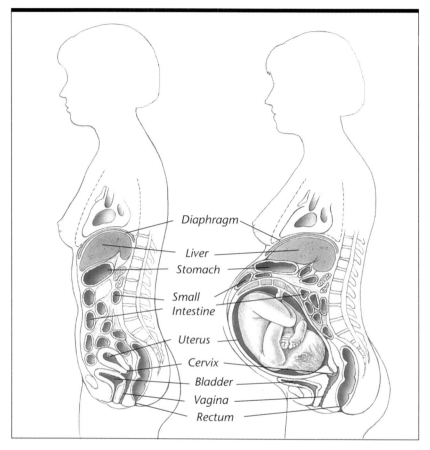

Diaphragm

Liver

Stomach

Small
Intestine

Uterus

Cervix

Bladder

Vagina

Rectum

In early pregnancy, shortness of breath occurs from hormonal changes. As the uterus grows from the beginning (*left*) to the end (*right*) of pregnancy, it takes up more and more room in your abdomen. This presses the digestive organs and the diaphragm up toward the lungs.

water-based cover-up, too. If you go to a dermatologist, be sure he or she knows you are pregnant. Some prescription drugs used to treat acne have been linked with severe birth defects.

- *Chloasma.* The "mask of pregnancy" gives some women brownish marks around their eyes and on their nose and cheeks. The deeper pigmentation (color) brought about by pregnancy hormones causes this to occur. Spending time in the sun can make chloasma worse. These marks will fade after delivery, when hormone levels return to normal. In the meantime, a good cover-up stick or foundation will cover the chloasma.

▶ *Linea nigra.* In many women, extra pigment in the skin causes the faint line running from the belly button to the pubic hair to darken during pregnancy. It will fade after delivery.

▶ *Red palms and spider veins.* You may have red, itchy palms and tiny red veins branching out under the skin of your face or legs. Again, the redness should fade after delivery.

▶ *Skin tags.* Your body's on growth mode, and that doesn't just include the baby you are making. You may find little flaps of skin on your breasts, neck, or armpits. They will not go away after the baby arrives, but they can be removed easily by a doctor.

▶ *Stretch marks.* As your belly and breasts grow, they may become streaked with reddish lines. These stretch marks happen when skin stretches quickly to support the growing fetus. Don't waste your money on any of the "miracle" creams or lotions sold to prevent stretch marks. There's little you can do to keep them at bay. Keeping your weight gain within the limits your doctor suggests may help. Once your baby's born, these red streaks will slowly fade. Some marks may remain.

▶ *Thicker hair.* This is one cliché about pregnancy that often—although not always—proves true. Your body's in a growth cycle, and so is your hair. As a result, you shed hair much more slowly than normal. (You may even sprout new hairs where you never had them before—on your bulging belly, for instance.) Chances are, your hair will thin out after the baby's born. Your hair should return to its normal cycle within a few months of birth.

Swelling

Some swelling (called **edema**) in the hands, face, legs, ankles, and feet is normal during pregnancy. It's caused by the extra fluid in your body. It tends to be worse in late pregnancy and during the summer.

For relief, put your feet up often and sleep with your legs propped up on pillows. This keeps fluid from pooling in the bottom half of your body. Also, standing neck deep in a swimming pool for 30 minutes a day may help reduce leg swelling. Don't take water pills or other medications to reduce swelling without your doctor's OK.

Let your doctor know if you are badly swollen or if you have sudden swelling in your face or hands (hint: your rings will be too tight). This could signal a problem such as high blood pressure.

Vaginal Discharge

Vaginal discharge often increases during pregnancy. A sticky, clear, or white discharge is normal, and it's nothing to worry about. Let your doctor know if the discharge has blood in it, is watery, has a bad odor, or has changed from normal. Also tell the doctor if you have pain, soreness, or itching in the vaginal area. Never douche when you're pregnant.

Varicose Veins

The weight of your uterus pressing down on a major artery can slow blood flow from your lower body. The result may be sore, itchy, blue bulges on your legs called varicose veins. These veins also can appear near your vulva, vagina, and rectum (see "Hemorrhoids"). In most cases, varicose veins are not a problem.

You are more likely to have varicose veins if someone in your family had them. You can't prevent varicose veins. However, taking these steps will help relieve swelling and soreness and may stop varicose veins from getting worse:

▸ If you must sit or stand for long periods, be sure to move around from time to time.

▸ Don't sit with your legs crossed.

▸ Prop up your legs—on your desk, a couch, a chair, or a footstool—as often as you can.

▶ Do exercise, such as walking, swimming, or riding an exercise bike.

▶ Wear support hose.

▶ Don't wear stockings or socks that have a tight band of elastic around the legs.

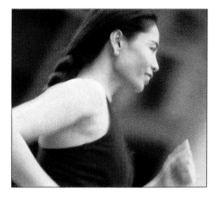

Emotional Changes

Your body's going through big changes now, and so are your emotions. Don't blame yourself if you are sad or moody. The emotions you are feeling—good and bad—are normal. Ask loved ones to support you and be patient. Rest and relax as often as you can. You'll feel better, emotionally and physically, if you do.

Anxiety

Pregnant women and their partners often have fears about pregnancy, labor and delivery, the effect a child will have on their lives, and whether they'll be good parents. Some people have strange or scary dreams during pregnancy. This is normal.

Most often, there's nothing to worry about. Still, there are things you can do to ease your mind. Here are some common fears and what you can do about them:

▶ "I'm worried that something will be wrong with the baby." Keep in mind that most children are born healthy. Calm your fears by doing all that you can to ensure that your baby is healthy: eat right, exercise, avoid risky behavior, and get early and regular prenatal care. If you smoke, stop.

▶ "I've never given birth before. I'm scared of the pain and afraid that I won't be able to stand it." Know what to expect during labor and delivery. Take a childbirth class to learn relaxation methods, ways to ease labor pain, and the pros and cons of pain medications. Even if you plan to give birth without pain relief, for instance, remind yourself that you won't "fail" if you decide you need some relief. Often, medication helps a woman relax enough to help labor along.

▶ "I'm worried that I'll forget the pain-management techniques I learn in class." Practice makes perfect. Rehearse the methods taught in childbirth class until they become second nature to you. Keep in mind, too, that your health care team will be there to support you.

▶ "I just know that something will go wrong in the delivery room." Remind yourself that having a baby is a natural event. Even if your birth doesn't go just as planned, chances are that you and your baby will be fine.

▶ "I don't know how to take care of a baby." Feeding, bathing, changing diapers, and dressing a baby are easy to learn. You may feel better prepared, though, if you take a newborn-care class before your due date. Many hospitals offer these 1- or 2- day courses. Also, read up on infant care before your baby arrives. To pick up a few tips, spend some time with a friend or family member who has just had a baby. After your baby is born, ask the nurses at the hospital to help you practice baby-care basics before you leave. Once you're home, ask family and friends for advice. There are good books at libraries and book stores that contain advice on caring for your newborn. Ask your doctor or your baby's doctor about the books they suggest. If you really need help with something, call your baby's doctor.

▶ "My life will never be the same again." You are right—but that doesn't have to be a bad thing. Having a baby means big changes. Your relationships will change. Hanging out with friends or spending time alone with your partner may be harder. Your interests may shift. Having a baby doesn't mean you have to give up everything you enjoy, though. You can still do many of the same things you did before. You just need to alter them to include your baby. Keep in mind, too, that a whole new world—with new people, new places, and new things to do—will open up to you now.

Body Image

Mixed feelings about your pregnant body are normal. Your growing body is a sign of a new life growing inside you. There may be days, though, when you'll feel fat and wonder if you'll ever get your figure back.

Eating a healthy diet and exercise will help keep these feeling at bay. Regular workouts will help you feel better about how you look. Eating right and keeping a healthy weight are an important part of health. If you're in good shape and don't gain more than the suggested weight during pregnancy, you'll have an easier time losing weight after delivery, too.

Depression

You may have heard of the "baby blues" or *postpartum depression.* Depression also can occur during pregnancy. More than 1 in 10 mothers-to-be has depression that doesn't go away.

A blue mood now and then is normal. If you feel sad most of the time, though, seek help. Women who are depressed may not take care of their health, and their baby may suffer.

The signs of depression often mimic the normal ups and downs of pregnancy. That's why depression can be hard to spot in mothers-to-be.

Your doctor may suggest counseling or certain medications for depression. A sadness that lasts for at least 2 weeks and having more than one of the following symptoms are signs of depression:

▶ Depressed mood most of the day, nearly every day

▶ Loss of interest in work or other activities

▶ Feeling guilty, hopeless, or worthless

▶ Thinking about death or suicide

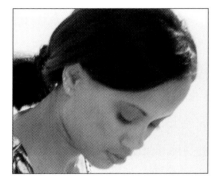

- Sleeping more than normal or lying awake at night

- Losing your appetite or losing weight (or eating much more than normal and gaining weight)

- Feeling very tired or without energy

- Having trouble paying attention and making decisions

- Having aches and pains that don't get better with treatment

Stress

Stress is a normal part of life. Although we often think of stress as bad, it has a good side, too. Stress can create energy to meet a challenge. Yet, too much stress—or stress that isn't managed well—can harm the health of you and your baby.

Pregnancy brings with it intense change. As a result, it can create a lot of stress. For day-to-day stress, try the "De-Stressing Tips" listed in Chapter 5.

Sometimes, though, stress is more serious. Get help right away if:

- You are a victim of abuse (see "The Abused Woman" in Chapter 5)

- You are turning to alcohol, cigarettes, or drugs for relief

- You are so stressed out that you are having trouble coping with daily life

- You feel the urge to take out your stress on your other children

Your doctor may advise stress-reducing methods that require you to get special training or visit an expert. These might include:

- Exercise

- Guided visual imagery

- Self-hypnosis

- Meditation or prayer

- Yoga

- Biofeedback

- Mental health counseling

Changes for Your Partner and Family

Pregnancy is a special time for a couple. It also can strain your relationship. Your old roles are shifting, and you need to adapt to new ones. You'll both spend a lot of time thinking about the baby, but try to make time for each other, too.

Try to understand what your partner's going through. Talk about your concerns and feelings and support each other. Be sure to include your partner in the pregnancy. Go to your prenatal visits and tests together. Attend childbirth and baby-care classes as a team.

Your partner may worry about the baby as much as—or even more than—you do. He's also anxious about his role in the birth. As if that isn't enough, he's worried about you, too. Remind him that you are in no danger, that you'll be in good hands during labor and delivery, and that most babies are born healthy.

Sex during pregnancy is a big issue for many couples. Unless your doctor has warned you not to, you can enjoy sex without

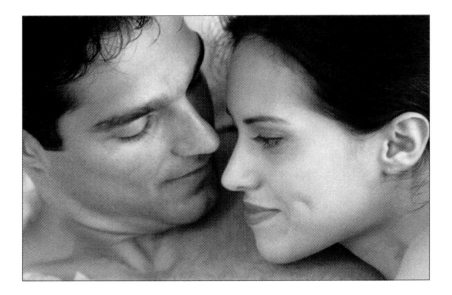

worry. (For details on the safety of sex during pregnancy, see "Sex" in Chapter 5.)

Some couples find that their desire cools during pregnancy. During the first and last months, for instance, nausea and fatigue may get in the way of sex. Your thoughts may center on the baby instead of sex. In that case, be open and honest with your partner. Talking can bring you closer and help avoid hurt feelings and loneliness.

You and your partner aren't the only people affected by your pregnancy. Your parents, siblings, and other children are also key players.

Pregnancy can trigger mixed feelings about your own childhood. It may bring you closer to your family. It may call up old childhood conflicts and cause you to push your family members away.

Whether your feelings about it are good or bad, you'll also find yourself thinking a lot about your relationship with your mother. This is all part of a normal process of figuring out what sort of parent you want to be. Put your own interests and need for privacy first, but try to involve your family in your pregnancy—and later, your baby's life—as much as you can.

The Second Time Around

Second-time (or third- or fourth-time) moms are one step ahead of their first-time peers. They know what to expect throughout pregnancy to labor and delivery. Still, this pregnancy may not be much like the last one. If your prior pregnancy was all smooth sailing, for instance, you may hit rough waters this time. Also, if you had problems before, they may not recur this time.

Keep in mind, too, that just as every pregnancy is different, so is every baby. This child may not be at all like your first. Also, the tricks and tips that worked the first time may not work with this baby.

Your Emotions During a Second Pregnancy

During your first pregnancy, you paid close attention to every detail. This time, you may not give the same attention to each movement. Don't feel guilty—this is normal. Many second-timers find that they are more interested in the product of their pregnancy (the baby) than the process. Also, your first child may be keeping you too busy to think about the daily changes in your body.

You may fear that you won't be able to love this child as much as your first. Rest assured, you will. And don't worry that the love you'll feel for this baby will take away from the love you have for your firstborn. You'll simply find extra stores of love that you didn't even know you had.

How Your Body May Change This Time

You may have sailed through your first pregnancy without a hint of nausea. That may not be the case this time. You may have been active right up until the end then, but you're barely able to drag yourself from the couch this time. There's no way to know ahead of time what a second (or later) pregnancy will be like.

One thing's a pretty sure bet, though: you'll be more tired this time. There are a few reasons for this. You are older than you were during your first pregnancy. You may not have had a chance to get back in shape after giving birth, so your energy may drop. Also, you have a child who needs care.

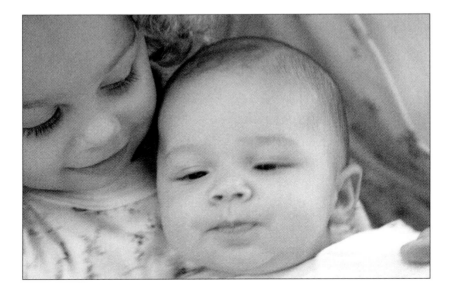

Second-time mothers often know they are pregnant sooner than rookie moms. They know just what to look for. They also recall what early pregnancy feels like.

You'll "show" earlier this time, too. In fact, you may need to start wearing your maternity clothes before your fourth month of pregnancy. That's because your abdominal muscles were stretched by your prior pregnancy. They may not have regained their former strength. As a result, these muscles won't hold the growing uterus in or up as well as they did the first pregnancy.

Chances are, you'll feel this baby move weeks earlier than you felt your first baby wiggle. The fetus isn't really moving sooner. You just know what to look for this time. You also may notice **Braxton Hicks contractions** sooner than you did during your first pregnancy. These "practice" contractions may show up during the second trimester rather than the third, for instance.

Women who have nursed a baby before may not notice the breast changes that first-timers do. That's because much of the work needed to prepare for breastfeeding has already taken place. Breasts that have been primed by prior nursing may begin to leak earlier in pregnancy, too. Your breasts may not be as tender or grow as much as they did in the first pregnancy. Some women, though, find that their breasts grow bigger and sag more in a second pregnancy. This may be because the tissue that supports the breasts is stretched out from prior growth and nursing.

Your first baby most likely dropped into your pelvis weeks before you went into labor. This time, though, lightening may not take place until delivery day. No one knows for sure why this is.

Although second-time moms more or less know what's going to happen next, it's still vital to listen to your body's signals. If something doesn't seem quite right to you, ask your doctor.

Your Baby May Be Born More Quickly

Although the pregnancy may seem longer, labor may be quicker. As long as you don't run into any problems during labor, your body knows just what to do to get the baby out. Your cervix has opened before, for instance. It won't take as long to dilate again.

The tissue around your vagina has been stretched, too. You're also less likely to feel the fear and anxiety that can slow labor down.

Your Other Children

Small children may have lots of questions about where babies come from. They may not want to talk about the baby at all. An older child may be eager to be a big brother or sister. He or she may resent losing center stage to a new sibling. A teen, busy with his or her own life, may not be very interested in the baby. He or she may be embarrassed by your pregnancy.

When should you share your news with them? That depends on your child, of course. Tell school-aged children before you tell anyone outside your family, though. (If you don't, they may resent being the last to know.) With younger children, it's a good idea to wait until they ask about your changing body. The idea of a baby growing inside you may be too hard for a small child to grasp before they can see your pregnancy.

No matter how your children act when you tell them about the baby, be sure to remind them that you love them and will always

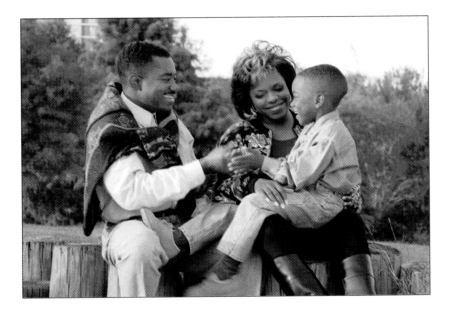

be there for them. Also assure your children that delivering the baby won't harm you. Let them know, too, that while you'll be in the hospital, it's not because you're sick.

To prevent your children from feeling left out, involve them in your pregnancy as much as you can. Ask your kids to help you get ready for the baby's arrival. Take them shopping and let them pick out items for their new brother or sister. Have them help you sort through hand-me-downs. Let them vote for the name they like best. The relationship between siblings is one of the longest and most important there is. Help promote this bond right from the start. When you're pregnant:

- Tell your child about the role he or she can play in guiding and teaching the new baby.

- Read books together about pregnancy, childbirth, babies, and being a big brother or sister.

- If "sibling prep" classes are offered in your area, sign your child up for one.

- Let your child feel the baby move.

- Take your child along on prenatal visits and let him or her hear the baby's heartbeat.

- Take your child on a tour of the hospital where you'll be giving birth.

- Show your child pictures and videos from when he or she was a newborn. Use images of you and your partner caring for your child to talk about how you'll need to take care of the new baby.

- Set up the baby's sleeping area well in advance. This way, your child won't feel displaced if he or she must share a room with the baby or give up his or her crib.

Some families even invite their children into the delivery room to witness a sibling's birth. Only you can tell if this option is right for your child—or for you. If you would like to make your baby's birth a family affair, talk to your doctor first. Also check to see what the hospital policy is on siblings at births. Arrange to have an adult look after your child during delivery. If your child isn't with you during delivery, there's no reason he or she can't meet a new sibling shortly after birth.

A Look Ahead

There is no question that your pregnancy is heading for its conclusion. Your baby is about to arrive. With your labor day so close at hand, the day-to-day changes that come with pregnancy soon will be a distant memory.

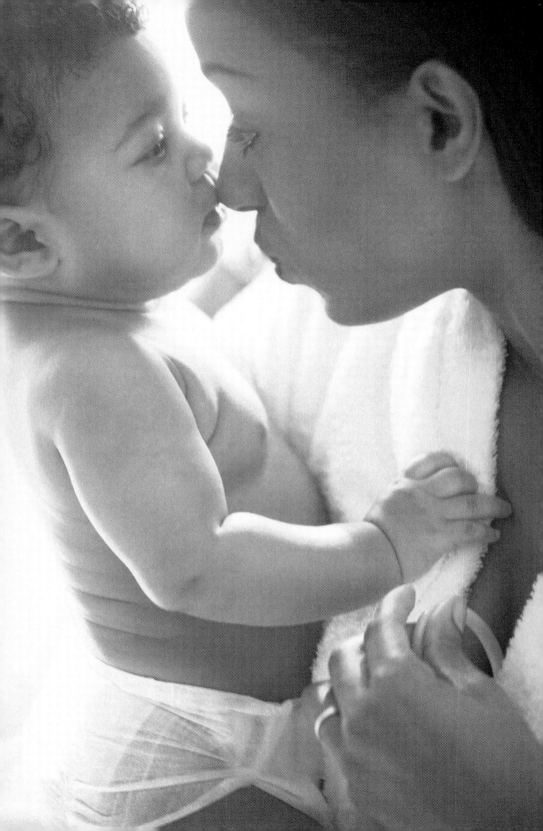

Labor, Delivery, and Postpartum

For the past 40 weeks, your body has been changing as your baby grows inside you. Now, as you near the end of pregnancy, you are eager to meet the product of all this change.

Still, you may be nervous about what's ahead and wonder what your life will be like after the baby arrives. Most women feel anxious about labor and delivery. This is even more true if they have never given birth before. Even seasoned mothers can't be sure what to expect from birth this time around.

No doubt, there are challenges ahead. Giving birth may be one of the hardest things you ever do. What's more, newborns demand love, care, and attention 24 hours a day. Looking after your own needs and getting support from those around you will help you cope during this great but tiring time.

The best way to confront the labor, delivery, and postpartum period is to arm yourself with information. Knowing what to expect and feeling ready to meet things head-on will help you get the most out of birth and being a new mother.

CHAPTER 8

Labor

After months spent waiting for your baby's birth, the big day is nearing at last. There's no way to tell for sure just when you'll deliver. However, most babies are born between 37 and 42 weeks of pregnancy. Birth often occurs as much as 3 weeks before or 2 weeks after your due date. Very few babies are born on their due date.

Your body's gone through some big changes during the last 40 weeks. It'll go through a few more as you prepare to give birth. Sometimes it's hard to tell if labor is starting or if you are simply having a false alarm. There may be times when you wonder, "Is this it?"

Rest assured, when "it" happens, you'll know. Plenty of women think they are in labor when they are not. Very few women think they are not in labor when they are, though.

Once labor starts in earnest, things will move quickly. Your water may break, your contractions will come faster and more often, and if all goes well your baby will be in your arms within hours. Get set for what may be the hardest work of your life—with the biggest payoff.

Getting Ready

Knowing what happens during labor will make it easier for you to relax, do what you can to help the process along, and focus on your baby's arrival when the time comes. If you plan for your baby's birth, you can take steps to help your labor go more smoothly. For instance, many mothers-to-be wonder how much time they should set aside for the trip to the hospital. That depends on a number of things. Because you may not be thinking very clearly once labor starts, consider these factors ahead of time:

▸ *Distance.* How far do you live from the hospital?

▸ *Transportation.* How will you get there? Is your car reliable? (Be sure to keep the tank filled.) Can someone drive you? Is there someone who can take you at any hour, day or night? How can you reach your partner or another driver if they are not at home or work when you need them?

▸ *Time of day.* If you are leaving for the hospital during the morning or evening rush hour, give yourself extra time to get there.

▸ *Time of year.* Don't forget to plan for bad weather. The trip to the hospital will take longer in the middle of a January snowstorm than it will in balmy July.

▸ *Other concerns.* Do you have children who you'll need to drop off at a friend's or a family member's home? If so, allow plenty of time to do that. Do you need someone to feed and walk a pet while you are in the hospital? Is there anything else that will need to be arranged?

Try a practice run to see how long it takes you to get to the hospital. Map out a backup route, too. It'll come in handy if you run into a delay.

Packing Your Hospital Bag

The last thing you want to be doing once labor starts is tossing items into a suitcase in a panic. To avoid this, pack your bag a few weeks before your due date. Leave it in a handy place, such as a hall closet or the trunk of your car.

You can't pack everything so far ahead of time. You may need things like your glasses and slippers in the meantime. Tape a note

Important Information

To plan for your baby's birth, think about these questions and get answers well before delivery day:

What number do I call if I have an emergency during pregnancy?

_____

What maternity benefits does my job offer? _____

_____

Have I filled out all the needed paperwork to begin my maternity leave and collect disability pay? _____

Do I need to register at the hospital before I check in for delivery?

_____

If so, have I done this? _____

Is there anything special I should—or shouldn't—do when I think labor has started? _____

When should I call if I think I'm in labor? _____

What number do I call when I go into labor?_____

At what point in my labor should I leave for the hospital? _____

_____

Should I go straight to the hospital or call the doctor's office first?

_____

Who will drive me to the hospital? _____

How will I get in touch with my driver when I'm ready to go?

_____

Where can we park the car? _____

What sort of birth experience do I hope to have? _____

_____

Will I breast- or bottle-feed my baby? _____

to your suitcase listing these last-minute items. That way, you won't forget them in the rush to the hospital.

You may want to pack two bags: a small one full of labor supplies and a larger one for your hospital stay. Then, you can grab the small bag on your way out the door. After your baby's born, someone can fetch the larger bag.

Don't worry if you forget something. The hospital will have most of the things you need. To find out what the hospital sup-

Some Things You May Want to Pack

For labor:

___Your health insurance card, ID, and hospital registration forms

___Lotion or oil for labor massage

___A picture or a treasured object to use as a focal point during contractions

___An old nightgown or nightshirt (if you don't want to wear a hospital gown)

___A pillow from home

___A bathrobe

___Slippers

___Socks

___A barrette or band to tie back your hair

___Glasses, if you wear them (you may not be allowed to wear contact lenses during labor)

___Lollipops or hard candies to keep your mouth moist

___A cassette or CD player and some soothing music

___A camera with fully charged batteries, if you plan to take pictures

For your hospital stay:

___Two or three nightgowns (be sure the gowns open at the front if you plan to nurse)

plies, call the nurses' desks in the labor/delivery and maternity wards or ask your doctor or childbirth educator.

How Labor Begins

Some women coast through the final days of pregnancy without a single sign of looming labor. Then all at once labor begins. Others have round-the-clock cramps for weeks. They may even make a few false starts to the hospital before true labor begins.

Some Things You May Want to Pack (continued)

___Two or three nursing bras and a dozen or so nursing pads

___A few pairs of socks

___Sanitary pads

___Shampoo

___Lotion, deodorant, lip balm, and other toilet items

___A toothbrush and toothpaste

___A hair brush or comb

___Barrettes or hair ties

___Contact lenses, if you wear them

___A notepad and pencil

___A camera, film, and batteries (check the hospital policy in advance if you plan to use a video camera during delivery)

___Change for the vending machine and pay phone

___A long-distance calling card

___Phone numbers of people you want to call after the birth

___Magazines or other reading material

___A baby book

___A receiving blanket and clothes for your newborn to wear home

___Loose-fitting clothes for you to wear home

___A car seat (see "Choosing an Infant Car Safety Seat" in Chapter 11)

No one knows for sure just what triggers labor. Hormones may play a role. Certain changes in your body also may give you a clue that labor isn't far off.

As labor begins, the cervix begins to thin out (efface) and open (dilate). During contractions, you may feel pain or pressure that starts in your back and moves around to your lower abdomen. When this happens, your belly will tighten and feel hard. Between contractions, the uterus relaxes and your belly softens.

These contractions are doing vital work. They open the cervix, which has been tightly closed since conception. They also help

TABLE 1. Signs That Labor Is Near

There's no way to predict just when you'll go into labor. But there are some signals that labor is close at hand:

Sign	What It Is	When It Happens
Feeling as if the baby has dropped lower in your belly	Lightening. The baby's head has settled deep into your pelvis.	From a few weeks (for first-time moms) to a few hours (for later births) before labor starts
More vaginal discharge (clear, pink, or slightly bloody)	**Show.** Thick mucus seals off the cervix during pregnancy. When the cervix starts to open, this mucus plug is pushed into the vagina.	A few days before labor starts or at the onset of labor
Fluid leaking from your vagina in a trickle or a gush	Rupture of membranes. The fluid-filled amniotic sac that surrounds your baby during pregnancy breaks (your "water breaks").	At the start of labor or during labor
Strong, rhythmic cramps that feel like a bad backache or menstrual cramps	Contractions. Your uterus tightens and relaxes. These contractions open the cervix and help push the baby into the birth canal.	At the onset of labor (although Braxton Hicks contractions can happen for weeks or even months before labor starts)

Labor Defined

Four terms are used to measure a woman's progress before and during labor:

Ripening—the softening of the cervix. Your cervix must be ripe before it can begin to thin or open.

Effacement—the thinning out of the cervix. It's measured in percentages, from 0% (no effacement) to 100% (fully effaced).

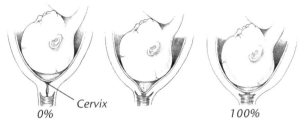

Cervix
0%   *100%*

Dilatation—the amount that the cervix has opened. It's measured in centimeters, from 0 centimeters (no dilatation) to 10 centimeters (fully dilated).

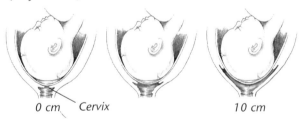

0 cm   *Cervix*   *10 cm*

Station—where the baby's head is in relation to the ischial spines, bony landmarks on either side of the pelvis. It's measured in numbers, from -5 (the baby's head is floating above the pelvis) to 0 (the baby's head has dropped into the pelvis) to +5 (the baby's head is **crowning** at the opening of the vagina).

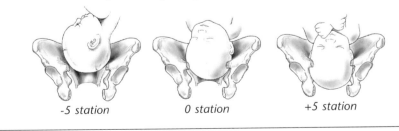

-5 station   *0 station*   *+5 station*

push your baby into the birth canal. As labor wears on, contractions will become more intense, last longer, and come closer and closer together.

What women tend to think of as "labor" is really just the first stage of labor. The baby's birth happens in the second stage. The placenta is delivered during the third stage. (For details on the second and third stages of labor, see Chapter 9.)

During each stage of labor, different things happen in your body. The way you feel during one stage won't be the way you feel during the next. You also won't get many clues about what to expect during labor from your mother or sisters. What they went through to deliver their children won't be just like what you go through. Each labor is unique, too—even in the same woman. No matter how many children you have, none of your labors will be alike.

Labor most often follows a fairly set pattern, though. Contractions open your cervix. They also help your baby move deeper into your pelvis. Later, they push the baby down into the birth canal. After birth, they help your body expel the placenta.

Your baby is an active player in its birth. The fetus moves its head and twists its body to find the best fit through your pelvis. Babies move into a head-down position to prepare for delivery.

The "average" labor lasts 12–14 hours for a first baby. The birth of second and later children is often much faster.

The first stage of labor is almost always the longest. It begins when your cervix starts to open and ends when it's fully dilated. Toward the end of this stage, contractions become longer and stronger. This stage is split into two phases: early labor and active labor. Some people believe there is a third phase that occurs as you near complete dilatation. It is called transition.

True Versus False Labor

Many women have periods of "false" labor. When this happens, your uterus knots up enough to make you think you're going into labor. False labor pains are called Braxton Hicks contractions. They do some of the early work—they help soften, thin, and perhaps even slightly open your cervix. They tend to occur more often as your due date draws near.

Sometimes, you can barely feel Braxton Hicks contractions. You may only notice a slight tightness in your belly. Other times, they can be painful. These contractions often show up in the afternoon or evening, after physical activity, and when you are tired.

If you have contractions, time them. Note how long it is from the start of one contraction to the start of the next. Keep a record for an hour and be sure to jot down how your contractions feel. You can walk around or do household tasks while you are timing your contractions. The time between contractions will help tell you if you are in true or false labor (see Table 2).

Don't feel silly if you go to the hospital, sure that the big day is here, only to be sent home again. It's easy to be fooled by false labor. Even a doctor or a nurse can have a hard time telling false labor from the real thing. He or she may need to observe you for

TABLE 2. Are You Really in Labor?

When you feel contractions, it's normal to think you're in labor. Don't head to the hospital just yet, though. You may be having false labor. This is a sort of practice labor. It helps your body gear up for birth, but it does not do much to open the cervix. Here's how to tell if you're really in labor:

Hint	False Labor	True Labor
Timing of contractions	Often irregular and don't get closer together as time goes on	Come at regular intervals and get closer together. Last 30–70 seconds
Change with movement	Contractions may stop when you walk, rest, or change position	Contractions keep coming no matter what you do
Strength of contractions	Often weak and tend to stay that way, or strong contractions are followed by weaker ones	Steadily get stronger
Pain of contractions	Usually felt only in the front	Usually starts in the back and moves to the front

The First Stage of Labor

Labor is often thought of as a single event, but the work that leads up to and follows your baby's birth happens in distinct stages.

Early Labor (your cervix dilates from 0–4 centimeters)

What's Happening:

▶ You may see a little blood-tinged mucus, or show, as this phase begins.

▶ Mild contractions begin. They are 15–20 minutes apart and last 60–90 seconds.

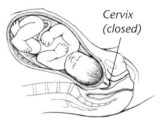

Cervix (closed)

▶ Contractions slowly become more regular. Toward the end of early labor, they'll be less than 5 minutes apart.

▶ You may feel relieved and excited that labor has started at last.

How Long It Lasts:

Stage 1

▶ The length of early labor varies quite a bit.
For some women, it's a few hours. For others, it's a day or more. But the average for first-time moms is 6–12 hours.

What You Can Do:

▶ Go for a walk with your partner or labor coach.

▶ Take a shower or bath (as long as your water hasn't broken).

▶ Try to rest and relax.

▶ Practice relaxation exercises or meditation.

▶ If you can, sleep.

Active Labor (your cervix dilates from 4–10 centimeters)

What's Happening:

▶ Contractions get stronger. They come as often as 3 minutes apart and last about 45 seconds.

▶ Your water may break. If it does, your contractions will get much more intense.

The First Stage of Labor (continued)

- You'll bleed from your vagina as your cervix opens.
- If the baby's head presses down on your backbone during contractions, you'll have a backache.
- Your legs may cramp.
- You may feel anxious and tired.
- You may have trembling legs, nausea, or vomiting.
- You may feel the urge to push.

How Long It Lasts:

- About 4–8 hours, on average

What You Can Do:

- If you feel like it and your doctor says it's OK, walk the halls.
- Use the toilet often. An empty bladder gives your baby's head more room to move down.
- Work with your labor coach through each contraction.
- Take your contractions one at a time. Focus on your breathing, and don't think about the next one.
- Try to relax between contractions.
- Use the pain-management methods you learned in childbirth class (or whatever happens to work).
- Ask someone to massage your back.
- If you have leg cramps, ask to have your feet flexed.
- Try different positions to find the one that works best for you.
- If you feel like lying down, lie on your side. Being flat on your back will add to your pain and cut down on the oxygen your baby gets.
- Ask for pain relief if you want it.
- If you feel the urge to push, tell your doctor. Don't give into the urge just yet—your cervix isn't fully dilated. Pant or blow to keep yourself from bearing down

a few hours to decide. A vaginal exam also will be done to see if your cervix is dilating.

One easy rule for telling true labor apart from false labor: as time goes on, true labor contractions get longer, stronger, and closer together. False labor contractions don't.

Keep in mind that painful contractions don't always signal true labor. Painless ones don't always mean false labor, either. The way one woman feels pain isn't the same as another. A few women feel only intense pressure during labor.

No matter what your stopwatch says about the timing of contractions, though, it's better to be safe than sorry. If you think you may be in labor, call your doctor's office or hospital. These other signs also should prompt a call:

▸ You have symptoms of labor before 37 weeks of pregnancy.

▸ Your water breaks (the fluid-filled amniotic sac that surrounds the baby during pregnancy breaks), even if you're not having contractions.

▸ You have vaginal bleeding.

▸ You have constant, severe pain with no relief between contractions.

▸ You have fever or chills.

▸ The baby seems to be moving less.

Helping Labor Along

Sometimes the baby needs a little urging to help labor along. Using medications or other methods to bring on labor is called labor induction. If keeping a pregnancy going is more risky than delivering the baby, then labor may be induced. Some of the methods used to induce labor also can speed up a labor that's not going well. Labor may be induced if:

▸ Your water's broken.

▸ Your pregnancy is *postdate* (more than 42 weeks).

> You have high blood pressure caused by your pregnancy.

> You have health problems such as diabetes or lung disease that could harm your baby.

> You have *chorioamnionitis* (an infection in the uterus).

Labor induction carries some risks. It should be done only to protect the health of the mother or the baby. Your baby may be monitored with electronic fetal monitoring if labor is induced (see "Monitoring"). There are four methods for starting labor:

1. *Stripping the membranes.* Your doctor inserts a gloved finger through your cervix. Next, he or she sweeps the finger over the thin membranes that connect the amniotic sac to the wall of your uterus. You may feel some intense cramping and have spotting when this is done. Stripping the membranes causes your body to release *prostaglandins.* These are hormones that ripen the cervix and may cause contractions.

2. *Ripening or dilating the cervix.* If your cervix is not ready for labor, steps can be taken to make it soft and able to stretch for labor. Certain medications or devices may be used to soften and dilate your cervix.

3. *Rupturing the amniotic sac.* If it hasn't broken already, breaking your water can get contractions started or make them stronger. Your doctor may make a small hole in the amniotic sac. You may feel discomfort as this is done. Most women go into labor within hours of their water breaking. Another method may be used if labor does not occur. That's because you and your baby are at risk for infection once the amniotic sac has broken.

4. *Oxytocin.* This is a hormone that causes contractions. When oxytocin is used to induce labor or make contractions stronger, it flows into your bloodstream through an intravenous (IV) tube in your arm. A pump hooked up to the IV controls the amount you are given.

The Support Person's Role

Many fathers want to be in the delivery room for the birth of their child. Some take an active role in the process. Your partner can help you use the relaxation and pain-management methods you learned in childbirth class. He can cheer you on when the going gets tough. He can be there for you to lean on—emotionally and physically. Many cut the baby's umbilical cord after birth.

Some fathers may not want to be in the delivery room during labor and birth. Even if your partner's not there for the big event, he still can give you support in other ways. He can come with you to prenatal checkups and take you to the hospital when you are in labor, for instance. He also can help care for you and the baby after delivery.

A labor coach doesn't have to be the father. A close family member or friend also can help you get ready for birth and be there with you when it happens.

There are even professional labor coaches, called doulas. They provide constant support and hands-on help to women in labor. (For details on doulas, see "Your Childbirth Partner" in Chapter 4.) Some of the things your support person can do during labor:

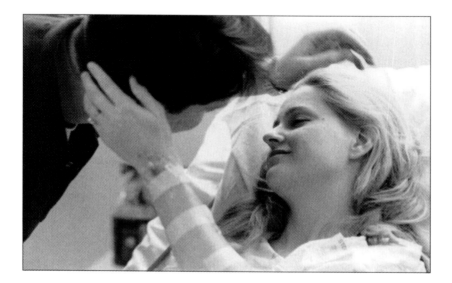

- Help distract you in early labor: play cards or other games with you, tell stories, read aloud, or take short walks with you

- Keep the room soothing by dimming the lights and keeping the noise level low

- Massage your back and shoulders, if that helps you relax

- Time your contractions

- Talk you through contractions

- Act as a focal point during contractions

- Guide you in breathing or other relaxation exercises

- Help you get into different labor positions

- Offer comfort and support

As your baby is being born, your coach may want to stand near the head of the bed. By standing at your shoulder, he or she can offer emotional and physical support as you push your baby into the world. From this spot, your coach will see your child being born just as you do.

Your birth partner may want to stand at the foot of the bed. From this vantage point, he or she can see the birth up close and take pictures of the big event. (If you plan to film it, check the hospital policy in advance to ensure video cameras are allowed during delivery).

If there's an emergency during labor or delivery, your support person may need to leave the room. There isn't always time to explain why. If your partner is asked to leave, he or she should do so right away. This is in the best interests of you and your baby. Your coach will be filled in later, when time permits.

Admission

Once you're in active labor, it's time to check into the hospital. After you're admitted to the labor and delivery unit, the next steps may vary. In most cases:

▶ You may be given a consent form to sign. (You may need to sign another one if a cesarean birth is needed.) These forms vary, but most spell out who will be taking care of you, why a procedure is being done, and the risks involved. Read this form and be sure to ask about anything that's not clear. Signing the consent form means that you understand your medical condition and agree to the care described.

▶ You'll be shown to a birthing or labor room. You may go through labor and delivery in the same room. Or you may be moved to a delivery room for the actual birth.

▶ You'll be asked to put on a special hospital gown. (If you'd rather wear your own nightgown or nightshirt, just ask. Know that it may get stained or ruined.)

▶ Your pulse, blood pressure, and temperature will be checked.

▶ A urine or blood sample may be taken.

▶ You'll be given a vaginal exam to see how much your cervix has dilated.

▶ An IV line may be started in your arm or wrist. A needle is placed in your vein, a small plastic tube is threaded over it, and the needle is removed. Medications and fluids can be given through the IV if you need them. An IV may limit your activity a bit during labor, though. If you'd rather not have an IV, talk to your doctor. He or she may be willing to wait and see if one is needed.

▶ You may be hooked up to an *electronic fetal monitor* to measure your contractions and check the baby's heart rate (for details, see "Monitoring").

Who will be with you during your labor? That depends on where you give birth and whether your doctor has other patients at the same time. A labor-and-delivery nurse will be checking on you from the time you check in until after your baby is born. (If your labor goes on for a long time or if a shift change happens in the middle of your labor, you may have more than one nurse.)

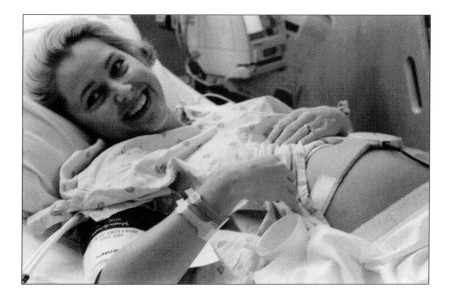

These nurses are well trained to help women through the physical and emotional demands of labor. In teaching hospitals, a resident doctor, student nurse, or medical student also may be a part of your birth team.

Your own doctor may be there from start to finish, or he or she may arrive shortly before you give birth. Even if your doctor is there only while you are pushing the baby out, he or she will check on your progress often during labor.

Your doctor or nurse will keep close tabs on you and your baby before delivery. He or she will:

▶ Check your heart rate and blood pressure. This will give clues to how well your body is handling the stress of labor.

▶ Time your contractions to monitor the progress of your labor. The doctor or nurse also will check your cervix from time to time to see how much it's dilating.

▶ Check your baby's heartbeat often during labor.

If you haven't done so, talk to your doctor about the sort of birth you hope to have. Also, inform your labor-and-delivery nurse.

You likely have many of the answers you need from reading about labor and delivery, taking childbirth classes, and talking to your doctor about birth ahead of time. Still, lots of new questions may occur to you now. Ask them. Your doctor and nurse are there to answer your questions.

Monitoring

To see how the baby is doing during labor, your doctor or nurse will check its heart rate often. (A normal fetal heart rate is between 110 and 160 beats a minute. A rate that's higher or lower than that or that doesn't stay fairly regular can signal a problem.)

Monitoring can't stop a problem from happening. It can alert your doctor or nurse to warning signs, though, and allow them to take steps to help the baby. These steps might include:

▸ Asking you to change positions

▸ Giving you oxygen through a mask

▸ Giving you IV fluids

▸ Putting extra fluid around your baby

▸ Giving you medication to weaken contractions and relax your uterus

Fetal monitoring is done by *auscultation* or with an electronic fetal monitor. Sometimes these methods can be used together. The method used in your labor depends on:

▸ The equipment on hand

▸ The number of nurses on duty

▸ The hospital's policy

▸ Your risk of problems

▸ How your labor is going

Auscultation

Auscultation means listening to the baby's heartbeat at set times. The timing depends on how well labor is going and whether there are any risk factors.

Two devices can be used to pick up the heartbeat: a *fetoscope* or an ultrasound.

1. A fetoscope is a type of stethoscope. Your doctor or nurse presses one end of the scope to your belly and listens to the baby's heartbeat through earpieces.

2. A *Doppler* ultrasound is a small, hand-held device that's placed on your belly. It uses sound waves to create a signal of the baby's beating heart (see "Ultrasound" in Chapter 17).

The fetal heart rate may be checked during and after a contraction. The doctor or nurse will place his or her hands on your abdomen to feel your uterus contract. You may be asked to lie in bed while this is done. During other times, though, you can move around as much as you want. Auscultation has no known risks.

Electronic Fetal Monitoring

The other type of monitoring measures the baby's heart rate with electronic equipment. It provides an ongoing record and often is used in high-risk pregnancies. Electronic fetal monitoring can be done from the outside (external), inside (internal), or both:

▸ For external monitoring, a pair of belts is wrapped around your belly. The belts hold two small devices in place. One device uses ultrasound to detect the fetal heart rate. The other measures the length of contractions and the time between them.

▸ For internal monitoring, a small device called an *electrode* is inserted through your vagina and placed on the baby's scalp. The electrode records the fetal heart rate. A thin tube called a *catheter* also may be put in your uterus to gauge the strength of contractions. Internal monitoring can be done only after the amniotic sac has ruptured. Most women report only minor pain when the devices are put in place—about the same as a routine pelvic exam.

▸ Sometimes, both methods are combined. The internal electrode records the fetal heart beat. The external pressure gauge records contractions.

No matter which type of electronic monitoring is used, the data the devices pick up is sent to a small machine and recorded.

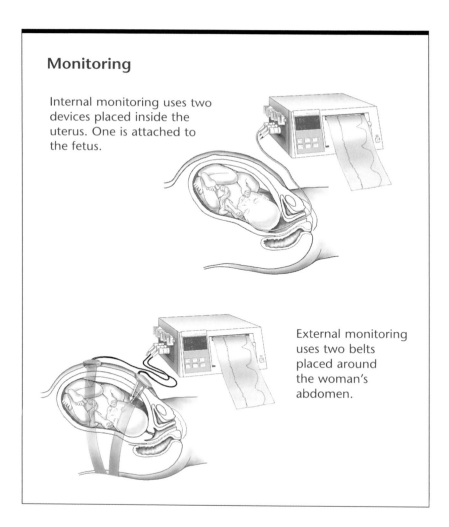

Monitoring

Internal monitoring uses two devices placed inside the uterus. One is attached to the fetus.

External monitoring uses two belts placed around the woman's abdomen.

The tracing from the machine shows how the fetal heart rate reacts to contractions.

One type of electronic monitoring may be more useful to you than the other. With the external monitor, the cervix doesn't have to be dilated and the sac around the fetus can be intact. Internal monitoring, though, may give a more precise picture of the baby's condition and the strength of contractions. Also, when an internal monitor is used, the spot where the electrode is placed on the baby's head can get injured or infected. This is rare, though.

Women who are monitored electronically often are asked to spend their labor in bed. This helps keep the monitor in place.

Pain Relief During Labor

There are two big questions women may ponder as their due date nears: "How much will labor hurt?" and "What can I do about it?" Each birth—and each woman's response to it—is unique. Different types of pain relief are available during childbirth. They should be discussed in advance with your doctor.

You should have an idea of what your prefer, but it often is best to keep your options open. Things can—and often do—happen in the delivery room that come as a surprise to both you and your doctor. You may not be able to get pain medication just when you need it, for instance. Not all types of pain relief are on hand at every hospital at all times either. The well-being of you and your baby is the main issue to keep in mind.

If you choose to use pain medication, an *anesthesiologist* or anesthetist (a doctor who's an expert in pain relief) will work with your doctor and nurse to choose the best *anesthesia* for you. If you know you want to use pain medication, let your doctor know during your prenatal care. That way, they can make sure it is available when you deliver.

Certain methods provide pain relief from labor right on through delivery. Others are used only while you're pushing the baby out or during a cesarean birth. No matter when they are used, you should be fully informed of your options in advance.

?

What Affects Your Feelings of Pain?

Why do some women recall the pain of labor as the worst they have ever felt, while others say it was no big deal? Because each woman feels pain in a way that's unique to her. No one's sure why this is.

Your state of mind also plays a role in how much pain you feel. Here are some factors that can make labor hurt more and what you can do about them:

▸ *Fear of the unknown.* Learn as much about childbirth as you can before delivery day: read about it, ask your doctor questions, and take childbirth preparation classes. The more you know about the birth process, the less scary it will seem.

▸ *Feeling helpless.* Learn ahead of time what your options are for labor and delivery. Practice the pain-management methods taught in childbirth class. If you do, you'll be a more active player in your baby's birth.

▸ *Fear of losing control.* Some women fear losing their cool as well as losing control of their body. Keep in mind that your body knows what to do, even if you don't. Do what your body tells you to, and don't worry about making a fool of yourself.

▸ *Being alone.* It's vital to have the support of your partner or a loved one during labor and delivery. The hands-on care of a labor-and-delivery nurse or doula also will help reduce your pain.

▸ *Fatigue.* Rest as much as you can in early labor. As labor wears on, rest after each contraction so you can cope with the next one.

▸ *Anxiety and tension.* Focus on your breathing during contractions. Use relaxation methods between them.

▸ *Expecting and fearing a lot of pain.* Don't focus on how much contractions hurt. Instead, try to distract yourself by using a focal point or doing breathing exercises. Remind yourself that each contraction is bringing you closer to your new baby. If you feel scared, go ahead and say so. Airing your fears gives others a chance to comfort you.

Epidural Block

Epidural block is an anesthetic that removes most feeling from the lower half of your body. An epidural numbs the pain of contractions. It also can numb the vagina as the baby's pushed out. In larger doses, an epidural controls pain during a cesarean birth. Just how numb you become depends on the exact medication given and how much of it is used. Here's what happens when you get an epidural:

▸ Your back is washed with an antiseptic.

▸ A small area of skin is numbed with a local anesthetic.

▸ You're asked to sit or lie on your side and curve your back outward. You'll need to stay this way until the injection is over.

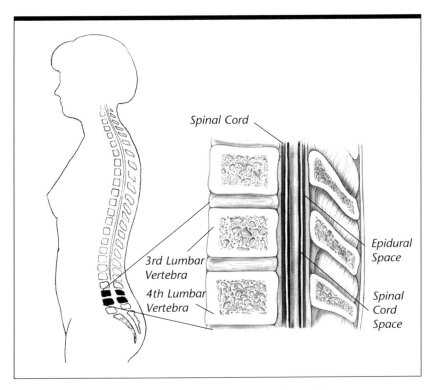

Area of the back where epidural or spinal anesthesia is inserted.

- An anesthesiologist inserts a needle into your lower back. The needle is placed in the epidural space near your spine. This is where nerves carry signals from the lower body to the spinal cord.

- After the needle is in place, a catheter is inserted through it and the needle is withdrawn. The catheter is left in the epidural space. This is so anesthetic can be given constantly or so small doses can be given later in labor or after delivery to help relieve pain.

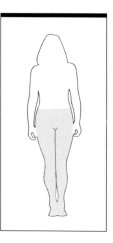

- Low doses of anesthetic are injected into the epidural space to numb your lower body. It may take a little while before the medication takes effect. Once it has, you'll be more comfortable. You still may be aware of your contractions. You're likely to feel them as pressure rather than pain, though.

- When more anesthetic is needed, more is injected. (In some hospitals, women in labor control the amount of epidural anesthetic they get by pressing a button on a special pump when they start to feel pain.)

- You can move once the epidural is injected. You may not be allowed to walk around, though.

Most women have epidurals with no problems. This pain relief method has some drawbacks, though:

- An epidural can cause your blood pressure to drop. This, in turn, can slow your baby's heartbeat. To prevent this, you'll be given fluids through an IV before the drug is injected. You may also need to lie on your side to improve blood flow.

- After delivery, your back may be sore from the injection.

- If the covering of the spinal cord is pierced, you can get a bad headache. If it's not treated, this headache can last for days. This rarely occurs.

▶ If an epidural is given too early, it may slow labor down. This, in turn, may mean that labor assistance may be needed. (However, if pain is making you very tense, an epidural might help you relax enough to speed labor along.)

▶ When an epidural is given late in labor or a lot of anesthetic is used, it may be hard to bear down and push your baby through the birth canal. If you can't feel what you're doing, you won't push as well as you could.

Serious complications are very rare:

▶ If the drug enters a vein, you could get dizzy or, rarely, have a seizure.

▶ If anesthetic enters your spinal fluid, it can affect your chest muscles and make it hard for you to breathe.

As long as your epidural is given by a highly trained and experienced anesthesiologist, there's little chance you'll run into trouble. If you are thinking an epidural may be the choice for you, bring up any concerns or questions you have with your doctor.

Systemic Analgesia

Systemic analgesia acts on the whole nervous system, rather than on just one area. These medications often are injected into a muscle or a vein. They lessen pain but let you stay awake. Sometimes other drugs are given with systemic analgesics to relieve tension or nausea.

Like any medication, analgesia can have side effects. You may feel drowsy, sick to your stomach, or have trouble focusing, for instance. Serious side effects are rare. In most cases, systemic analgesia is often not given right before delivery because it may slow the baby's reflexes and breathing at birth. These problems can be treated with medications.

Pain Relief During Birth

If you think you'll want pain relief for labor, think about options to ease the pain of delivery as well. Even if you go through labor without medication, you may want some form of pain relief during the pushing stage. You'll also need anesthesia if you get an episiotomy, if your doctor uses *forceps* or *vacuum extraction*, or if you have a cesarean birth.

Local Anesthesia

Just as your dentist uses medication to numb your mouth before filling cavities, your doctor can use *local anesthesia* to ease pain during delivery. Local anesthetics numb a small area. They are injected into your skin and muscle in most cases.

If you have an episiotomy, for instance, local anesthesia will numb your *perineum* before the cut is made. If you tear during delivery, your doctor will give you anesthetic before stitching the tear closed.

Local anesthesia rarely affects the baby. After the anesthetic wears off, effects will not linger in most cases.

Pudendal Block

Pudendal block is an anesthetic that's injected through the wall of the vagina and into the pudendal nerve. It's given shortly before delivery to block pain in the perineum.

Pudendal block is one of the safest forms of anesthesia. Severe side effects are rare.

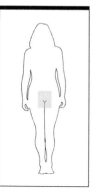

Spinal Block

Like an epidural block, a *spinal block* is an injection of anesthetic into your lower back. It numbs the lower half of your body.

Unlike an epidural, though, a spinal block usually is given only once during labor and lasts just an hour or two. Because of this, it's often given just before delivery.

While you sit or lie on your side, an anesthesiologist or nurse anesthetist will inject a small amount of anesthetic into the fluid around your spinal cord. After the shot is given, you'll need to stay in bed.

A spinal block causes total numbness and prevents the muscles used to push the baby out from working. It's most often used only if a baby needs to be helped out of the birth canal with forceps or vacuum extraction. A spinal block also can be used to numb pain during a cesarean birth.

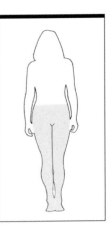

A spinal block sometimes can cause the same side effects as an epidural block. These side effects are treated in much the same way.

A saddle block is a type of spinal block. It affects a smaller area, though. The part of your body that loses feeling is the part that sits in a saddle—your buttocks, perineum, and vagina.

General Anesthesia

General anesthesia makes you lose consciousness (puts you to sleep). If you are not awake during delivery, you will not feel pain.

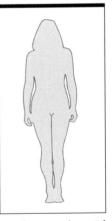

General anesthetics are given through an IV, inhaled through a mask, or both. Most of the time, general anesthesia is used only for an emergency cesarean birth, for cesarean delivery when an epidural isn't safe, or when the baby must be delivered quickly. General anesthesia is not used to relieve the pain of labor.

The baby often is born before the drug enters his or her system. Sometimes, though, general anesthesia can sedate the baby as well as the mother. If this happens, it can slow his or her breathing and reflexes.

Another rare but severe side effect of general anesthesia occurs when food or acid from the stomach enters the windpipe and lungs and causes injury. To be on the safe side, your doctor may ask you not to eat solid food or drink fluids once you're in labor.

Even if you haven't had anything to eat or drink, stomach acids still may get into your lungs. If it looks like general anesthesia may be needed, your nurse will give you medicine (such as antacid) to reduce these acids.

The Home Stretch

You have waited for months, endured many changes, and powered through many hours of labor. At last, the moment is nearing that will make it all seem worthwhile—the birth of your baby.

CHAPTER 9

Birth

Forty weeks of pregnancy and hours of labor are about to pay off. Still, many women are nervous about the prospect of delivery. Try not to worry about it too much. Chances are, your baby's entry into the world will come off without a problem (in fact, most do). Babies sometimes run into a few problems on their way out of the uterus, though.

Special procedures may be required to help your baby exit the birth canal, for instance. If the baby's health is at risk, a cesarean delivery may be needed. Keep in mind: no matter how your birth goes, a healthy baby is the main goal.

Delivery

Once you get to the delivery stage, you'll be amazed by your strength and what your body can do. Your pelvis is designed to allow babies to fit through it. Your vagina is a very elastic organ. It can easily stretch to make way for a 7- or even a 10-pound newborn.

Here's what happens during the second stage of labor, as the baby's birth is called: once your cervix has opened fully, you'll notice a change in the way your contractions feel. With each one, you'll have an urge to bear down. This can feel like the urge to move your bowels, but it's much stronger.

The Second and Third Stages of Labor: Delivery and Afterbirth

This is the home stretch of labor. Once your cervix is fully dilated, you can begin to push your baby out. After your baby is born, your body will expel the placenta.

The Second Stage

What's Happening:

Stage 2 (early)

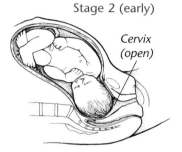

Cervix (open)

- Contractions may slow down. They are 2–5 minutes apart and last 60–90 seconds.

- Contractions usually are regular.

- You feel the urge to push or bear down with each contraction. Pushing may feel good.

- You feel great pressure on your rectum from the baby's head.

Stage 2 (late)

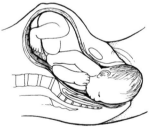

- You feel pressure and stinging in your vagina as the baby's head crowns.

- Your doctor may do an episiotomy to widen the opening of the birth canal.

- The baby's head emerges.

- Your doctor helps guide the baby's shoulders and body out of the birth canal.

How Long It Lasts:

- 20 minutes to 3 hours or more

What You Can Do:

- Ask for a mirror so you can see your baby being born.

- Find a pushing position that works for you.

- If you are not comfortable or pushing has stalled, change positions.

The Second and Third Stages of Labor: Delivery and Afterbirth (continued)

- Push when you feel the urge or when you are told to.
- Work closely with your support person.
- Rest between contractions.
- Ask the nurse to hold a warm cloth to your perineum. This will focus your pushing efforts and help your skin stretch.
- As soon as your baby's born, hold your son or daughter to your skin and look into his or her eyes. This is the moment that will make all of your effort seem worth it.

The Third Stage

What's Happening:

- Contractions keep coming. They are less painful, though.
- The placenta peels away from the wall of the uterus.
- The placenta and amniotic sac are pushed out through the vagina.
- Contractions cause the uterus to get smaller.
- Your doctor or your labor coach cuts the umbilical cord.
- If you had an episiotomy or tear, it's stitched closed.
- You may shake or shiver.

Stage 3

Uterus

Placenta

How Long It Lasts:

- From a few minutes to half an hour

What You Can Do:

- Push when you feel the urge or you are asked. This will help expel the placenta and amniotic sac.
- Ask for a warm blanket if you are cold.
- Enjoy your baby. Cuddle your newborn or try breastfeeding.

Tell your doctor or nurse as soon as you feel like pushing. He or she will need to check your cervix to make sure it's dilated all the way. (If you start pushing before you are fully dilated, you can damage your cervix as well as exhaust yourself.)

To avoid pushing, control your breathing. Blowing air out in short puffs, for instance, stops many women from bearing down. If you took a childbirth class, you may have learned controlled breathing methods from the instructor. If not, your nurse will guide you in breathing exercises.

If you have been in a standard labor room, you'll be moved to a delivery room now. If you are in a labor/delivery/recovery room, your doctor and nurse will help you get into a good delivery position.

Many women deliver their baby while propped up in bed, with their legs braced against foot rests. As long as your doctor OKs it, though, there are other good birth positions you can try.

Once your doctor gives you the go-ahead, bear down with each contraction or when he or she tells you to push. As the baby moves down the birth canal, your doctor will track the progress and tell you how to help your baby along.

Sometimes, a few good pushes is all it takes before a baby is born. Other times, a woman may work for hours before her baby emerges.

When the baby's head appears at the opening of your vagina, you'll feel a burning or stinging feeling there as the perineum stretches and bulges. This is normal.

Your doctor may perform an episiotomy. This is a small cut to widen the opening of your vagina. The doctor also may do

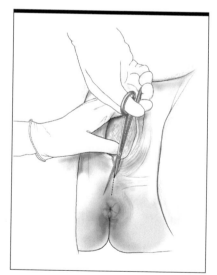

For an episiotomy, a small cut is made in your vagina and perineum to widen the opening of the vagina.

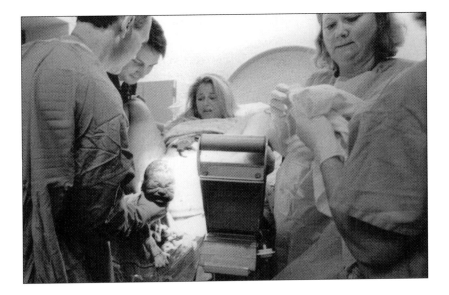

an episiotomy if he or she needs to get the baby out quickly. The area is numbed with a local anesthetic before the cut is made, so you shouldn't feel a thing. (An episiotomy will hurt as it heals, though.)

Delivering the baby's head may take some time. After the head emerges from the birth canal, the baby's body turns. First one shoulder slips out, and then the other. After the shoulders are delivered, the rest of the baby's body follows quickly.

Afterbirth

Many women think that once their baby is born, labor's over. There's a bit more work to be done. The good news: this last stage of labor is the shortest of all.

After your newborn is delivered, the placenta peels away from the wall of your uterus. Contractions move the placenta and the empty amniotic sac (often called the afterbirth) down into the birth canal. Once there, a push or two by you will help expel them from the vagina.

Just as they cause the placenta to separate from the uterine wall, contractions help your newly empty uterus return to its smaller size. As the uterus shrinks, the blood vessels that brought nutrients and oxygen to the placenta and took waste products away are sealed.

The contractions felt after delivery are often milder than those felt during labor. Still, they can be painful.

Forceps and Vacuum Extraction

Sometimes a woman sails through labor with no problems. When it's time to push, though, she may bear down for hours without making much progress. Other times, the baby's heartbeat may become slow or erratic. Still other times, the baby's position makes delivery harder. Also, a woman may become too tired to push.

In such cases, a doctor may need to help delivery along by using forceps or vacuum extraction. This is done in about 1 in 10 vaginal deliveries.

Forceps look like two large spoons. Forceps are inserted into the vagina. Next, the doctor places the forceps around the baby's cheeks and jaw (the fat there provides a nice cushion). Then the doctor uses the forceps to gently guide the baby's head out of the birth canal.

Vacuum extraction is much like forceps delivery. Instead of forceps, a plastic cup is inserted into the vagina and applied to the baby's head. Suction holds the cup in place. A handle on the cup allows the doctor to pull the baby through the birth canal.

Forceps and Vacuum Extraction

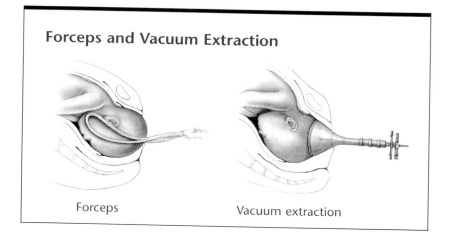

Forceps   Vacuum extraction

In most cases, using special tools to help delivery causes no major problems. Still, both forceps and vacuum extraction can bruise the baby's head or tear the vagina or cervix.

Cesarean Birth

Most babies enter the world through the birth canal. In about 1 in 5 cases, though, a baby is born by cesarean birth. This means the baby is delivered through an incision in the mother's abdomen and uterus.

A cesarean birth may be planned ahead of time because of certain problems. Also, issues may come up in labor that make a cesarean birth a safer choice than a vaginal birth.

You may need a cesarean birth if:

▸ You gave birth by cesarean before. Sometimes, a prior cesarean birth means that you'll need cesarean delivery this time, too. (Many women who have had a past cesarean birth can try to deliver vaginally. For details, see "Vaginal Birth After Cesarean Delivery.")

▸ You have certain medical conditions. An active genital herpes infection may make a vaginal birth risky, for instance, but most women with these conditions don't need cesarean birth.

▸ You have a multiple pregnancy. Many women having twins can give birth vaginally. The risks of vaginal birth go up with the number of fetuses. As a result, women carrying more than two babies often have a cesarean delivery.

▸ You have a large baby or a small pelvis. Sometimes, a baby is too big to pass safely through a woman's pelvis and vagina. This is called *cephalopelvic disproportion.*

▸ Your baby is in an unusual position. If you are in labor and your baby is *breech* (buttocks- or feet-down), your doctor may feel that a cesarean birth is the safest. (Some doctors perform vaginal deliveries for breech babies.) If the baby is *transverse* (lying sideways in the uterus rather than head-down), a cesarean birth is the only choice for delivery.

Breech Presentation

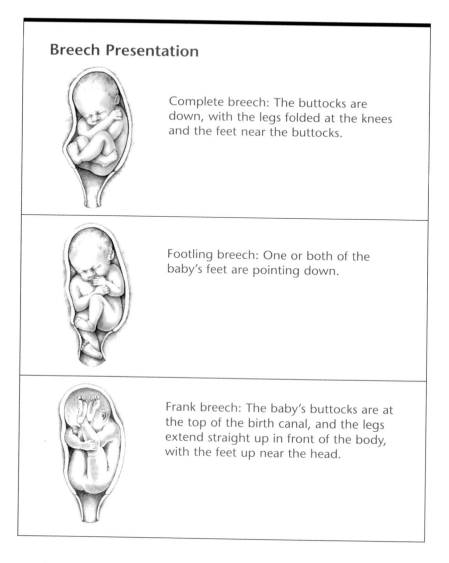

Complete breech: The buttocks are down, with the legs folded at the knees and the feet near the buttocks.

Footling breech: One or both of the baby's feet are pointing down.

Frank breech: The baby's buttocks are at the top of the birth canal, and the legs extend straight up in front of the body, with the feet up near the head.

▶ There are problems with the placenta. Placenta previa means the placenta covers all or part of the cervix. This blocks the baby's exit from the uterus. Another problem that may occur is abruptio placentae. It happens when the placenta tears away from the wall of the uterus before birth. This cuts off the baby's oxygen supply. Both of these conditions can cause heavy bleeding. In both cases, a cesarean birth may be the safest choice.

▶ There's a problem with the umbilical cord. Sometimes, the umbilical cord becomes pinched or compressed. If this happens, the baby may not get enough oxygen. An emergency cesarean delivery may be done.

▶ Your labor fails to progress. About 1 in 3 cesarean births is done because labor slows down or stops. You may have contractions, but they don't open the cervix enough for the baby to move through the vagina, for instance. If medication doesn't speed things up (see "Helping Labor Along" in Chapter 8), a cesarean birth may be needed.

▶ Labor is too stressful for your baby. Cesarean births often are done in cases where monitoring picks up signs of problems.

What happens during a cesarean birth? That depends on how urgent the surgery is. In most cases, though, a cesarean birth goes something like this:

1. To numb pain during surgery, an anesthesiologist gives you an epidural, a spinal block, or general anesthesia if you haven't already been given it. The anesthesiologist will talk to you about your pain relief choices and take your wishes into account.

2. Once that's done, the anesthesiologist hooks you up to monitors that track your breathing, heart rate, and blood pressure. He or she also covers your nose and mouth with an oxygen mask or places a tube in your nostril to make sure you get plenty of oxygen during surgery.

3. Your labor coach puts on a sterile mask and gown so he or she can be at your side in the operating room. (If an emergency cesarean birth is needed, your partner most likely won't be allowed to join you.)

4. Your nurse prepares you for surgery. You may be given medication to dry the secretions in your mouth and upper airway and to reduce acid in your stomach. Your abdomen will be washed and any hair between your pubic bone and navel may be shaved. A catheter will be inserted into your bladder. This

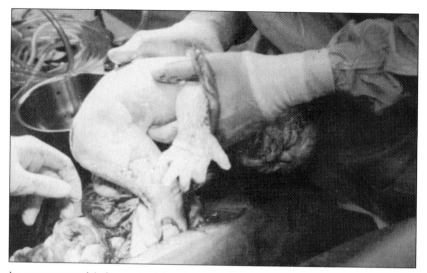

In a cesarean birth, an incision is made in the mother's abdomen and uterus. This makes an opening for the baby to be delivered.

keeps the bladder empty so that it's not injured during surgery. An IV line will be started in a vein in your arm or hand. This allows you to get fluids and medications during the surgery. Last, your abdomen will be swabbed with an antiseptic, and sterile drapes will be placed around your belly.

5. Your doctor makes a 4- to 6-inch incision through your skin and the wall of your abdomen. This cut may go from side to side, just above your pubic hairline (transverse). Or it may go up and down, from your pubic bone to your navel (vertical).

6 The doctor gently spreads apart your abdominal muscles and cuts through the lining of your abdominal cavity. Your abdominal muscles are not cut.

7. When he or she reaches your uterus, the doctor makes another cut in the uterine wall. This also can be transverse or vertical. In most cases, a transverse incision is made. This type of cut is done in the lower, thinner part of the uterus. It causes less bleeding and heals with a stronger scar. A vertical incision may need to be done if you have placenta previa or if the baby is in an unusual position. (After delivery, be sure to ask which

type of cut was made. This affects how you'll deliver your next child. For details, see "Vaginal Birth After Cesarean Delivery.")

8. The baby is delivered through the incisions. The umbilical cord is cut, and the baby is passed to the nurse. The placenta is removed from the uterus.

9. The uterus and abdominal wall are closed with stitches that dissolve in your body. Stitches or surgical staples are used to close the incision in your skin. A dressing is placed on it.

Like any surgery, a cesarean birth involves risks. The special risks of cesarean birth include:

▸ Infection in your uterus, pelvic organs, or abdominal incision

▸ Blood loss, but rarely enough to require a blood transfusion

▸ Blood clots in your legs, pelvic organs, or lungs

▸ Injury to your bowel or bladder

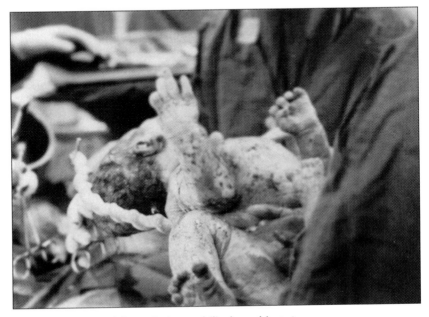

Once the baby is delivered, the umbilical cord is cut.

Vaginal Birth After Cesarean Delivery

It was once thought that if a woman had one cesarean birth, all other children she had should be born the same way. Today, many women who have had a cesarean delivery can give birth through the vagina in a later pregnancy. This is called vaginal birth after cesarean (VBAC) delivery. VBAC is an option for many women. There are some risks, though.

Of women who try VBAC, about 60–80% succeed and are able to deliver vaginally. Other women may try VBAC but need to switch to a cesarean birth.

There are some good reasons to try VBAC. Advantages to a vaginal birth include:

▸ No abdominal surgery

▸ Shorter hospital stay

▸ Lower risk of infection

▸ Less need for blood transfusions

▸ Faster recovery

In deciding if you can try VBAC, a key factor is the type of incision you had in your uterus for your previous cesarean birth. For cesarean birth, one incision is made in your abdomen and another in your uterus. Any incision makes a scar. Certain types of incisions of the uterus have a higher risk of rupture or tearing during the next birth.

You can't tell what type of scar you have on your uterus by looking at the scar on your skin. Your medical records should show which type of incision was used. There are three types of incisions:

▸ Low transverse—A side-to-side cut made across the lower, thinner part of the uterus

▸ Low vertical—An up-and-down cut made in the lower, thinner part of the uterus

▸ High vertical (or classical)—An up-and-down cut made in the upper part of the uterus

Uterine Incisions

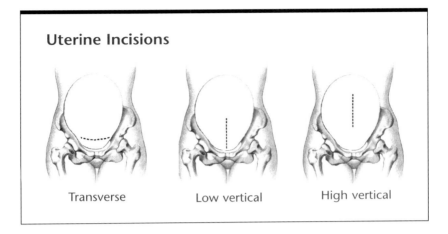

Transverse   Low vertical   High vertical

Women with high vertical (classical) scars on the uterus have a higher risk of rupture. Women who have had more than one cesarean delivery also may have an increased risk of rupture. Although it does not occur often, a rupture of the uterus may be harmful to you or your baby. If your doctor thinks you are at high risk for rupture of the uterus, VBAC should not be tried.

Other factors may affect whether VBAC is an option for you. It may not be a good choice in some cases:

▸ Small pelvis/large baby—the baby is too large to pass safely through your pelvis during delivery

▸ Problems for the baby—there are signs that the baby may have problems during labor or vaginal delivery

▸ Problems with the placenta—includes abruptio placentae or placenta previa

▸ Certain conditions—includes certain serious medical or obstetric conditions

If problems arise or worsen during labor, or if labor is taking too long to progress, cesarean delivery may be needed. The facility where you deliver your baby should be equipped to handle an emergency cesarean delivery with doctors on hand to give emergency care. There is a higher risk for infection in the mother and baby in women who try VBAC and then give birth by cesarean.

No labor or delivery is risk free. When considering VBAC, you need to know the risks. Weigh those risks against the benefits before you decide. Your doctor will guide your decision to do what's best for you and your baby.

After Delivery

Once your baby's born, your doctor and nurse keep a close eye on you and your baby to make sure there are no problems. If you had a vaginal delivery:

▸ The doctor will examine your vagina, cervix, and perineum to make sure that it all looks normal. If you had an episiotomy or a tear, it will be repaired.

▸ Your nurse will take your blood pressure, pulse, and temperature often. He or she will massage your uterus. Your nurse also will check for heavy vaginal bleeding or signs of infection.

▸ You should move around—with the nurse's help—as soon as you can.

If you had a cesarean delivery, you will be taken to a recovery room or straight to your hospital room. There, nurses will:

▸ Give you medicine to relieve pain or nausea (the anesthetic used for surgery may leave you feeling sick to your stomach).

▸ Check your incision, vaginal bleeding, blood pressure, pulse, breathing, and temperature often.

▸ Bring your baby to you for cuddling and nursing. If you don't feel up to being with your newborn just yet, though, there's plenty of time for that later.

▸ Take your IV out when you are ready to eat and drink again.

No matter how your baby is born, the next steps follow pretty much the same course:

▸ Your baby will be held with his or her head down to keep amniotic fluid, mucus, and blood from getting into the lungs. The baby may be placed on your belly while these fluids drain.

Recovering From a Cesarean Delivery

If you had a cesarean delivery, it may take a while for you to feel like yourself again. You are not just recovering from labor and delivery. You also are recovering from major surgery.

On top of all the normal postpartum aches and pains (see Chapter 12 for details), you'll have a few more symptoms that need care. Here's what to expect after a cesarean birth:

▸ You may be very tired. Why? You lost blood during surgery. This can sap your energy for a few days or weeks. You may be even more tired if you went through hours of labor before the surgery began.

▸ You have to stay in bed for a day or so after the surgery. When you are ready to get out of bed, you'll need help.

▸ The incision in your abdomen will be very sore for the first few days or even weeks. Your doctor can give you medication to ease the pain. (It is safe to use over-the-counter pain relievers, even if you are breastfeeding.) You may need to nurse your baby while lying on your side. You have to avoid heavy lifting and driving for a few weeks, too. This keeps excess pressure off the incision while it heals.

▸ You may have painful gas and constipation. Anesthesia and surgery slow digestion. This causes your bowels to get bloated from trapped food gasses. Walking should get things moving again.

▸ You may stay in the hospital for about 4 days after a cesarean birth. Even after you check out, you will have to take it easy for awhile. You will need extra help at home for a few weeks. Ask someone to bring the baby to you for feedings and help change the baby's diaper. Be sure to ask friends and relatives to help with cooking, cleaning, errands, or older children, too.

▸ You should be on the lookout for fever or incision pain that gets worse. Both can signal an infection.

▸ Aside from being physically wiped out, you may feel a little down after a cesarean birth. Having a cesarean birth is not a failure. Sure, you may have had your heart set on a natural birth. But the way your child comes into the world isn't nearly as important as your baby and you being healthy.

▶ The baby's mouth and nose are suctioned with a small bulb syringe.

▶ The umbilical cord is clamped and cut.

▶ One minute after delivery, the baby's *Apgar score* will be checked. This is used to assess a newborn's health and to see if extra care is needed. The test is done again at 5 minutes after delivery. (Chapter 11 has details on Apgar scoring.)

▶ The baby is dried and wrapped in blankets (heat lamps or a heated bassinet sometimes are used).

▶ As long as you are up to it and there are no major medical problems, you can hold your newborn right away. Cradle your baby next to your skin. Look into his or her eyes. If you are going to nurse, put your baby to your breast. Some newborns don't want to nurse right away. Others latch right on.

▶ When you are ready to part with your son or daughter for a few minutes, the nurse will weigh and measure the baby, give him or her a bath, slip identification bands around the baby's ankle and wrist, and perhaps take tiny handprints and footprints.

▶ Within a few hours of birth, your baby will have a head-to-toe exam and a few standard newborn procedures.

Your Hospital Stay

Hospitals vary in how mothers and their babies are cared for after delivery. Your baby may "room-in" with you until you go home. This is a good way to get to know your new baby. It's also a good way to get started breastfeeding. Many hospitals allow your partner to stay with you, too.

If you are too tired to have the baby in your room, your newborn can stay in the nursery and be brought to you for feedings. It depends on how you feel.

If you feel unsure about newborn care (and many new parents do), now is the perfect time to get tips and advice from the hospi-

Bonding With Your Baby

For many women, love doesn't come at first sight. A baby may be whisked away shortly after birth to get special medical care. A woman may be tired from hours of labor, fuzzy from pain medication, or sidelined by a cesarean birth. Lots of new moms are simply too overwhelmed by the responsibility that's just been thrust into their arms to feel much emotion at all. This is normal, and it doesn't mean you won't form a loving bond with your baby.

If you feel up to it, take time after birth to cradle your newborn in your arms and hold him or her against your skin. But don't feel guilty if your first moments—or even days—with your baby aren't as close as you thought they would be.

Bonding takes months—not minutes. Give yourself time to warm up to your baby. Your connection may take a little while, but it'll be strong enough to last a lifetime.

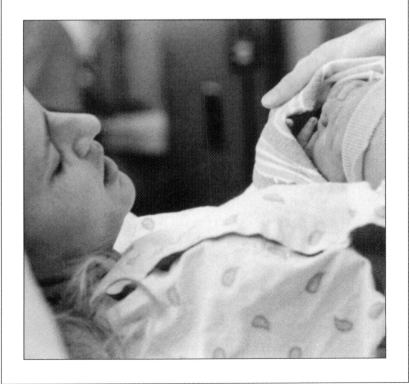

tal staff. Ask your nurse to help you with breastfeeding, teach you the best ways to soothe your baby, or show you how to diaper or swaddle your newborn—whatever advice you need. Maternity nurses are experts at infant care. This is a good chance to learn from them.

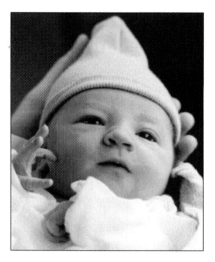

Before you gave birth, you may have pictured yourself cradling a plump, rosy-cheeked infant. The way your newborn really looks can come as quite a surprise. Most of the time, nothing is wrong. If something about the way your baby looks or acts worries you, though, be sure to ask about it. The doctors and nurses at the hospital are there to answer your questions and can set your mind at ease.

If you have other children, they'll be eager to meet their new brother or sister. They can visit you and the baby in the hospital. The more involved siblings feel, the better they'll respond to the new baby.

Before an older child's visit, be sure to check the hospital's policies and hours for visitors. Also make sure that:

▶ Your child hasn't been exposed to any known viruses, such as chickenpox.

▶ Your older child is healthy. If your child has a fever, a cough, or other symptoms, wait until he or she is feeling better before meeting the new baby.

▶ Your partner or a family member has talked to the child about the visit and told him or her how to behave and what to expect.

▶ An adult (other than you) can keep an eye on the child during his or her visit.

Keep your well-being in mind, too. Having your children and other close relatives drop by is fine. But you may want to hold off

? How Long Will You Stay in the Hospital?

A federal law called the Newborns' and Mothers' Health Protection Act says that managed care plans and health insurers that offer hospital childbirth coverage must pay for at least 48 hours in the hospital after a vaginal delivery, and at least 96 hours after a cesarean birth. The 48- or 96-hour period applies independently to women and their newborn children. A mother's length-of-stay may not be the same as her child's. Length-of-stay for the mother and infant is determined by the doctor in consultation with the mother. Some women may need to stay longer if problems come up during labor or after delivery. Talk to your doctor and your baby's doctor about what's best in your case.

If a woman is discharged early, she may be able to have follow-up home care. It depends on her insurance plan. Many insurance plans pay for a nurse to visit you at home a day or two after your hospital discharge. The home care nurse:

▶ Gives you and your baby a thorough exam to make sure you are both doing well.

▶ Finds out how you are recovering from delivery and checks you for signs of infection.

▶ Looks your baby over for conditions such as newborn *jaundice*. This often doesn't show up until a few days after birth.

▶ Makes sure your milk has come in if you are breastfeeding, your baby is latching on, and nursing is going well.

▶ Finds out how you are doing with the basics of newborn care and asks how you and your baby are settling in.

If a home visit is an option for you, don't pass it up—even if all seems to be going fine.

on other visits so you have more time to rest and get to know your baby. After all, the last thing you need when you are trying to recover from birth is a crowd of friends, neighbors, and coworkers in your hospital room. Greeting visitors can be tiring. There will be plenty of time for people to wish you well and to see the new baby after you are settled in at home. Suggest that well wishers visit you at home after a few weeks.

Going Home

The idea of leaving the hospital after your baby's birth may make you a little nervous. After all, for the last few days expert help has been just a call-button away.

If you really don't feel ready to go home or if you are worried about your baby, speak up. What if you just have some new-mom jitters? Know that you can (and should) call your doctor, the hospital nursery, or your baby's doctor with any questions that arise.

Before heading home, your doctor will want to make sure you are well enough to care for yourself and your baby. You should be able to answer yes to these questions before checking out:

____Do you know how to hold, bathe, diaper, and dress your baby?

____Do you know the best ways to put your baby down to sleep?

____Do you know how to care for the baby's umbilical stump?

____If your son was circumcised, do you know how to care for his penis?

____If you are breastfeeding, has your baby latched on and nursed well at least twice?

____Do you know how to tell if your baby is getting enough milk?

____Do you know how to get in touch with a lactation consultant (breastfeeding expert) if you run into nursing problems?

____If you are bottle-feeding, has your baby taken at least two bottles?

____Has your baby urinated and passed stool?

____If you are checking out within 48 hours of giving birth, have you arranged for a follow-up home visit (within the next couple of days)?

____Has your baby had all of his or her newborn tests, procedures, and vaccines?

____Do you know how to spot signs of common problems, such as jaundice?

Going Home (continued)

_____Do you know the warning signs that should prompt a call to your baby's doctor?

_____Have you scheduled your newborn's first visit to the pediatrician (within a few weeks of birth)?

_____Have you filled out the paperwork for your baby's birth certificate and Social Security card?

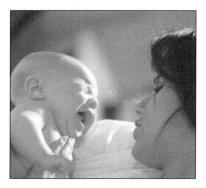

_____Do you have a rear-facing infant safety seat correctly installed in the back seat of your car?

_____Do you know how to care for yourself (such as keep stitches clean and manage pain)?

_____Is your blood pressure normal?

_____Have you urinated?

_____Can you walk without help?

_____Can you eat and drink without trouble?

_____Do you know the warning signs that should prompt a call to your doctor?

_____Have you asked your doctor when it's safe to resume sex?

_____Have you picked a birth control method (see Chapter 12 for details on postpartum birth control)?

_____Have you scheduled your postpartum visit (often 4–6 weeks after delivery)?

_____Do you have help (from your partner, family, friends, a postpartum doula, or a baby nurse) lined up for your first few days at home?

Leaving Your Baby Behind

If your baby has health problems, he or she may need to stay in the hospital after you go home. It may be hard to leave your newborn behind. Keep in mind, though, that this is the best place for your baby to be cared for until his or her health improves.

In most cases, you'll be able to spend much of each day in the hospital nursery. If you are breastfeeding, the nurses there can set you up with a breast pump and teach you how to express milk to leave for your baby when you go home.

Some hospitals may allow you to remain with your newborn around the clock after you have been discharged. If your baby needs to stay in the hospital for a while, find out what you can do to spend time with him or her.

Your New Family

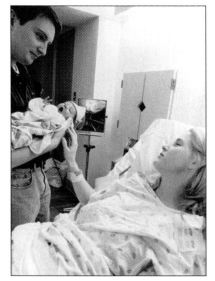

When you were pregnant, you focused on your changing body and your baby's birth. In fact, you may have been so wrapped up in pregnancy and the "big event" that you didn't have much chance to think about the biggest issue of all: what things would be like after delivery. Now that your son or daughter is here, all the new duties may be overwhelming.

Know that help is there for you—the hospital staff, your doctor, your baby's doctor, friends, family, and parents' groups—if you need it. Also, remind yourself that caring for your baby will soon become second nature.

Most of all, try to rest as much as you can during the hours and days after your little one's arrival. You worked hard to bring your baby into the world. Now relax and enjoy the fruit of your labor!

CHAPTER 10

Breastfeeding

Often, one of the most treasured experiences in a mother's life is breastfeeding her baby. How you feed your newborn is a personal choice. Bottle-fed babies can be well nourished and well loved. Still, the experts agree: breastfeeding is best.

Before you choose to breastfeed or bottle feed, talk to your doctor, your baby's doctor, your partner, family members, and friends who have breastfed their babies. You also may find it helpful to talk with a lactation specialist. They can tell you more about such things as methods of breastfeeding and pumping your breast milk. You can find one of these breastfeeding experts through your doctor or hospital. Ask any questions you have. Also, find out if your local hospital or parents' resource center offers breastfeeding classes for mothers-to-be.

Even if you are not sure breastfeeding (also called nursing) is right for you, think about giving it a try. You can always switch to formula later. You also can feed your baby with breast and bottle. Many women who aren't sure about breastfeeding find that, once the baby arrives, they love the special feeling of closeness it gives them.

The Benefits of Breastfeeding

Why should you think about nursing your baby? There are many reasons why breastfeeding is best for your baby:

215

▶ The colostrum that your breasts make for the first few days after birth helps your newborn's digestive system grow and function. Colostrum is thick and yellow. It's rich in protein and is all your baby needs for the first few days of life.

▶ Breast milk is nature's perfect baby food. Your milk has just the right nutrients, in just the right amounts, to nourish your baby completely.

▶ The protein and fat in breast milk are better used by the baby's body than the protein and fat in formula.

▶ Breast milk has growth factors, enzymes, hormones, and other things that help a baby grow and develop the way he or she should. As the baby grows and his or her needs change, breast milk changes.

▶ Breast milk has **antibodies** that help your baby's **immune system** fight off sickness, such as colds or ear infections. Breastfeeding also lowers the risk of asthma, allergies, and colic.

▶ Breastfed babies are at lower risk for sudden infant death syndrome (SIDS).

▶ Breast milk is easily digested. Infants who are breastfed have less gas, fewer feeding problems, and often less constipation than those given formula.

▶ Babies who are breastfed may be smarter. Breastfeeding helps your baby's brain develop. This may improve his or her IQ.

Breastfeeding isn't just good for babies—it's good for mothers, too.

▶ Breastfeeding releases the hormone oxytocin, which makes the uterus contract. This helps it return to its normal size more quickly and cuts down on bleeding after delivery.

▶ Nursing burns calories. It may help you lose those pregnancy pounds faster than you would if you were bottle feeding.

▶ Breastfeeding lowers your risk of osteoporosis and some forms of breast and ovarian cancer.

Dealing With a Lack of Support

What if your partner isn't so keen on the idea of you breastfeeding? That's a big stumbling block.

The support of your partner is key to your breastfeeding success. A man who envies the special bond between a nursing mother and her baby or who thinks that breastfeeding is ugly or indecent is likely to hinder a woman's attempts at nursing.

To avoid this problem, talk to your partner about why you want to breastfeed. Explain it is good for the baby's health.

Also, ask your partner to come with you to a prenatal breastfeeding class. The more he knows about the benefits (and challenges) of nursing, the more likely he is to support you in your efforts.

What if your partner's on board, but some of your friends or family members don't approve of your choice to breastfeed? Simply tell them that your doctor says it's best for the baby. After all, there's nothing like saying "doctor's orders" to quiet someone's concerns.

If you are going to succeed at breastfeeding, you need to feel that you have support. If your loved ones don't offer this support, find it elsewhere. Join a new mothers' group that has lots of nursing moms. Seek out a local La Leche League chapter or other breastfeeding support group. There's no better place to find like-minded moms (and good breastfeeding advice) than at these meetings.

▶ Breastfeeding is easier and cheaper than bottle feeding. You don't need to run out to the grocery store to pick up formula or to stock up on bottles and nipples. You also don't have to worry about heating a bottle when your baby's hungry or keeping bottles cool when you go out for the day.

▶ Nursing helps you bond with your baby. Many women find breastfeeding to be a loving and natural way to feed their babies. When you nurse, you hold your baby close to you. You also learn to pick up and respond to his or her signals. Both of these things help strengthen the bond between you.

Facts About Breastfeeding

Breasts are glands. Inside them are tiny sacs. These sacs contain cells that, given the right cues from your hormones, will start to make milk. The sacs are clustered together into lobes. Each lobe has a single milk duct that carries milk to the nipple. There are about 14–16 of these ducts.

During pregnancy, your nipples may start to drip a little colostrum. After you deliver, your body sends a signal to your breasts to start making milk. Within a few days, colostrum gives way to mature milk. It is normal for milk to take a few weeks to become mature. When your milk lets down, you may feel engorgement (see "Engorgement").

During a feeding, the first milk that flows out of your breasts is thin, watery, and sweet. This quenches the baby's thirst and provides sugar, proteins, minerals, and the fluid he or she needs. As the feeding goes on, the milk changes. It becomes thick and creamy. This milk will satisfy hunger and give your baby the nutrients he or she needs to grow.

When your baby suckles at your breasts, the nerves in your nipples send a message to your brain. In response, your brain releases hormones that tell the ducts in your breasts to "let down" their milk so that it flows through your nipples. This is called the **let-down reflex**. Some women bare-ly notice let-down. Others have a pins-and-needles feeling in their breasts 2–3 minutes after their baby starts nursing.

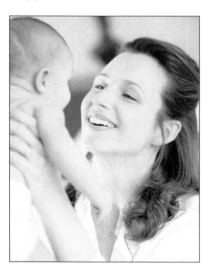

Sometimes, let-down is slowed if you are embarrassed, in pain, or feeling anxious or stressed. Other times, it's triggered simply by looking at your baby, thinking about your baby, or hearing your baby cry. For some women, hearing any baby cry will trigger the let-down reflex.

Mothers With Special Problems

Most women can breastfeed, given support and guidance. Still, some women need special advice to nurse their babies.

Women Who Can Breastfeed

In most cases, you can nurse if you have a chronic illness (for exceptions, see "Women Who Shouldn't Breastfeed"). You may need to make certain changes, though.

Sometimes it's not the illness itself that's cause for concern. Rather, it's the medications a woman takes to control a health problem. Certain prescription and over-the-counter medications can pass through breast milk and harm the baby. In such cases, a woman's doctor may advise her to switch to another medicine or lower her dosage until her baby is no longer breastfeeding (weaned). Most of the time, medications are not harmful.

If you have a chronic illness or take medication for an ongoing health condition, before your baby is born talk to your doctor about breastfeeding. Also, be sure to tell the doctor that you are breastfeeding if you need to be treated for an illness or health condition after giving birth.

Surgery to remove cysts and other benign breast lumps rarely causes problems with future breastfeeding. If you have had surgery on your breasts, talk to your ob-gyn or surgeon before your delivery date to help plan for breastfeeding.

Many women who have had their breasts enlarged or reduced are able to nurse their babies. Women with **breast implants** may have problems if the implants rupture. This may cause scarring that affects milk production and release. If you are worried about your breast implants, talk to your doctor.

Likewise, women who have had surgery to reduce the size of their breasts may have breastfeeding problems. That's because breast-reduction surgery can cut into milk ducts and prevent a nursing mother from making enough milk. If you have this surgery, talk with your doctor to be sure your nipple, areola, and ducts were left intact.

?

Common Questions About Breastfeeding

Mothers-to-be often have lots of questions about nursing. Here are answers to a few of the questions asked most often. If you have a question that isn't addressed here, be sure to ask your doctor or a lactation specialist.

Are my breasts too small for breastfeeding?

It might seem logical that well-endowed women would make more milk than their flat-chested peers. But breast size doesn't matter. The amount of milk your breasts make has to do with your health and how well your breasts are stimulated. It has nothing to do with their size or shape.

Will nursing make my breasts sag?

Breastfeeding alone won't cause your breasts to sag. Aging is mostly to blame for that. Your breasts will get heavier during pregnancy and nursing as they enlarge and make milk. This extra weight can stretch the ligaments that support them. Wearing a good support bra will help.

How do I get ready to nurse my baby?

You don't need to do anything to prepare. If you are concerned about your nipples or breasts, discuss it with your doctor. You may be referred to a lactation consultant.

Women Who Shouldn't Breastfeed

As good as breastfeeding is, it's not for every woman. Women should not nurse if they:

- Have infections that could be passed to the baby through breast milk. These include human immunodeficiency virus (HIV) and active tuberculosis (TB) that is not treated. If TB is treated, the baby can be breastfed. (Chapter 16 has details on the infections that can be passed to your baby.)

- Take certain medications. In rare cases, women who must take medications to treat a health problem (and who can't

Common Questions About Breastfeeding
(continued)

Will I be able to make enough milk?

In most cases, making enough milk to nourish your baby is a simple matter of supply and demand. In other words, your body supplies as much as your baby demands. Nurse as often as your baby needs to and for as long as he or she wants. That way, your body will respond by making just the right amount of milk. Supplementing with formula to make up for a shortfall may cause you not to make as much milk. That's because skipping feedings tells your body to cut down on milk production. You also can prevent a milk shortage by getting enough to drink each day, eating well, and getting plenty of rest.

What if I couldn't breastfeed last time?

If you have given birth before and had trouble breastfeeding, that doesn't mean you can't nurse now. Whatever caused the problem last time most likely won't happen again. Even if it does, getting expert help early on will boost your chance of nursing success. To help prevent problems, talk about your prior breastfeeding experience with your doctor, childbirth educator, a lactation specialist, and other nursing mothers. Sometimes a change in technique is all it takes to solve the problem.

switch to a safer drug) may need to bottle feed. Many medications are safe for the baby. In other cases, so little medication gets into a woman's breast milk that her baby does not receive it. Still, some prescription drugs can pass into breast milk and harm a baby (see box). These include ergotamine (used to treat migraine headaches), lithium (used to treat mental illness), some drugs used to treat high blood pressure, and chemotherapy drugs (used to treat cancer). If you are taking any medication, check with your doctor to find out if breastfeeding is safe or how the dosage can be altered to make breastfeeding possible.

Harmful Medications

Women who are taking these drugs or medications should not breastfeed:

- Bromocriptine
- Cocaine
- Cyclophosphamide
- Cyclosporine
- Doxorubicin
- Ergotamine
- Lithium
- Methotrexate
- Phencyclidine (PCP)
- Phenindione

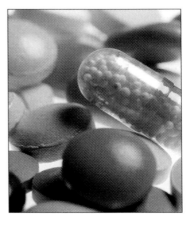

▶ Use illegal drugs, abuse alcohol, or smoke. Drug use and heavy drinking (more than two drinks a day on a regular basis) may be harmful to the mother and baby. These substances can be passed to the baby through breast milk. If you smoke one or two cigarettes every now and then, it's most likely safe to breastfeed. In this case, the benefits of breastfeeding may outweigh the dangers of a cigarette or two. However, if you chain smoke or smoke regularly, breastfeeding may harm your baby. Never smoke around your baby or other children.

Breastfeeding Know-How

Breastfeeding is the natural way to nourish your newborn. Not all mothers and babies get the hang of it right away. It takes learning, practice, and plenty of patience for both of you to master this skill. Some pointers will give you a good start.

Be prepared. Take a breastfeeding class before your baby is born. These classes are offered at many hospitals and parents' cen-

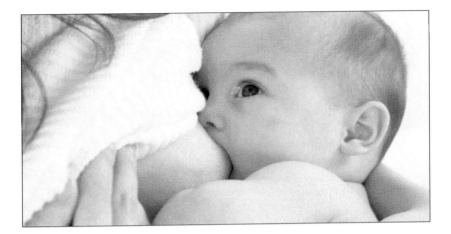

ters. A breastfeeding class will teach you what you need to know to get started. It'll also help you avoid some common problems.

Share the news. During your pregnancy, tell your doctor that you plan to breastfeed your baby. He or she can give you advice and answer any questions you may have. When you get to the hospital, remind the doctor and nurses that you want to nurse. That way, they can help you get started right after delivery.

Nurse soon after your baby is born. If you are up to it, put your baby to your breast shortly after he or she is delivered. This is a great way to greet your new baby. This is also the time that your newborn is most alert and ready to suck. Later, your baby may be too sleepy to nurse well.

Find a good position. If you are positioned right, you'll be able to hold the baby for some time without feeling cramped or stiff (see box). Also, the baby will be able to get a good grasp on your breast. No matter which position you use, make sure the baby's whole body (not just his or her face) is turned toward you. To avoid back and neck strain, use pillows or folded blankets to place the baby at the level of your breast. Tuck pillows behind your back, under your arms, and on your lap for extra support. You may want to prop your feet on a stool to raise your knees and help bring your baby closer to your breast if you are sitting.

Get the baby latched on. A baby is born with the instincts he or she needs to nurse. Take the rooting reflex, for instance. This

Good Breastfeeding Positions

When you are just getting the hang of breastfeeding, finding a good position is key.

Cradle hold. Sit up as straight as you can and cradle your baby in the crook of your arm. The baby's body should be turned toward you and his or her belly should be against yours. Support the baby's head in the bend of your elbow so that he or she is facing your breast.

Cross-cradle hold. As in the cradle hold, nuzzle your baby's belly against yours. Hold him or her with the other arm. This way, the baby's bottom rests in the crook of your arm and your hand supports the baby's head and neck. This position gives you more control of the baby's head. You may need to support the baby's head with pillows. It's a good position for a newborn who is having trouble getting the hang of nursing.

Football hold. Tuck your baby under your arm like a football. Sit the baby up at your side, level with your waist, so he or she is facing you. Support the baby's back with your upper arm and hold his or her head level with your breast. The football hold is good for nursing twins. It's also good for women who had cesarean births because the baby doesn't lie across your abdomen.

Side-lying position. Lie on your side and nestle your baby next to you. Place your fingers beneath your breast and lift it up to help your baby reach your nipple. This position is good for night feedings. It's also good for women who had a cesarean birth because it keeps the baby's weight off the incision. Put your lower arm forward to hold your head and place a pillow between your knees to keep you from rolling over.

is a baby's natural instinct to turn toward the nipple, open his or her mouth, and suck. When you and your baby are ready to begin nursing, cup your breast in your hand and stroke your baby's lower lip with your nipple. The baby will open his or her mouth wide (like a yawn). Quickly center your nipple in the baby's mouth, making sure the tongue is down, and pull him or her close to you. Keep in mind: you need to bring your baby to your breast—not your breast to your baby.

Check the baby's technique. If the baby is latched on right, he or she will have all of your nipple and a good deal of the areola— the dark area around it—in his or her mouth. The baby's nose will be touching your breast. The baby's lips also will be curled out around your breast. The baby's sucking should be smooth and even. You should hear him or her swallow. You might feel a slight tugging. You may feel a little discomfort for the first few days. You shouldn't feel any severe pain, though.

Keep trying. If the baby grasps only your nipple in his or her mouth, the baby's lips are curled under, you hear clicking sounds as he or she sucks, or nursing hurts, start over. A newborn who doesn't latch on well won't get a good meal. To break the suction, gently insert one of your fingers (make sure they are clean) between your breast and your baby's gums. When you hear a soft

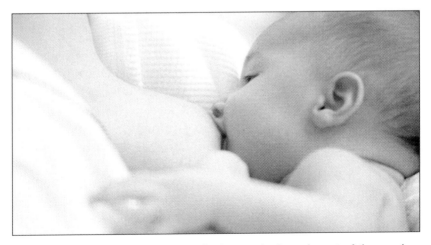

When your baby is breastfeeding, all of your nipple and most of the areola should be in his or her mouth.

pop, carefully pull your nipple out of his or her mouth. Keep trying until your baby is latched on well. Getting your baby onto
your breast may take some practice, but it's worth the effort.

Don't watch the clock. Experts used to think that newborns
should nurse for just a few minutes at each breast. They now
know that this may cut babies off before they get their fill.
Cutting back on nursing time also keeps your breasts from making enough milk. Let your baby set his or her own nursing pattern. Many newborns nurse for 10–20 minutes on each breast. (A
baby who wants to nurse for a very long time—say, 30 minutes
on each side—may be having trouble getting enough milk. If this
happens each time you breastfeed, tell your doctor.) When your
baby's full, he or she will let go of your breast. If not, gently break
the suction.

Switch sides. When your baby empties one breast, offer the
other. Don't worry if he or she doesn't latch on, though. You
don't have to nurse at both breasts in one feeding. You may want
to put a safety pin on your bra strap to mark the side your baby
nursed from last. At the next feeding, offer the other breast first.

Nurse on demand. When your baby's hungry, he or she will
nuzzle against your breast, make sucking motions, or put hands
to mouth. Crying is a late sign of hunger. (Rooming in with your
baby at the hospital will help you pick up on these cues.) Follow
your baby's signals—not the clock. You may eat your meals at
set times, but don't expect your baby to do the same. Putting a
newborn on a feeding schedule will deprive him or her of nourishment and tell your body to make less milk. During the first
few weeks, your baby should be fed at least 8–12 times in 24
hours (every 1–2 hours). Some newborns are happy to go 3
hours between feedings. Others need to nurse once an hour for
the first few weeks. Over time, you and your baby will set your
own schedule.

Don't supplement. The colostrum your breasts make for the
first few days after birth is all your baby needs. Your newborn has
extra stores of fat and body fluids to draw on until your milk
comes in. Even if you plan to combine breast and bottle when your
baby is older, breastfeed alone for at least the first 6 months of

How Can I Get Help?

If you and your baby are having trouble nursing, don't give up—get some help. Ask your postpartum nurses to assist you with nursing positions or getting the baby latched onto your breast. Let your doctor know if you are worried the baby isn't getting enough to eat. Also seek help if nursing hurts. Breastfeeding may be a little uncomfortable at first, but it should never hurt.

Find out if the hospital or your pediatrician's office employs a licensed, certified lactation specialist. These breastfeeding experts offer telephone advice or hands-on help for a small fee (some health insurance companies will cover this cost).

Even if nursing seems to be going fine, don't leave the hospital without getting a phone number to call for breastfeeding help. If you forget, call:

▶ The International Lactation Consultant Association at 919-787-5181 or www.ilca.org. This group can direct you to certified lactation specialists in your area.

▶ La Leche League International at 1-800-525-3243 or www.lalecheleague.org. This support network for breastfeeding mothers can help with questions and concerns. Local chapter leaders offer free phone advice and run support groups for nursing moms.

▶ Women, Infants, and Children (WIC) federal program at 703-305-2746 or www.fns.usda.gov/wic. WIC helps low-income, nutritionally at-risk pregnant and breastfeeding women (through pregnancy and up to 6 weeks after birth or after pregnancy ends). One in four new mothers participate in WIC.

your baby's life if you can. This will help you make enough milk. It also won't confuse your baby about which nipple is being used. (Sucking from a bottle isn't the same as sucking from a breast. If a baby gets used to bottle nipples, he or she may forget how to draw milk out of your nipples.) For the same reason, it's best not to give your baby a pacifier until he or she is used to nursing.

Is Your Baby Getting Enough Milk?

When an infant is fed formula, it's simple to figure out how much he or she is drinking. All you have to do is add up those empty bottles. Not so with breastfeeding. There are other ways to tell if your baby is well-nourished:

▸ Your baby nurses often. A newborn should nurse at least 8–12 times in 24 hours. The bigger your baby is, the more his or her stomach will hold and the less often he or she will need to eat. Even so, a newborn shouldn't go more than 3 hours without nursing (even at night). Each nursing session should last 20–45 minutes.

▸ Your baby is full after nursing. A baby who's just had a good meal will be drowsy and content.

▸ Your breasts fill and empty. Your breasts should feel full and firm before feedings. After, they should be less full and feel softer.

Warning Signs

Call the doctor right away if your baby:

▸ Has trouble latching onto your breast or staying latched on

▸ Cries when you offer your breast or cries after 1–2 minutes of nursing

▸ Often falls asleep after only a few minutes of nursing or is often too sleepy to nurse

▸ Has fewer than 6 wet and 3 soiled diapers a day

▸ Has dark green stools or stools with mucus in them

▸ Has a sunken soft spot on the top of his or her head (this can be a sign of dehydration)

▸ Feeds less than 6 times in 24 hours in the first month of life

▸ Looks yellow (jaundice) below the navel and is groggy

▸ The baby goes through lots of diapers. After your milk comes in, your baby should soak at least six diapers a day. His or her urine should be nearly clear. During the first month, your baby should have at least three bowel movements a day. (In fact, most breastfed newborns pass a stool after each feeding.) The stool should be soft and yellow.

▸ Your baby is gaining weight. Most newborns lose a little weight at first. After 2 weeks, your baby should be back up to his or her weight at birth. The doctor will weigh your baby at each visit and let you know if he or she isn't gaining enough weight. If you are worried that your baby isn't getting enough milk, tell the doctor.

Clothes for Women Who Are Breastfeeding

Unlike bottle feeding, breastfeeding requires little in the way of supplies. Still, buying a few good nursing bras and a couple of nursing shirts or dresses is well worth it. You can find nursing bras, pads, and clothes in maternity shops, baby supply stores, and mail-order catalogs. You can save money by asking friends or relatives to lend you their nursing clothes or by shopping for used clothing at exchange or consignment shops.

Nursing bras have cups that open (with snaps, hook-and-eye closures, or peel-away elastic bands) for easy access at feeding time. Some cups open from the top. Others open from the side.

No matter which style you choose, you should be able to open the cups quickly and with one hand (the other hand will be holding your baby). Be sure to test this feature before you buy the bra.

Some nursing bras also have cups that can be made bigger or

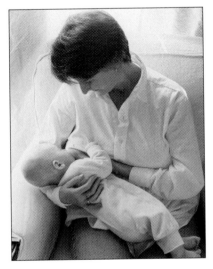

smaller. These bras allow you to adjust the size by hooking the cup closed at a higher or lower point. Why? Your cup size will grow and shrink as your breasts fill with milk and your baby empties them. Your breasts also will be larger in the early weeks of nursing, and smaller once the breasts adjust to nursing. By 3 months of nursing, there may seem to be little change between feedings, but you still will have plenty of milk.

It's a good idea to pick up a nighttime nursing bra as well. These bras give breasts a little support while you sleep. The cups can be opened for feedings.

When you are choosing nursing bras, stock up on plenty of nursing pads, too. Many women find that their breasts leak between feedings. One nipple also may dribble a little milk while your baby nurses on the other side. Wearing pads inside your bra will soak up the excess.

You can wear just about anything to breastfeed—as long as you can lift it up or unbutton it. Clothes that are designed for nursing mothers will help you feed your baby quickly. They also cover you when you are nursing in public. These clothes have hidden openings that you can spread apart to get your baby latched on, then arrange to cover your breast once your baby's nursing. Nursing clothes make many breastfeeding mothers feel comfortable feeding their babies in restaurants, at the mall, or even during religious services.

Nutrition for Moms Who Breastfeed

When you are pregnant, your body stores extra nutrients and fat to prepare you for breastfeeding. Even so, once your baby is born you need more food and nutrients than normal to fuel milk production. Don't panic if your diet isn't always perfect. Your baby still can get the nutrients he or she needs. When you are nursing:

▸ Eat more. During breastfeeding you need about 200 calories a day more than you did during pregnancy. That's 500 more calories than you needed before you got pregnant. (A government program called the Special Supplemental Food Program for Women, Infants, and Children—WIC for short—provides vouchers so that low-income nursing mothers can get the extra food they need).

▸ Eat a well-balanced diet. Eat a variety of healthy foods, as outlined in the Food Guide Pyramid (see Chapter 6). That means daily servings of fruits and vegetables, whole-grain breads and cereals, milk and milk products, and high-protein foods such as fish, beans, meat, and poultry.

▸ Get the right nutrients. Nursing moms need 1,000 mg of calcium a day, for instance. You can get that by eating plenty of dairy products like milk, yogurt, and cheese. If you can't digest milk products, ask your doctor about taking a calcium supplement. When you are nursing, you also need an extra serving of protein each day—four servings instead of the three you needed during pregnancy. Be sure to get folic acid each day, too. This will help you maintain good health and ensure that you have plenty of folic acid stores. Your doctor may suggest that you keep taking a daily prenatal vitamin until your baby is weaned. (The "Recommended Dietary Allowances for Nonpregnant, Pregnant, and Breastfeeding Women" table in Chapter 6 has detailed guidelines on your nutrition needs during breastfeeding.)

▸ Skip foods that bother the baby. Some nursing infants are sensitive to certain foods in their mothers' diet. If your baby acts fussy or gets a rash, diarrhea, or congestion within a couple hours of nursing, let his or her doctor know. This can signal a food allergy. Cut out that food for a few days and see if your baby seems better. You also might want to keep a food diary. This will help you spot links between what you eat and how your baby reacts.

▸ Drink up. You need at least eight glasses of liquid a day. Breastfeeding uses up lots of fluid. That's why nursing mothers often are thirsty. If you get dehydrated, it can affect your milk supply. To prevent this, make sure you have a drink within easy reach each time you sit down to nurse. Do not force fluids, though.

▶ Don't diet. Be patient about losing the weight you may have gained during pregnancy. If you eat a well-balanced diet, you'll be close to your normal weight within a few months. Start an exercise routine once your doctor gives you the go-ahead. This will keep your muscles toned.

Breastfeeding and Birth Control

Breastfeeding has pros and cons when it comes to your sex life. On the downside, round-the-clock nursing may reduce your desire for sex. Other breastfeeding women notice an increase in desire. In some cases, you may have the desire, but prefer a hands-off policy during lovemaking to protect sore or leaking breasts.

Breastfeeding causes a drop in estrogen levels, too. The vaginal dryness that results can make sex less than fun. An over-the-counter lubricant, as well as plenty of time and tenderness, will help with these problems. (See Chapter 12 for more tips on post-baby lovemaking.)

When you are breastfeeding, you are less likely to get pregnant. You may not ovulate or have your period for as long as you breastfeed. To become pregnant, ovulation (the release of an egg to be fertilized) must occur.

It's best not to rely on breastfeeding as birth control, though. Because women's periods return at different times after delivery, it is hard to predict when you will begin to ovulate again. You could get pregnant before you even know you are fertile. If you are not ready for another baby right away, talk to your doctor about which method of birth control is good for you. What you were using before pregnancy might not be a good choice now.

Good choices for hormonal birth control are the minipill, implants, or injections. These are progestin-only, so they won't affect your milk supply. (See Chapter 12 for more details on post-baby birth control.)

Combination birth control pills contain the hormone estrogen and **_progestin_**, a synthetic version of the hormone progesterone. Estrogen can cut down on your milk supply. As a result, combination pills should not be used until milk flow is steady. This occurs about 3 months after delivery. Until then, use progestin-only birth control pills or barrier methods such as condoms or a diaphragm with spermicide.

Breastfeeding and Work

Going back to work—whether it's a few weeks or many months after your baby is born—doesn't have to mean the end of breast-feeding. Many mothers keep nursing their babies after their maternity leave ends.

If you want to breastfeed when you go back to work, have a plan. Practice with the pump a few weeks before your first day back on the job. Pump any milk that's left in your breasts after a feeding. Give some of this milk to your baby in a bottle. (You may want to have someone else do it. Breastfed babies often do not want to take a bottle from their mothers.) This will help your baby get used to drinking your milk from something other than your breasts. Also, store a few bottles of milk in the freezer for later use. Talk to your doctor about when to start trying the bottle.

Storing Breast Milk

You can keep pumped milk in the refrigerator—in clean glass or plastic bottles or special milk collection bags—for up to 2 days. Be sure to mark the bottles or bags with your baby's name and the date the milk was pumped.

If you don't have a refrigerator at work, keep the milk you have just pumped in a small cooler with a few ice packs. Don't leave breast milk at room temperature for more than 8 hours—the enzymes will begin to digest the fat.

If you need to store milk longer than a week, keep it in the freezer for up to 3 months. If you store it in a deep freezer, you can keep it there up to 6 months. To thaw frozen milk, put the bottle in a bowl of warm water. Don't heat bottles in boiling water or in the microwave. This destroys breast milk's disease-fighting qualities. What's more, it can make the milk hot enough to scald your baby. You also can let frozen milk slowly thaw in the fridge. Once milk is thawed, use it within 24 hours.

Choosing a Breast Pump

Not every woman who breastfeeds will need a pump. Many nursing mothers learn how to express breast milk by hand. This is a good skill for any breastfeeding mom to have. Still, most women find it easier to use a breast pump to empty their breasts for storing milk. This is even more true for working mothers who need to express milk several times a day.

There are dozens of breast pumps on the market, with many features to choose from. How do you know which one to pick? That depends on your needs. If you plan to stay home with your baby until he or she is weaned, a simple manual pump may be fine. If you are going back to work full-time soon after your baby is born, an electric pump likely is the best choice.

Talk to your doctor or a lactation specialist before you rent or buy a pump. Some pointers:

▸ If you plan to pump only for a short time, you may want to rent. You can rent a high-quality breast pump from a medical supply store or hospital for as little as $1 a day. Some WIC programs also loan out breast pumps. If you rent, you'll need to buy a kit with tubing for the pump, cups that fit over your breasts, and collection bottles.

▸ If you think you'll pump for more than a few months, buying a breast pump is a good idea. Compare rental costs to purchase price before you decide.

▸ If the cost of renting or buying a pump seems high, just think about all the money you'll save by not having to buy formula or not having to buy as much. You'll also help maintain your baby's health.

▸ Pick a pump that has two tubes and kits. This cuts your pumping time in half by letting you empty both breasts at once.

▸ You may want to choose a pump with automatic cycling. This closely mimics a baby's natural sucking rhythm as it draws milk out of your breasts. It also means you don't have to keep pushing a button or lift or roll your finger over a hole, as semi-automatic pumps require you to do.

Choosing a Breast Pump (continued)

▸ Look for quick cycling times. The more often a pump cycles (or sucks), the less time it takes to empty your breasts and the more milk you'll get. Cycling times range from about 12 to 60 cycles per minute.

▸ Choose a pump that lets you adjust the suction level. Otherwise, you may find the suction so strong that it hurts your breasts or so weak that you can't get much milk out.

▸ Look for a lightweight, portable model if you are going to be on the road for work or if you need to bring your pump home with you each night.

▸ If you want a manual pump to use at home, avoid the kind with a rubber bulb at one end. Why? Your milk can flow back into the bulb. This type of pump is hard to clean and can harbor bacteria.

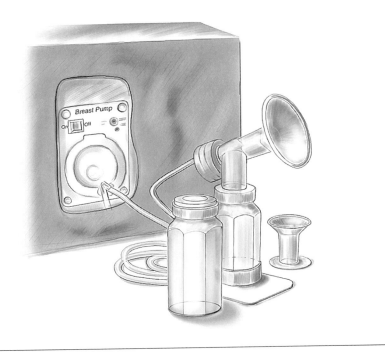

Some women breastfeed when they are home and have their baby's caregiver use formula for other feedings. Women who work close to home or childcare can try to arrange breaks and lunch hours around their baby's feeding times. Other women pump their breast milk before they leave for work or during the work day. This allows them to leave milk with the baby's caregiver while they are away.

If you want to keep nursing after you go back to work, ask your doctor, your lactation consultant, and other working women who have breastfed for tips and advice. Look into buying or renting a breast pump.

Before you go back to work, talk to your boss about your plans to pump milk on the job. Ask if there's a clean, private place for you to pump—such as a pumping room, an empty office, or a meeting room that's rarely used.

Be sure to let your boss know that pumping takes just a few minutes a day. It may even cut down on the amount of work you'll miss. Breastfed babies have fewer illnesses than infants who are given formula. That means you'll need less time off to care for a sick baby or to take him or her to the doctor.

It helps to wear two-piece outfits or clothes that button in the front to work. Express your milk at least twice a day.

It takes a while to get used to your new routine. Give yourself time. Once you get it down and fit pumping into your workday, it doesn't take much time or effort.

Breastfeeding Problems

For some women, nursing comes off without a hitch. Others may have to deal with a few minor problems. Most often, though, they are easy to treat.

Engorgement

Engorgement may occur when your milk comes in a few days after delivery. Engorged breasts feel full and tender. You may even run a low fever. If the fever exceeds 101°F or if you are in severe pain, call your doctor. If you are very engorged, it can be hard for your baby to latch on.

Once your body figures out just how much milk your baby needs, the problem should go away. This often takes a week or so. In the meantime:

▶ Increase feedings. This will help drain your breasts.

▶ Express a little milk with a pump or by hand to soften your breasts before nursing.

▶ Before feedings, massage your breasts, take hot showers, or apply hot packs to your breasts. This will help your milk flow.

▶ After feedings, apply cold packs to your breasts to relieve discomfort and reduce swelling.

▶ Between feedings, place chilled cabbage leaves around your breast. The leaves of the cabbage are soothing and fit nicely around your breast.

Sore Nipples

It's normal for your nipples to feel a little tender during the first few days of nursing. If breastfeeding is painful or your nipples are cracked or bleeding, though, get expert help. To relieve soreness and prevent it from getting worse:

▶ Learn proper nursing technique.

▶ Make sure your baby has your entire nipple and a good portion of your areola in his or her mouth.

▶ Check that the baby's lips are curled out around your breast and that his or her tongue is beneath your nipple.

▶ Before you remove your breast from your baby's mouth, use your finger to break the suction.

▶ Change positions at each feeding so the baby's mouth doesn't always put pressure on the same part of your nipple.

▶ Gently pat your nipples dry with a clean cloth after feedings. You might also want to expose them to air and dry heat (such as a hairdryer on low or sunlight streaming through a window).

▸ Use only cotton bra pads, and change them as soon as they get wet.

▸ Apply a few drops of breast milk to your nipples after feeding.

▸ Don't wash your nipples with harsh soaps or use perfumed creams.

▸ Check for thrush. This is a yeast infection in your baby's mouth that can spread to your breasts. Suspect thrush if your baby has diaper rash and white patches in his or her mouth. Other signs of thrush include a cracked, itchy, red, and burning nipple or shooting pains in your breasts during or after nursing. In this case, call your doctor.

▸ Nurse often. If your baby's really hungry, he or she will suck harder. This can make sore nipples hurt even more.

▸ If one nipple is tender, offer the other breast first. Save your sore side for when your baby is less hungry.

Blocked Ducts

If a duct gets clogged with unused milk, a hard, tender knot will form in your breast. Call your doctor if the knot doesn't go away within a few days or if you run a fever. In the meantime, try these methods to drain the duct:

▸ Let your baby nurse long and often on the plugged side.

▸ Offer the breast with the blocked duct first.

▸ If there's any milk left in your breast after a feeding, pump it out or hand express it.

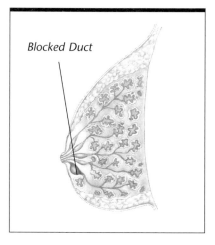

Blocked Duct

▶ Take a hot shower or apply a hot pack to the lump before nursing.

▶ Massage the lump while your baby nurses to help the milk drain.

Mastitis

If a blocked duct doesn't drain, it may become inflamed. A breast infection, called *mastitis*, can result.

If your breast is swollen, painful, streaked with red, and feels hot to the touch, you may have mastitis. Women with mastitis often feel like they are coming down with the flu. They run a fever and feel achy and tired.

If you think you have mastitis, call your doctor right away. He or she will take steps to treat the infection. You should feel better within a day or two of starting treatment, but keep taking the treatment for the full prescription.

Until then, do the same things you'd do to treat a plugged duct. Get plenty of rest and drink lots of fluids. Your doctor may suggest you take ibuprofen to ease your discomfort, too.

Don't stop nursing. Breastfeed your baby often to help drain your breast. (The baby cannot catch the infection.) If you stop nursing, the plugged duct will get more inflamed, your milk supply will go down, and recovery will take longer.

When to Wean?

You can breastfeed for as long as you and your child want. Any amount of breastfeeding is good for the baby. Still, the longer you stick with it, the better off your baby will be. Mothers should try to nurse their babies for at least 6 months. Although not every woman can do that, it's a good goal.

Breastfeeding doesn't have to be an all-or-nothing thing. Some women give their baby only breast milk for the first few weeks or months and then combine breastfeeding and bottle feeding.

Whatever you choose, make sure it's a choice that feels right to you. Only you and your baby know when the time is right.

As for how to go about weaning, there are a few ways to do it. Some women let their baby take the lead. They slowly drop feedings as their baby eats more food and starts drinking from a cup. This can be a long process. It's a gentle change for both of you, though.

Other women decide to wean their baby when he or she reaches a certain age. In this case, it's still best to take it slow. An abrupt stop in breastfeeding can cause you physical pain as your breasts fill with unused milk. It also can be hard for your baby.

Instead, replace one nursing session with a bottle or cup feeding every few days. Start by cutting out the feedings your baby seems to enjoy the least. Slowly work your way up to the more important ones. Most often, the feeding before bedtime is the last to go—and the hardest to give up. As you reduce the amount you nurse, your milk supply will decrease slowly.

A Unique Bond

No matter how long you nurse, you'll look back on this time in your child's life with fondness and pride. Even if you nurse for only a short while, you'll know that you gave your baby a healthy start in life. You'll also know that your baby got something very special—something only you can give.

CHAPTER 11

The Newborn Baby

You'll never forget the first time you lay eyes on your new baby. This moment is the start of a new life—for you and your baby.

For 40 weeks, you sheltered and nurtured the fetus growing inside you. Now, you must learn to care for this life in a new way. Your baby, nestled safely in your uterus for so long, also must learn to adapt.

Your baby's body goes through big changes in the minutes, hours, and days after birth. Some risk goes along with these changes. Most of the time, though, babies do just fine as they become used to the outside world. Your doctor and nurses will keep a close eye on your newborn to make sure all is going well.

As a new mother, you may have lots of questions about the way your newborn looks and acts. Chances are, you'll also wonder how to best care for him or her.

Knowing what's normal and what to expect from this time in your baby's life will help you relax and enjoy watching your baby grow. Relish this special time in your baby's life—it will be over before you know it.

At Birth

How well did your baby fare during labor and delivery? To find out, your doctor will look over your newborn at 1 minute and 5 minutes after birth. Then the nurse will assign the baby a score to measure his or her well-being. The score—called the Apgar score—is named after Dr. Virginia Apgar. She had a strong interest in babies' responses to birth and life outside the uterus.

The Apgar score rates five things:

1. Heart rate

2. Breathing

3. Muscle tone

4. Reflexes

5. Skin color

Each is given a score of 0, 1, or 2. The total of all scores is the Apgar score. Most babies have an Apgar score of 7 or more at 5 minutes. Few babies score a perfect 10.

The Apgar score is a good measure to check the baby's condition right after delivery. It's also a good way to see how the baby adjusts to the outside world in the minutes after birth. On its own, though, the Apgar score doesn't show how healthy your baby was before birth or what the future will hold.

Your doctor also may check your baby's health at delivery by testing the umbilical cord blood. In this test, a sample of blood is

TABLE 1. The Apgar Score

Component	Score		
	0	1	2
Heart rate	Absent	Fewer than 100 beats per minute	More than 100 beats per minute
Respiration	Absent	Weak cry or hyperventilation	Good, strong cry
Muscle tone	Limp	Some flexing of arms and legs	Active motion
Reflexes	No response	Grimace	Cries or withdraws feet
Color*	Blue or pale	Body pink; hands and feet blue	Pink all over

*In babies with dark skin, the mouth, lips, palms, and soles are examined.

Newborn Tests and Procedures

Before your baby leaves the hospital, a doctor or nurse will:

▸ Take a blood sample from his or her heel to check for certain diseases. One of these is phenylketonuria (PKU). A baby with this defect can't break down a substance in food called phenyl-alanine. Another disease the heel-stick will check for is hypothyroidism (low thyroid hormone). Both conditions can cause mental retardation. They can be avoided if they are found and treated early. Yet another condition your baby will be tested for is *hypoglycemia* (low blood sugar). Your baby also may be tested for sickle cell anemia and rare metabolic conditions (it depends on which state you live in).

▸ Give him or her a shot of vitamin K. A newborn's body can't make vitamin K on its own for a few days. Without it, blood won't clot. A vitamin K shot helps protect against a rare but severe bleeding disorder.

▸ Put a medicated ointment or liquid in your newborn's eyes. This guards against infection from germs that can get into the eyes during birth.

▸ Give your baby a complete physical exam. A doctor or nurse will look your baby over from head to toe, listen to his or her breathing and heartbeat, check the pulse, feel his or her belly, and look for normal newborn reflexes.

▸ Perhaps test your baby's hearing. Many hospitals do routine hearing tests on newborns. First, tiny earphones are placed over your baby's ears. Then special sensors attached to his or her head measure brain-wave responses to soft sounds.

▸ Possibly give your baby the first of three immunizations against hepatitis B. This virus can lead to severe illness and liver damage. Ask your baby's doctor about the pros and cons of giving the vaccine to your newborn.

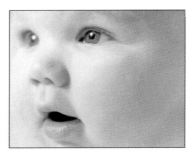

taken from the umbilical cord. The balance of chemicals in the blood (pH level) is checked. This test can show whether a baby needs special care right after birth.

Your Baby's First Breath

During pregnancy, your baby got oxygen through the placenta and umbilical cord. In the moments after birth, your newborn takes his or her first breath of air.

This is a huge step. It's not just the lungs that must be able to fill with air seconds after delivery. All the related structures—such as muscles around the lungs and airways leading from the mouth and nose—also must be ready to start working.

What triggers this first breath? Instinct plays a role. Breathing is a vital step in the move from the uterus to the outside world.

Newborns are meant to gasp for air after delivery. After birth, there's more pressure outside the lungs than there is inside them. This pressure causes the lungs to expand and fill with air. As a result, the baby draws breath and may start crying.

Movies and TV programs often show the doctor slapping a newborn's bottom to cause that first wail. Don't expect to see this in the delivery room, though. Many babies cry on their own at birth. Others don't cry right away. Instead, they simply start breathing. (That doesn't mean these babies won't cry later.)

After birth, your doctor and nurses watch your baby's breathing closely. If the baby isn't breathing well, they take steps to help. Often, this simply means rubbing the baby's body to wake him or her up a bit.

Your Baby's Blood System

While your baby was in your uterus, his or her blood moved to and from the placenta through blood vessels in the umbilical cord. At birth, the placenta peels away from the inside of the uterus and is expelled.

When your baby's lungs are filling with air right after birth, the doctor or nurse may listen to your newborn's chest with a stethoscope. This device detects sounds linked with normal changes in blood flow after delivery.

The doctor or nurse also may feel your baby's pulse in the arm or groin. These exams are part of the normal routine to check your baby's well-being.

Your Baby's Temperature

The temperature inside your uterus is fairly stable. There, your baby was kept warm by your body. At birth, your baby enters a place that's much cooler. Your newborn also is wet with amniotic fluid. As a result, the baby can lose a lot of heat as the moisture on his or her skin evaporates. To prevent this, your nurse will dry off your baby and snugly wrap him or her in a blanket just after birth.

Just like you, your newborn has controls to keep body temperature even. These controls don't work as well as yours do, though. A newborn can easily get too hot or too cold.

To keep your newborn warm, dress him or her in a cotton shirt or gown and wrap a light blanket around his or her body. Make sure the room is free from drafts and the temperature stays around 70–75 degrees.

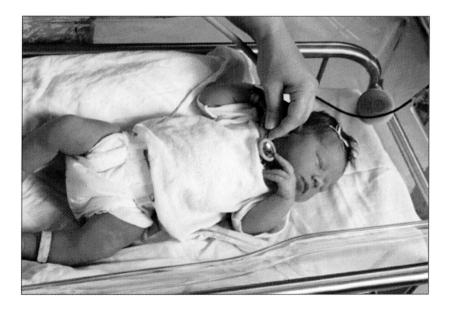

Your Baby's Nervous System

Right from birth, your newborn responds to people, sound, light, and touch. You may not pick up on all of these responses right away. As your baby matures, they'll become easier to notice.

Your baby also is born with certain reflexes, or automatic responses. These include:

▶ *The Moro (startle) reflex.* This happens when your baby's head falls backward, there's a loud noise, or someone nearby makes a sudden movement. In response, your baby will throw out his or her arms, extend his or her neck, and then draw his or her arms back to the chest.

▶ *The rooting (sucking) reflex.* This is an instinct to search for the breast. If you stroke your baby's cheek or lip, he or she will turn toward you with pursed lips, ready to suck. This helps the baby find your nipple at feeding time. A newborn also will suck when he or she feels pressure on the roof of the mouth, behind the upper gums.

▶ *The grasp reflex.* If you stroke your baby's palm, his or her fingers will close tightly around yours.

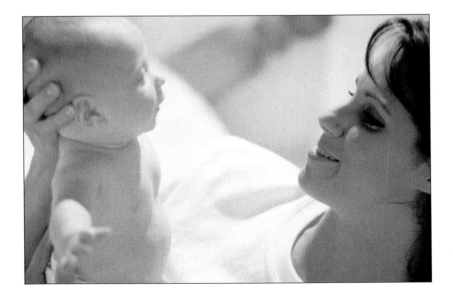

Your Baby's Digestive System

For 40 weeks, the placenta was your baby's main food source. Nutrients from your blood crossed the placenta and entered your baby's bloodstream through the umbilical cord.

After birth, your baby eats his or her meals the way the rest of us do—by mouth. Shortly after delivery, your baby can suck and swallow milk. This milk moves through the digestive tract, where carbohydrates, proteins, and fats are broken down and absorbed into your baby's blood.

Once the milk gets to your baby's intestines, it mixes with *meconium*. This is the greenish-black, sticky substance that formed in the baby's bowels during pregnancy. In most cases, you see meconium in the baby's first bowel movement. This often occurs within 24 hours of birth. During the first few days of your baby's life, the color of his or her stools will slowly change as the gooey green meconium is replaced by yellowish digested milk.

How Your Newborn Looks

At birth, babies often look different than they will a few weeks or months later. Magazines and TV shows often use babies who are a few months old to depict newborns. Unless you have seen a real newborn, you may be surprised by the way your baby really looks:

▸ Your newborn's body may seem scrunched up. That's because a new baby draws his or her arms and legs up close, into the so-called "fetal position." This is the way he or she fit into the close confines of your uterus. Even though the baby has more room now, it'll take a few weeks for him or her to stretch out a bit.

▸ Your baby's face may be slightly swollen, and his or her eyes may be a little puffy for a few days. The baby's head also may look long and pointy at first. Why? Babies have two soft spots on the top of their head. This is where the skull bones haven't yet joined. These soft spots make the head flexible enough to fit through the birth canal. Your baby's head will round out in

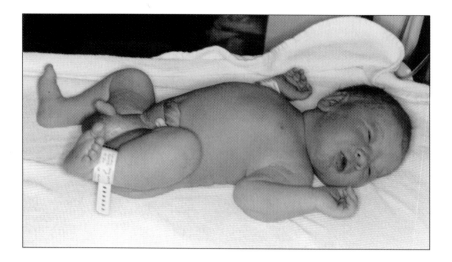

a few days or weeks. (A baby born by cesarean birth can look the same way if you went through labor before delivery. If you went straight to the operating room, though, your baby's head and face will look like those of babies a few days old.)

▸ Your newborn's genitals may look swollen or very large for such a small body. In boys, the scrotum may be red. Girls may have a slight bloody, clear, or white discharge from their vagina. Both boys and girls may have puffy-looking breasts. Some babies' nipples may leak a few drops of milk. These signs are the result of the high levels of hormones your baby was exposed to in the uterus. They go away a few days after birth, once the hormones work their way out of your baby's system.

Your Baby's Skin

A baby who has just been born is often covered with a greasy, whitish coating called vernix. There also may be traces of blood and other material on your baby's skin. After he or she is cleaned up, your baby's skin may:

▸ Look very delicate. (It is, so don't use harsh soaps or scented creams on it.)

▸ Peel slightly after the protective layer of vernix is washed away.

‣ Be covered with fine hair called lanugo. Lanugo often appears on a baby's shoulders and back. It will shed within 1 or 2 weeks.

‣ Be blotchy. The skin on some newborns' hands, feet, and mouth area has a bluish or grayish cast. This is caused by early changes in the baby's circulation. Most often, it goes away. A baby's skin color may change somewhat as he or she grows older, too. This is even more true of babies whose racial or ethnic groups tend to have dark skin. Hair and eye color often change, as well.

‣ Look a little yellow. This is called jaundice. Jaundice is caused by a buildup of *bilirubin* in the blood. This greenish-yellow substance forms when old red blood cells break down. During pregnancy, the placenta (and then your liver) removes bilirubin from your baby's blood. The baby's liver won't start removing bilirubin until a few days after birth. This causes the yellowish tint to the skin. Although too much bilirubin can be harmful, normal levels won't cause a problem. If your baby has jaundice, the doctor will check the level of bilirubin in his or her blood. If it's high, special treatment will bring the level down.

Your Baby's Weight

One of the first questions people ask after a baby arrives is how much he or she weighs. In fact, that's one of the first things doctors and nurses at the hospital want to know, too.

There's no such thing as a "right" weight for a newborn. Even so, there is a range that is thought to be normal for most babies. The hospital staff notes your baby's weight in grams:

2.2 pounds = 1,000 grams = 1 kilogram

They'll give you the figure in pounds and ounces, though. Most full-term babies weigh between 5 1/2 and 9 1/2 pounds. The average weight is 7 1/2 pounds (about 3,400 grams).

The weight often depends on how close a baby is born to his or her due date. Babies born early tend to weigh less than those born at term (37–42 weeks after your last period). Babies born late tend to weigh more.

How Your Newborn Acts

Most newborns' basic needs and responses to the outside world are the same. Even so, each baby has a unique personality right from the start.

The way one baby behaves and interacts with people can be very different from the way another newborn acts. Some babies are quiet and calm. This is likely to be true of babies who seemed quiet in the uterus. Other babies are bundles of energy from the start. They cry and kick with vigor and demand round-the-clock attention.

After the stress of birth, most newborns are very alert for the first hour or so. This is a good time to nurse, talk to, or just cuddle your new son or daughter.

When this alertness fades, the baby will get sleepy. Don't worry if your newborn seems very drowsy or sleeps a lot for the next few hours or even days. After all, you are not the only one who needs to recover from birth.

Many babies do little else besides sleep at first. Most newborns spend 14–18 hours a day sleeping—although not all in a row. Short stretches of sleep broken up by brief alert periods are normal. But again, it depends on the baby. Some newborns sleep less and are fussy when they wake up. Others sleep for long stretches and are quiet and calm when they are awake.

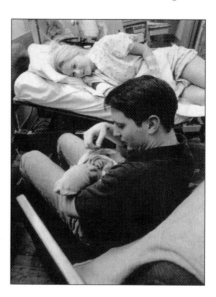

Some mothers fall head-over-heels in love with their newborns the minute they set eyes on them. For others, this love takes time to form. If a woman feels unsure or nervous around her new baby, for instance, it may take longer to feel a bond. It also can be harder to connect if the baby doesn't look the way she expected him or her to or if the birth process was stressful.

Don't worry if you don't bond with your baby right away. You and your newborn will grow closer as you get used to each other. Forming an attachment to your baby over the long run is more important than having an instant bond. Think of bonding as love at first sight, and attachment as slowly building a loving relationship. How your relationship starts matters less than what it becomes. (For more on bonding, see "Bonding With Your Baby," Chapter 9.)

Stocking Up for Baby

Many couples are so thrilled at the prospect of a new baby that they start shopping as soon as the pregnancy test is positive. Friends and family, too, often shower parents-to-be with dozens of gifts.

Sure, it's hard to resist all the cute clothes, cuddly toys, and high-tech baby gear sold today. What do you *really* need, though?

You don't need very much—at least at the start. You can't do without basics like clothes, diapers, a car seat, a baby carrier, and a place for your newborn to sleep. You can wait until later to get most other items.

A newborn's needs are simple: food, warmth, and love. The thing that he or she needs most is you—and as much time, attention, and love as you can give.

Baby Clothes

When choosing clothes for your new baby, be practical. If your newborn arrives in July, for instance, you won't need a thick blanket sleeper or bunting right away.

Don't buy many newborn outfits. A newborn grows so fast that these clothes may last just a few weeks. Buy baby clothes a little big. They'll last

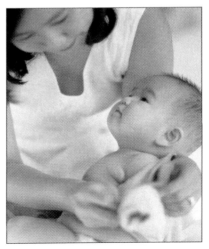

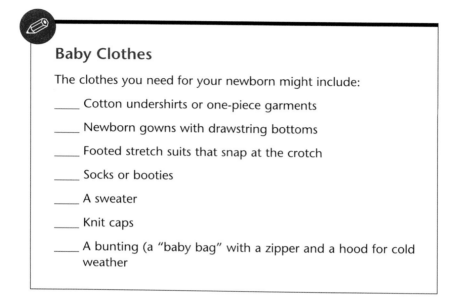

Baby Clothes

The clothes you need for your newborn might include:

_____ Cotton undershirts or one-piece garments

_____ Newborn gowns with drawstring bottoms

_____ Footed stretch suits that snap at the crotch

_____ Socks or booties

_____ A sweater

_____ Knit caps

_____ A bunting (a "baby bag" with a zipper and a hood for cold weather

much longer this way. You can always roll up sleeves and hems. It's best to stick to a basic wardrobe.

How many of each item you need depends on how often you can do laundry. You may need to change your baby's outfit two or three times a day at first.

Baby Supplies

Whether you buy new baby gear, purchase it secondhand, or get hand-me-downs, be sure furniture and other supplies are clean, safe, and sturdy. Cribs made since 1989 must meet strict safety standards. If you buy a new crib, be sure it has a Juvenile Products Manufacturers Association seal. If you use an older one, make sure it has certain safety features:

▸ Slats are no more than 2 3/8 inches apart and none are missing or cracked (the baby's head or body could slip through).

▸ There are no cutouts or crossbars in the headboard or foot-board (the baby's head could get trapped).

▸ There are no corner posts (the baby's clothing could get caught and strangle him or her).

- Latches are secure and can't be opened by a baby or a toddler.

- There are no rough edges, sharp points, or loose screws or bolts.

- The paint is lead-free and isn't chipping or peeling.

- There are at least 9 inches between the top of the side rail and the mattress when it's in the highest position, and at least 26 inches when it's in the lowest position.

No matter what kind of crib you pick, make sure:

- The mattress is firm and fits snugly. No more than two fingers should fit between the mattress and the crib on all four sides.

- The mattress is waterproof. Don't use a plastic or rubber mattress cover—the baby could get trapped under it.

- The bumper pads fit snugly, go all the way around the crib, and are tied or strapped on tightly. Bumper ties should be no

Other Baby Supplies

Other supplies you also should have on hand:

_____ Diapers (cloth or disposable)

_____ Cloth diapers (to use as burp pads or to wipe up after your baby)

_____ Receiving blankets for swaddling your newborn

_____ Baby washcloths and hooded towels

_____ Bedding (fitted sheets and a light blanket)

_____ A large diaper pail that closes tightly

_____ A front carrier (so you can "wear" your baby when you go out for walks or even around the house)

_____ A diaper bag

_____ A rear-facing car safety seat

longer than 6 inches. Remove the bumper when your baby can pull to standing.

Bassinets and cradles also are good to use for the first few months. One feature is they are easy to move from room to room. If you use a bassinet or a cradle, make sure:

▸ The bottom is sturdy and the base is wide. This will prevent the cradle or bassinet from tipping over.

▸ Folding legs lock firmly in place.

▸ The surfaces are smooth. Staples or other hardware that sticks out could hurt the baby.

▸ The mattress is firm and fits snugly.

Be aware: older babies can tumble out of a bassinet or a cradle. Once your baby's sitting up, move him or her into a crib.

Choosing—and Using—A Car Safety Seat

No single item will do as much to protect your baby as a car safety seat. In a crash, car safety seats:

▸ Prevent injury 50 percent of the time

▸ Prevent death 71 percent of the time

▸ Reduce the need for hospitalization 67 percent of the time

The worst place for your baby to be in a car is in someone's arms—even yours. Here's why: during a crash, you can be thrown forward with enough force to crush the baby against the dashboard or windshield. Even if you're wearing a seat belt, the force of a crash can throw the baby from the car. If you wrap a seat belt around both of you, your baby could be crushed between the belt and your body.

Also, it's illegal in all 50 states and the District of Columbia to drive a baby or a small child in a car without a safety seat. Most hospitals won't let you take your new baby home unless you have a car seat. Practice putting it in and out of the car to be sure you know how to install it when the time comes.

If you can't afford to buy a seat, you may be able to rent one. Check with your doctor, hospital, local baby stores, car dealers, or consumer safety council about buying or renting a car seat before your baby is born.

Caring for Your Newborn

Newborn babies can function well in the outside world. Even so, they need lots of help to get nourishment and to stay clean, warm, safe, and healthy.

Keeping Your Baby Safe

New parents often worry about their baby's safety. Taking the following steps will keep your baby safe and help put your mind at ease.

Things You May Need to Buy for Your Baby

Many parents buy or borrow these items, although you can manage without them, too:

___ A changing table with safety straps

___ A plastic baby bathtub

___ A rocking chair or a glider to sit in while you feed or soothe your baby

___ A baby seat with a safety belt (this allows your baby to get a look at the world while you do dishes, pay bills, or take a shower)

___ A stroller with a reclining seat (a baby shouldn't be propped up in a stroller until he or she can sit up)

___ A baby swing

___ A baby monitor

___ A cool-air humidifier to moisten the air when your baby has a cold (steam vaporizers can cause burns)

Pointers on Choosing and Using a Car Seat

▶ Don't confuse a plastic baby carrier with a safety seat. Even if a seat belt is placed around it, a carrier can shatter in a crash.

▶ Look for a seat that's safe. The best seats have straps that hold the baby's body at each shoulder and hip and between the legs. This cuts down on the impact during a crash by spreading the force over more of the baby's body—much like a lap–shoulder belt does for an adult.

▶ Choose a seat that's easy to use. Some seats are harder to use than others, with a complex system of straps and buckles.

▶ Pick a seat that's made for a baby. Choose either an infant seat (for newborns to babies who weigh 20 pounds) or a convertible seat (for newborns to children who weigh 40 pounds). If your baby is preterm or very small, ask his or her doctor about the best seat to use. Each type of seat has pros and cons. Most infant seats are made to pop out of a base. That way, you can carry the seat by its handle or place it in a special stroller base. You'll need to replace an infant seat when your baby hits 20 pounds. A convertible seat will last longer. It's made to hold newborns, but also has restraints that can be adjusted for a larger baby or child. These seats aren't as portable as infant seats, though.

▶ Don't buy a used car seat. A used seat may look fine. If it's been in an crash, though, it won't work the way it should. You also won't know if the seat meets current safety standards or if it's been recalled. (A car seat rented from a reliable source is safe.)

▶ Try before you buy. Before you settle on a car seat (or at least before you take it home), make sure the seat fits in the back seat of your car and works with your car's seat belts.

▶ Send in the registration card that comes with the seat. That way, you'll be informed if the seat is recalled.

▶ Install the seat in a reclined, rear-facing position in the back seat of your car (the center of the back seat is best). In a head-on crash, the baby is pressed backwards into the safety seat, with less risk of harm. In a rear-end crash, the back seat acts as a buffer to hold the car seat tightly. (Once your baby's a year old *and* weighs 20

Pointers on Choosing and Using a Car Seat
(continued)

pounds, turn a convertible seat around or move him or her into a front-facing toddler seat.)

- Never use a rear-facing seat in the front seat of a car with a passenger-side airbag. In a crash, the airbag could inflate with enough force to harm or even kill your baby.

- When you install the seat, be sure to follow the instructions. The seat won't do much good if it's not put in the right way. Also check your car owner's manual for details on installing and using a car seat in your model.

- Check the instructions and owner's manual to see if you need to secure the seat with a special locking clip. (New car seats come with these clips.)

- If you need to, wedge a rolled-up towel under the car seat to keep the base level. Otherwise, if the seat of your car slopes down in the back, it can cause the car seat to tilt so much that your baby's head flops forward.

- Strap the seat in as tightly as you can. Pressing down on the seat with your knee while you tighten the seat belt will help. Once the seat's installed, make sure that it doesn't move from side to side or forward and backward.

- Use a special car-seat headrest to keep your newborn from slouching in the seat. Rolled-up cloth diapers or blankets placed on either side of your baby's body work well, too.

- Dress your baby in clothes that let you thread the car seat straps between his or her legs.

- Adjust the seat straps so they fit snugly. If the straps are loose, the baby could slip out or be thrown from the seat.

- Make sure the straps lie flat and aren't twisted.

- Fasten the seat's retainer clip at the level of your baby's armpits. This will keep the straps from slipping off of his or her shoulders.

For more details, contact National Highway Traffic and Safety Administration at 400 Seventh Street, SW, Washington, DC 20590.

Lay your baby down to sleep on his or her back. This greatly lowers the risk of sudden infant death syndrome (SIDS). In the United States, nearly 5,000 babies younger than age 1 die from SIDS each year. No one knows for sure what causes SIDS. Experts think that putting babies down to sleep on their stomachs is the cause in some cases. (If your baby has health problems, talk to his or her doctor about the best sleeping position.)

If you lay your baby down to sleep on his or her side, make sure your baby's arm is forward. This will stop the baby from rolling over onto his or her stomach. Side sleeping doesn't offer as much protection against SIDS as back sleeping. It's safer than stomach sleeping, though. Make sure that relatives and babysitters follow this advice, too. Until a few years ago, parents were told to put their babies to sleep on their stomachs. Explain to family members and caregivers that this advice has changed.

When you put your baby down to sleep, place him or her on a firm mattress. Don't let the baby sleep on a waterbed, sofa, sheepskin, or other soft surface. Remove pillows, quilts, comforters, toys, and stuffed animals from his or her crib. They can smother the baby.

You may want to dress your baby in a warm sleeper and not use a blanket when he or she goes down to sleep. If you use a blanket, tuck it snugly under the crib mattress and make sure that it goes up only as far as your baby's chest.

Always use a car safety seat when your baby rides in a car, van, or truck. These are designed to protect babies and small children in a crash. (See "Choosing—and Using—a Car Safety Seat.") Always use the safety straps that come in infant seats, strollers, and high chairs.

Never leave your baby alone in a car. The temperature in parked cars can soar to more than 100 degrees in just a few minutes.

Never leave your baby alone—even for a second—in the bathtub or on the changing table, bed, sofa, or anywhere he or she could fall or drown. Have all that you need within arm's reach. Keep a hand on your baby at all times. If you have to answer the phone or the doorbell, take your baby with you.

Check your baby's toys and clothing for ribbons, buttons, or other small parts that can be pulled off and swallowed. Also, keep older children's toys, coins, and other small objects out of your baby's reach. These can lodge in the baby's throat and block his or her airway.

Don't let anyone smoke around your baby. Infants and young children who are exposed to secondhand smoke have more colds and respiratory infections and are at higher risk of SIDS.

Don't warm your baby's bottle in the microwave. This creates hot spots that can burn his or her mouth. Also, don't drink hot drinks or cook while you are holding your baby.

Feeding Your Baby

Whether you choose to breastfeed or bottle feed your new baby, be sure to do it often. A newborn's tummy is about the size of his or her fist. Your baby can take in just a little breast milk or formula at a time. As a result, he or she needs to eat at least every few hours. For how-tos on breastfeeding, see Chapter 10.

If you are bottle feeding, the first thing you need to do is choose a formula. Formulas are often made with nonfat cow's milk and fat from soy, coconut, or corn. They also have vitamins, minerals, and other elements that closely mimic those found in breast milk. Most formulas have extra iron as well. Ask your doctor which type of formula he or she sug-

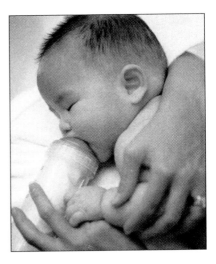

gests. A government program called the Special Supplemental Food Program for Women, Infants, and Children—WIC for short—provides formula for mothers who can't afford it.

Some babies are allergic to cow's milk or have trouble digesting it. If your baby reacts badly to formula, talk to his or her doctor about switching to a formula made with soy protein instead of milk.

Formulas come in powdered, condensed, or ready-to-serve form. Water must be added to powdered and condensed formulas. If you buy either of these, follow the directions. Formula that's too weak or too strong isn't good for your baby.

Next, choose the type of bottles you'll use. Baby bottles come in lots of designs. Bottles can be upright or angled. They either are made to use over and over or to hold special bags that are thrown away after each feeding.

No matter which type you choose, stock up on a supply of 4-ounce bottles for your newborn. Your baby's tiny tummy won't be able to handle a feeding from a standard 8-ounce bottle until he or she is older.

Now, pick nipples for the bottles. Nipples can be standard, orthodontic, flat-tipped, or elongated.

For a baby who's fed only formula, a standard or orthodontic nipple may be fine. If you are combining breastfeeding and bottle feeding, though, a flat-tipped or elongated nipple may be the best choice. These nipples are made to prompt a type of sucking that's close to the sucking used to draw milk from the breast. This way, your baby is less likely to be confused about what he or she needs to do.

Before feeding your newborn, be sure the bottle and nipple have been cleaned well in hot, soapy water. Special bottle brushes help you scrub the hard-to-reach inside of your baby's bottles.

Give your newborn his or her first feeding within 6 hours of birth. Formula takes longer to digest than breast milk. That's why bottle fed babies often can go for longer stretches—3 to 4 hours—between feedings. Still, follow your baby's cues, not the clock. If he or she seems hungry, offer a bottle.

When you're ready to start feeding, hold your baby in the crook of your arm. The baby's head and chest should be higher than his or her feet. Tilt the bottle so the nipple fills with formula. This will cut down on the amount of air your baby swallows and help prevent gas.

Don't "prop" the bottle in your baby's mouth. This can lead to choking or ear infections because the formula pools at the back of the baby's throat.

Your newborn needs contact with you, too. At feeding time, hold your baby close and look into his or her eyes. Relax and enjoy this time together.

Bathing Your Baby

You should keep your baby clean, but there's no need for a daily tub bath just yet. Your newborn will get a good wash in the hospital after birth. Wait until your baby's umbilical stump has

Your Baby's First Tub Bath

Your baby's first real bath is a milestone. It can be a little scary, too. Don't worry—you'll get the hang of it in no time. A bath every few days (with spot cleanings in between) is more than enough to keep your baby clean. Here's how to tackle that first dip:

1. Gather your supplies. You'll need mild soap, baby shampoo, cotton balls, a washcloth, and a hooded towel.

2. Use a sink lined with a foam pad or a special basin made for babies. Don't bathe your baby in the bathtub until he or she is old enough to sit up.

3. Fill the basin with 2 inches of water. Test the heat of the water with your wrist before putting your baby in. The water should be warm—not hot.

4. Start by wiping your baby's eyes and face clean with a wet cotton ball or washcloth.

5. Work your way down his or her body, ending up at the diaper area.

6. To keep your baby from getting chilled, wash his or her hair (or scalp) last and rinse with clean water.

7. If your baby seems to enjoy the bath, don't rush it. Let him or her relax, splash, and explore the water. Young infants don't need bath toys—the water itself is fun enough.

8. When the bath is over, wrap your baby snugly in a hooded towel.

dried up and fallen off before you give him or her another bath.

In the meantime, sponge baths a few times a week will do. Here's how to keep your newborn's skin and scalp clean:

1. Undress your baby and wrap him or her in a hooded towel.

2. Gently wipe your baby's eyes clean with a moist cotton ball.

3. Use a wet washcloth (no soap) to gently wipe your baby's face.

4. Undress one part of your baby's body at a time to prevent him or her from getting cold.

5. Wipe each body part clean with a washcloth that's been dipped in warm water and a few drops of mild baby soap.

6 Pay close attention to the folds of skin in your baby's neck, arms, and legs. You'll be surprised by how much milk and stool find their way into these creases.

7. Rinse and pat dry.

8. Wash the diaper area last.

Many mothers are nervous about bathing their newborns. If you have questions about how to do it, ask the nurses at the hospital to show you.

Caring for Your Baby's Umbilical Stump

In most cases, the stump of the umbilical cord dries up and falls off within 7–10 days of birth. The spot beneath the stump becomes your baby's belly button. Many parents wonder if the way the stump looks has anything to do with their baby's navel being turned in or out. It doesn't.

While the stump's drying out, keep the area clean and dry. This will speed healing and prevent infection. Expose the stump to air and protect it from urine and stool by folding down the top of your baby's diaper. Don't cover the stump with gauze or bandages.

Your doctor may suggest you use ointment or rubbing alcohol around the base of the stump for the first week or so. Call the doctor if the stump looks infected or the skin around it is red.

Diapering Your Baby

Most newborns empty their bladder and bowels within a day of birth. It may occur in the delivery room. Some babies wait more than 24 hours. If your baby takes more than 1–2 days to urinate

Choosing Diapers

A baby goes through about 65 diapers a week. That's more than 3,000 diapers a year. Cloth diapers and disposables each have pros and cons when it comes to cost and convenience. Here's a look at your options:

▶ Disposable diapers. These are the easiest to use. They cost the most, though. Disposable diapers don't breathe as well as cloth diapers, so they can sometimes cause diaper rash. If you use disposables, try a number of brands until you find one you like. Don't use disposable diapers that shred when they are wet. Your baby could swallow loose pieces.

▶ Cloth diapers that you buy, wash, and reuse. This is the cheapest option, but it takes the most time and energy. Cloth diapers come in two styles: flat and prefolded. Flat diapers can be adjusted to fit your growing baby. They may be hard to find, though. Diapers with the fold stitched in place are faster to put on. No matter which type of cloth diaper you choose, start with at least three dozen of them. You'll also need at least three cotton diaper wraps. These hold the diaper in place and close with snaps or fasteners (so no diaper pins are needed). They also cut down on leaks and help keep clothes and bedding dry. They breathe better and are easier to use than rubber diaper covers, too.

▶ Cloth diapers from a diaper service. This is cheaper than using disposables. It's more costly than buying and washing your own diapers, though. Diaper services often pick up dirty diapers and drop off clean ones once or twice a week. They give you a choice of diaper sizes and often provide diaper wraps and a diaper pail for dirty diapers. Some parents use a diaper service for the first few months, when babies tend to go through the most diapers. Afterwards, they wash their own diapers or switch to disposables.

How to Diaper Your Baby

Before you change your baby's diaper, make sure you have the things you need within reach. Never leave your baby alone on a changing table or any other raised surface. He or she could roll or slide off.

Things you'll need:

▶ A clean diaper

▶ A diaper wrap (if you use cloth diapers)

▶ Alcohol-free diaper wipes or a washcloth and a basin filled with lukewarm water

▶ Diaper-rash ointment (if your baby has a rash)

▶ Cornstarch (for hot weather or if your baby has a rash)

What to do:

1. Remove the dirty diaper.

2. Have an extra cloth diaper handy. Babies often urinate when their diaper comes off. While you are changing your baby, place the extra diaper under the diaper area (for a girl) or on top of the diaper area (for a boy).

3. Gently wipe your baby's genitals and bottom clean. (If your baby's skin is irritated by baby wipes, use a wet washcloth instead.)

4. Be sure to wipe from front to back. This keeps bacteria from the baby's stool away from the urethra or vagina, where it can cause infection.

5. Pat the diaper area dry.

6. Apply diaper-rash ointment to irritated skin if your baby has a rash.

7. Apply a light dusting of cornstarch if it's very hot out or your baby has a rash. (Babies can inhale powder, which irritates the lungs. Don't use baby powder made with talc. Also, be careful not to shake out the powder near your baby's face. Never leave a container of powder within your baby's reach.)

8. Put on the new diaper as shown in the "Types of Diapers" box.

or pass stool, his or her doctor will try to find out why. Most newborns urinate 6–18 times and pass stool as often as 7–8 times a day. It may be hard to tell if your baby is urinating (especially with super absorbent diapers). Placing a tissue in the diaper is a good test to check.

To protect your baby, you can use either cloth or disposable diapers. No matter which type you choose, change your baby's diaper each time he or she wets or soils it. This will help prevent diaper rash. You may go through nearly six dozen diapers a week at first. Have a good supply of clean ones on hand.

Dressing Your Baby

Although babies should be kept warm, there's no need to pile on layer after layer of clothing unless it's really cold. Your baby needs about the same amount of clothes as you do—plus one layer because he or she doesn't move around as much. Add a knit cap if it is cold when you and the baby go outside. Newborns can lose a lot of heat through their heads.

When it comes to choosing clothes, let the climate, the season, and the ease of dressing your baby be your guide. For the early weeks, footed one-piece baby suits are a good choice. Just make sure they are made with a soft material that breathes and doesn't irritate your baby's skin. Easy access to the diaper area also is vital. A zipper or snaps in the front are easier to deal with than closures in the back.

If it's chilly, layer an undershirt beneath the baby suit and a sweater or a bunting on top. If it's warm, a diaper and a one-piece garment may be all your baby needs.

Caring for Your Son's Penis

If your son was circumcised, a light dressing of gauze with petroleum jelly was placed over the head of your baby's penis after the procedure. This keeps it from rubbing against the diaper while it heals.

Keep the area clean. Wash your son's penis with soap and warm water each day. Change his diaper often so urine and stool

Types of Diapers

For both types of diapers, make sure it isn't too loose or too tight. The diaper should be snug, but allow you to fit two fingers between the diaper and your baby's skin.

Disposable diaper:

1. Use one hand to grasp your baby's ankles and gently lift up his or her legs and bottom.

2. With the other hand, slide the back of the clean diaper under your baby's bottom. The top of the diaper should be level with your baby's belly button.

3. Lower your baby's legs.

4. Bring the front of the diaper between your baby's legs and up over the genitals.

5. If your baby still has his or her umbilical stump, fold the top of the diaper down so the stump is exposed.

6. Unfasten the tabs on the back of the diaper. Stick them down on the front of the diaper.

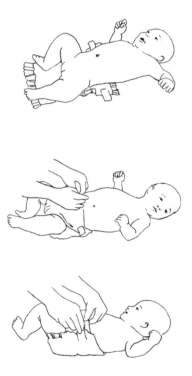

Types of Diapers (continued)

Cloth diaper:

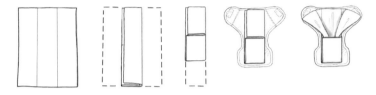

1. Lay the diaper so the short end faces you.

2. Fold the sides of the diaper over the middle so you have one long strip.

3. Fold the bottom third of the diaper up.

4. Lay the folded diaper inside a diaper wrap.

5. Unfold the top of the diaper so it fans out.

6. Slide the back of the diaper and the diaper wrap under your baby's bottom.

7. Bring the front of the diaper between your baby's legs and up over the genitals. (If your baby still has his or her umbilical stump, the top of the diaper and diaper wrap should be beneath the stump.)

8. Bring the sides of the diaper and the wrap over your baby's hips and attach them to the front.

don't irritate the tender tissue or cause infection. Dab the tip of your baby's penis with a little petroleum jelly to keep it from sticking to his diaper.

With one type of circumcision, a plastic ring is left on the penis. The ring will slip off on its own when the circumcision is fully healed. This takes about 7–10 days.

If you didn't have your son circumcised, you don't need to do anything special to care for his penis. Just wash the outside of the penis with soap and water when he takes his bath.

Don't try to pull back your son's foreskin. The foreskin may not retract over the head of his penis until he's between 3 and 5 years old. Once this happens, you can teach your son how to clean under his foreskin.

Taking Your Baby Home

In most cases, you and your baby can leave the hospital within a few days of delivery. At this early stage, you're both still recovering from birth and getting used to life together.

You more than likely found a doctor for your baby before he or she was born. If you haven't chosen a doctor yet, ask the hospital staff for leads.

Be sure to set up a doctor's visit for your baby before you are discharged. The timing of this visit depends on how long your baby stays in the hospital, whether there are any special problems (such as jaundice or trouble breastfeeding), and what the doctor prefers.

The first visit can be planned for a few days or a few weeks after delivery. If you and your baby left the hospital less than 48 hours after a vaginal birth, ask about getting a home visit from a nurse. You also can arrange to have an exam with your baby's doctor within a day or so of discharge. (For more on early discharge, see "How Long Will You Stay in the Hospital?" in Chapter 9.)

Don't be shy about asking the doctor questions. Doctors and nurses are used to lots of questions from new parents and wel-

When to Call Your Baby's Doctor

Call the doctor if your newborn:

▶ Has trouble breathing (the baby has to work hard to get air in and out)

▶ Has skin that looks blue or very pale

▶ Has a seizure (shaking arms and legs)

▶ Has a fever higher than 100°F

▶ Doesn't want to wake up after sleeping for a few hours

▶ Doesn't seem as alert as normal when he or she wakes up

▶ Cries much more than normal and doesn't respond to comforting

▶ Moans as if in pain

▶ Acts very fussy

▶ Seems weak or cries more quietly than normal

▶ Has mucus, blood, or blood clots in his or her urine or stool

▶ Has diarrhea (a large, very watery bowel movement)

▶ Has fewer than six wet diapers a day

▶ Has dark or strong-smelling urine

▶ Has no stool for 48 hours

▶ Has stool that's not yellowish by day 5 if you are breastfeeding

▶ Vomits (not spits up) more than once a day

▶ Nurses poorly or doesn't want more than half a bottle for two feedings in a row

▶ Has very yellow skin or eyes

▶ Has bleeding or discharge from his or her eyes, nails, navel, or genitals

▶ Has diaper rash that doesn't go away or gets worse

▶ Has white patches in his or her mouth

▶ Just doesn't seem "right" to you

come the chance to help. Some doctor's offices even have special call-in times for questions. Call right away if you're really worried about something.

Once you and your baby are settled in at home, don't try to do too much. You may want to ask for extra help from your partner, relatives, or friends. If your employer doesn't offer paid maternity leave, find out if state or local agencies can give you help and support.

Keep in mind: newborns need time to get used to the outside world. Avoid loud noise, intense light, or lots of people. Instead, give yourself and your baby a couple of weeks of peace and quiet. Keep trips around town short. Limit visits from well-wishers. Use this time to rest, get to know your new baby, and settle into life as a family.

Remember, too, that each baby is unique. Some adapt well to their new surroundings. Others have a harder time at first.

Your biggest task during these early days with your baby is to learn how to read his or her signals. Chances are, these signals won't be the same as the ones used by your neighbor's baby, or a friend's baby, or even your last baby if you are a veteran mom.

No matter how your baby tells you that he or she is hungry, tired, or needs to be held, respond to these signals. Feed a baby who's hungry. Gently rock a baby who's tired. Pick up a baby who cries. Meet your baby's needs quickly and lovingly. If you do, you'll foster feelings of trust and security that will help your baby grow into a healthy child.

A Family Is Born

The days and weeks after your baby arrives can be among the most challenging in your life. You may be tired and overwhelmed. Your baby may fuss a lot, be hungry around the clock, and have trouble settling into a regular sleep pattern.

Even so, this time with your newborn is special. Savor it while you can. Keep in mind that your main job right now is to nurture your new baby and welcome him or her into your family.

Give yourself time to master all the skills you'll need to take care of your baby, too. You become a mother the moment your baby is born. Mothering your child won't be second nature right away, though. Pretty soon, as you watch your baby grow, you'll wonder how you ever managed without him or her in your life.

CHAPTER 12

Postpartum Care

You became a mother the moment your baby was born. Yet it can take time for this new status to really sink in. It may be hard to believe that childbirth is over and that this baby is really yours. At first, your focus may be less on your newborn and more on what happened during labor and delivery. It is a life-changing event, after all. It's normal to want to talk about it with others, write about it in a journal, and relive it in your mind.

Once your thoughts turn to your new baby, you may be surprised by how anxious and stressed you feel. You may wonder whether you'll be a good mother. Tasks that you once did with ease seem harder. You are tired from birth and sleep deprived from caring for your new baby. You may feel a little down, despite having this precious new person in your life. If you know what's happening to your body and your emotions, you can better face the ups and downs of the first few months of being a mother.

Taking care of your physical and mental well-being is key. A good diet, exercise, and lots of rest boost your energy level and help your body get back to normal. Having people who support you nearby helps you ease into your new role. Joining a group for new mothers provides a place to share your feelings, get useful tips, and make new friends.

As you resume your daily life, you'll be faced with choices about going back to work, choosing childcare, and planning your family. Don't feel you have to make all of these choices alone. Your doctor as well as your partner and other loved ones can help. Remind yourself that there are no "right" choices. Each mother must do what's best for her and her family.

Your Changing Body

While you were pregnant, your body worked round-the-clock for 40 weeks to help your baby grow. Now that your baby is here, there's more work to be done as your body recovers from pregnancy, labor, and delivery. It may take another 40 weeks or more for things to get back to normal.

Your Uterus

After delivery, your uterus is hard and round and can be felt behind your navel. It weighs about 2 1/2 pounds. Six weeks later, it weighs only 2 ounces. You can no longer feel it when you press on your belly. The opening of your uterus—the cervix—also shrinks quickly.

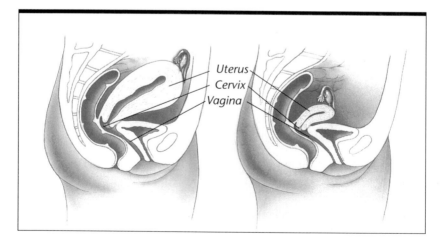

Just after birth, the uterus measures about 7 inches long and weighs about 2 1/2 pounds (*left*). It can be felt just below the navel. In 6 weeks, it has returned to normal size (*right*). The normal size is about 3 inches long, weighing about 2 ounces.

Lochia

Once your baby is born, the blood and tissue that lined your uterus is shed. This vaginal discharge is called *lochia*.

For the first few days after delivery, lochia is heavy and bright red. It may have a few small clots. Soak up this discharge with sanitary pads—do not use tampons.

As time goes on, the flow gets lighter in volume and color. A week or so after birth, lochia is often pink or brown. Bright red discharge can come back, though. You may feel a gush of blood from your vagina during breastfeeding, when your uterus cramps down. By 2 weeks postpartum, lochia is often white or yellow. After that, it slowly goes away. How long the discharge lasts differs for each woman. Some women have discharge for just a couple of weeks after their baby is born. Others have it for a month or more.

Return of Menstrual Periods

If you are not breastfeeding, your period may return about 6–8 weeks after giving birth. It could start even sooner, though.

If you are nursing your baby, your periods may not start again for months. Some nursing mothers don't have a period until their baby is fully weaned.

Be aware: your ovaries may release an egg before you have your first post-baby period. This means you can get pregnant before you even know you are fertile again. If you don't want another baby right way, start using birth control as soon as you resume having sex. (For details, see "Family Planning.")

Once menstruation returns, it may differ from what you are used to. Periods may be shorter or longer than they were before your pregnancy, for instance. Chances are, they'll slowly return to normal. Some women notice that menstrual cramps are less painful than they were before they got pregnant.

Your Abdomen

After delivery, chances are you still look like you are pregnant. During pregnancy, the abdominal muscles stretched out little by

little. They won't just snap back into place
the minute your baby is born.

Give it time. Consistent exercise will
help. Doing a few exercises at least
three times a week will get you started (see "Postpartum Exercises").

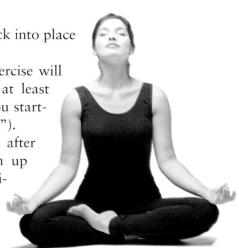

You may have backaches after
delivery, too. Until they firm up
again, those stretched abdominal muscles don't help your
back muscles support your
weight. To prevent a sore
back, practice good posture,
support your back when you breastfeed, and try not to lift anything heavier than your baby for awhile. Also, exercises to
strengthen back and abdominal muscles will help.

Postpartum Discomforts

When you imagined the days and weeks after your baby's birth,
chances are you gave little thought to how your body would feel:
sore. Most aches won't last. Following are some ways to relieve
postpartum aches and pains.

Afterbirth Pains

Your uterus contracts and relaxes as it shrinks back to its normal
size after delivery. These cramps are called afterbirth pains. If you
have given birth before or you are breastfeeding, they may be
more painful. They'll go away in just a few days. In the meantime,
take an over-the-counter pain reliever.

Painful Perineum

The perineum, the area between your vagina and rectum, stretches during delivery. You may have had an episiotomy, an incision
to widen the vaginal opening during delivery. Your perineum may
have torn as your baby emerged from the birth canal. As a result,

this area may feel a bit numb at first. Once the numbness wears off, it may feel swollen, bruised, and sore.

This tender tissue needs time to heal. During the weeks after birth, the perineal muscles will slowly start to regain some of their tone. You can help this process by doing Kegel exercises (see "Postpartum Exercises"). Start them soon after birth. Do them as often as you can, anytime and anywhere.

To ease discomfort and speed healing:

▸ Ask for a cold pack right after delivery. Applying this to your perineum will cut down on swelling and help lessen soreness and stinging.

▸ During the days that follow, keep using cold packs. Apply chilled witch-hazel pads to the area.

▸ Ask your doctor about using a numbing spray or cream to ease pain.

▸ If it hurts to sit down, cushion the area with a pillow.

▸ Take sitz baths. Soaking your perineum in a few inches of warm water will bring relief.

▸ Keep stitches clean to prevent infection. The nurses at the hospital will show you how after you deliver.

▸ Use a water bottle you can squeeze to wet the area in a soothing stream of warm water after you urinate.

▸ Always wipe from front to back after you use the toilet. This will prevent a healing episiotomy or tear from getting infected with germs from your rectum.

Hemorrhoids and Vulvar Varicosities

If you had hemorrhoids or varicose veins in your vulva during pregnancy, they may get worse after delivery. These sore, swollen veins also can show up for the first time now because of the intense straining you did to push your baby into the world.

For relief, try medicated sprays or ointments, dry heat (from a heat lamp or hairdryer turned on low), sitz baths, and cold witch hazel compresses. If hemorrhoids make bowel movements painful, be sure to eat a diet rich in fiber and drink plenty of fluids. In time, hemorrhoids and vulvar varicosities will get smaller or go away.

Bowel Problems

It may be hard to have bowel movements for a few days after delivery. There are lots of reasons for this: stretched abdominal muscles, bowels made sluggish from surgery or pain medication, and an empty stomach because you haven't eaten. You also may be afraid to move your bowels because of pain from an episiotomy or hemorrhoids.

The result: constipation and painful gas. To solve this problem:

▸ Take short walks as soon as you can. This will get your bowels moving again.

▸ Eat foods high in fiber and drink plenty of fluids to ease constipation.

▸ Ask your doctor about taking a stool softener.

▸ Try not to strain when you have a bowel movement. This can worsen hemorrhoids.

Some new mothers can't control their bowel movements. This is called fecal *incontinence*. It is caused by stretching of the nerves and tissues in the perineum during birth. The urge to have a bowel movement may not feel the way it used to, or you may pass stool between bowel movements. If this happens, talk to your doctor.

Urinary Problems

In the first days after delivery, you may feel the urge to urinate but can't get anything out. You may feel pain and burning when you urinate. That's because during birth, the baby's head put a lot of pressure on your bladder, your urethra (the opening where urine comes out), and the muscles that control urine flow. This can cause swelling and stretching that gets in the way of urination.

To lessen swelling or pain, try a warm sitz bath. When you are on the toilet, spray warm water over your genitals with a squeeze bottle to help trigger the flow of urine. Running the tap while you are in the bathroom may help, too. Be sure to drink plenty of fluids as well. Your doctor may give you medication to ease the pain.

Just as some women have trouble with fecal incontinence, many new mothers have another problem: urinary incontinence. This means you can't stop the flow of urine—even when you are not trying to go to the bathroom.

In most cases, with time, the tone of your pelvic muscles will return and the problem will go away. Kegel exercises also will help tighten these muscles. If urinary problems persist more than a few weeks, let your doctor know. There are treatments he or she can offer.

Sweating

In the weeks after birth, many new mothers find themselves drenched with sweat. This happens most often at night. Don't worry about it. Your body is adjusting to changing hormones. To keep your sheets and pillow dry at night, you can sleep on a towel until the sweating eases up.

Swollen Breasts

Your breasts fill with milk about 2–4 days after delivery. When this happens, they may feel very full, hard, and tender. The best relief for this engorgement is breastfeeding. Once you and your baby settle into a regular nursing pattern, the discomfort will go away. (Chapter 10 has details on easing breastfeeding discomforts.)

If you are not nursing your baby, severe engorgement should not last more than about 36 hours. Until then:

▸ Wear a good-fitting support bra, sports bra, or chest binder.

▸ Apply ice packs to your breasts to reduce swelling.

▸ Don't express any milk. This sends a signal to your breasts to make more.

▸ Take pain medication if you need it.

Fatigue

No wonder you are tired. You just finished a very hard task—childbirth. You also lost blood during delivery. Your new baby may be keeping you up all night, too.

Fatigue goes hand-in-hand with being a new mother. You can't really avoid it. You can take steps to ensure that you are rested during the days and weeks after giving birth, though:

▸ Ask for help. Your family and friends are more than likely eager to pitch in. Let them. Be specific when someone wants to know what they can do. Ask a friend to bring something for dinner, stop at the grocery store, start a load of laundry, or watch the baby or an older child for a couple of hours so you can take a nap.

▸ Sleep when your baby sleeps. Use your baby's nap time to rest—not to tackle household chores.

▸ Suggest quiet play. If you have an older child, set him or her up with a few puzzles, picture books, or other quiet activities so you and the baby can rest.

▸ Take it easy. Keep trips out of the house short. Save big household projects for later, too.

▸ Only do what must be done. Know that some things will have to wait. It's important that you get the rest you need.

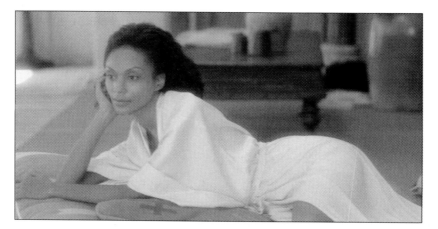

- Limit visitors. There will be plenty of time for people to meet your new baby when you are feeling rested. Until then, the last thing you need is a constant stream of well-wishers.

- Eat a healthy diet. It may be hard to find time to eat when you are caring for a new baby. Even so, it's vital that you do. Foods rich in protein and iron help fight fatigue.

- If you feel really weak or the fatigue continues, talk to your doctor. Sometimes women have a change in thyroid function after pregnancy, especially if they had a thyroid problem before or during pregnancy or someone in their family has thyroid problems.

When to Call Your Doctor

Postpartum discomforts are normal. Some can signal a health problem, though. Call your doctor if you have any of these symptoms:

- Fever more than 100.4°F (38°C)
- Nausea and vomiting
- Pain or burning during urination
- Bleeding that's heavier than a normal menstrual period or that increases
- Severe pain in your lower abdomen
- Pain, swelling, and tenderness in your legs
- Chest pain and cough
- Red streaks or painful new lumps on your breasts
- Pain from an episiotomy, perineal tear, or abdominal incision that doesn't go away or that gets worse
- Redness or discharge from an episiotomy, tear, or incision
- Vaginal discharge that smells bad
- Severe depression

Postpartum Sadness

Although this is a special time, taking care of a newborn is stressful. Hormone levels decrease quickly after delivery. Lack of sleep takes its toll, too.

Many women have *postpartum blues* after delivery. This sadness also is called the "baby blues" or "maternity blues." Most often, it's mild. The blues should go away within a few weeks. In some cases, though, such feelings are intense and don't go away. This can signal a more severe condition called postpartum depression.

The Baby Blues

Many new mothers are surprised by how fragile, alone, and drained they feel after the birth of a child. Their feelings don't seem to match their expectations. They wonder, "What have I got to be depressed about?" Also, they fear that being less-than-joyful means they are bad mothers. These emotions are normal. In fact, about 7 out of 10 new mothers get the baby blues.

These feelings are baffling and scary. They fade quickly, though. The baby blues tend to last from a few hours to a week or so. Most often, they go away without treatment.

When you feel blue, remind yourself that you have just taken on a huge job. Feeling sad, anxious, or even angry doesn't mean you are a failure as a mother. It also doesn't mean you are mentally ill. It simply means that your body is adjusting to the normal changes that follow the birth of a child.

Keep in mind, too, that things will soon start looking up again. Until then:

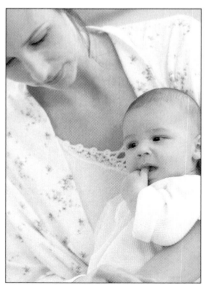

- Talk to your partner or a good friend about how you feel.

- Get plenty of rest.

- Ask your partner, friends, and family for help.

- Take time for yourself.

- Get out of the house each day, even if it's only for a short while.

- Join a new mothers' group and share your feelings with the women you meet there.

Postpartum Depression

For some women, new motherhood brings with it more intense feelings. Postpartum depression is marked by feelings of despair, severe anxiety, or hopelessness that get in the way of daily life.

Women are more likely to have postpartum depression if they:

- Suffered from mood disorders before pregnancy

- Have a family member with a mood disorder

- Have a lot of stress in their lives

If you are prone to depression, seek professional help and enlist support from your loved ones before your baby arrives.

Treatment and counseling will help relieve postpartum depression. Talk to your doctor right away if you have any of these signs of depression:

- Baby blues that last for more than 2 weeks

- Deep depression or anger that appears 1–2 months after birth

- Feelings of sadness, doubt, guilt, or hopelessness that get worse with each passing week and get in the way of day-to-day life

- Not being able to sleep, even when you are tired

- Sleeping most of the time, even when your baby's awake

- Eating much more or much less than normal

- Constant worry about the baby

- Lack of interest in or feelings for the baby or your family

- Panic attacks

- Thoughts of harming the baby or yourself

Return to Daily Living

Having a baby will change the way you live your daily life. Your relationship with your partner will be affected. Your old routines may no longer work. If you know this in advance and try to accept these changes rather than fighting them, you'll be a lot more relaxed as you start your new life together.

Keep in mind, too, that a new baby touches the lives of the whole family. Each person has a role and should take part in the baby's care. There will be some tension as you all adjust to having a baby around. Talk about it. Share your feelings with your partner, your parents, and your children. Listen to their concerns, as well.

Talk to other new moms, too. Just hearing that your family isn't the only one feeling the effects of the birth of a baby can help you cope during this stressful time. The support of other mothers also can make you feel more comfortable in your new role.

If the stress of parenting seems like too much to handle, get some help. Talk to your doctor or call a local crisis hot line. (These hot lines are listed in the community pages of the phone book.) All new parents reach the end of their rope from time to time. This is even more true if you don't have a lot of support or if your baby is fussy.

No matter what triggers them, never take out your emotions on your child. A baby can get injured easily, even if you don't intend to hurt him or her. Shaking a baby for just a few seconds, for instance, can do enough harm to cause brain damage or even death.

If you ever fear that you are going to lose control and hurt your baby, hand him or her to your partner or another loved one and walk away. If you are alone, put your baby in a safe place, such as the crib. Then go into another room (if you can, one that's out of earshot of your baby's cries) until you calm down.

Once the episode has passed, ask yourself what you can do to prevent it from happening again. Tell your partner you need more help from him, for instance. Call in backup from friends and relatives when you have been on baby duty for too long without a break. Find out what sort of community services—such as counseling, respite care, or financial help—are available to you.

You and Your Baby

First-time moms often think that knowing how to care for their newborn will come naturally. In fact, women have to learn mothering skills just as they learn other skills. Keep in mind during these early weeks that mastering baby care takes time, patience, and practice.

You also may feel bad about yourself if you don't have a "perfect" baby or don't measure up as the "perfect" mother. Rest assured—there's no such thing. First, babies have distinct characters right from birth. The fact is, some are just easier to care for than others. Also, it's very hard to juggle taking care of a new baby, running a household, caring for other children, and having a job.

Your Partner

Your partner, too, is going through a lot of changes right now. Often, a new father's needs and concerns aren't given much thought. A new dad gets lots of advice about how to help the mother, for instance. But getting used to a new baby can be just as hard for him.

A father may have mixed feelings about being a parent. Some dads plunge into family life with gusto. Others throw

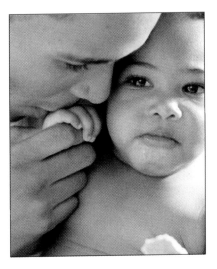

themselves into work to provide for their child. Still others, unsure about their new role, withdraw. They may even start spending more time away from home.

To enhance father–baby bonding, make sure your partner gets a chance to help. As a new mom, it may be hard to hand your baby to someone else. Most often, this is due to your own desire to do everything "right." Even so, not letting your partner help sends the message that you doubt his ability. If he doesn't help with the baby now, he won't learn how and will feel even more unsure of himself as time goes by. To prevent this, give the father plenty of chances to hold, care for, and get to know his new son or daughter.

It's also vital that he has a chance to spend time alone with you. Many men feel left out after a baby arrives. They even may be jealous of the baby for getting what seems to be all of your time, attention, and love.

Try to make time each day to spend together. Once you feel ready to leave the baby with a trusted sitter for an hour or two, make a "date" with each other. Go for a walk, catch a movie, or grab a bite to eat.

What if your baby's father is not involved in your baby's life? In that case, don't try to shoulder the entire burden of raising a baby by yourself. There are many forms of family that help to enrich a child's life. Surrounding yourself with friends and family is good for you and good for your baby.

Your Other Children

If you have other children, they can react to a new baby in many ways:

▸ They may feel let down that the baby isn't an instant playmate or that he or she is the "wrong" sex.

▸ No matter how well you prepare your children, they may be annoyed that all the baby does is eat, sleep, and cry.

▸ They may be jealous and insecure. As a result, they may try to get your attention by throwing temper tantrums, asking to nurse or be given a bottle, wetting their pants, changing their sleeping or eating patterns, or getting mad at you for paying so much attention to the baby.

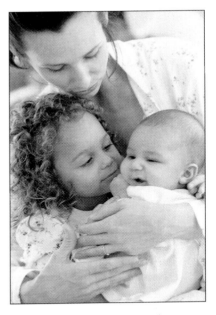

▶ They may show anger toward the baby by hitting, biting, or throwing things.

When a new brother or sister comes home from the hospital, it's a perfect time for your partner to strengthen his relationship with your other children. Don't send your child to stay with someone else while you settle in at home. No matter how good your intentions, this may send your child the message that you no longer want him or her now that you have the baby. Instead, ask a relative or friend to stay with you and pay extra attention to the new big brother or sister. After your baby is born:

▶ Give your child a new doll so he or she has a "baby," too.

▶ Spend time alone with him or her. Do this when the baby's sleeping or when your partner can take over on baby duty. Just 15 minutes a day spent talking, playing, reading, or simply snuggling with you helps remind your child how special he or she is.

▶ Listen to your child and respond to any questions, even if your hands are full with the baby.

▶ Ask your child to help you dress, bathe, feed, or burp the baby. Let a sibling amuse the baby by singing, talking, or making faces. If a big brother or sister wants to keep his or her distance from the baby, that's OK, too. Make sure you don't leave your baby alone with a young sibling.

Your Baby's Grandparents

When a grandchild is born, some grandparents hold back. They may want to give new parents some space and not interfere. You may welcome this distance or be hurt by it. If you'd like your parents or in-laws to be more involved, invite them to see the baby. Call and ask how they dealt with a certain problem when they were new parents.

Other grandmothers and grandfathers are eager to jump into their new role. They may visit often and give lots of advice. You may be thankful for this or see it as a nuisance. If you feel grandparents have overstayed their welcome, gently tell them that you need time alone as a family, and set a date for their return home.

What if your parents or in-laws don't approve of something you are doing—such as breastfeeding your baby, picking the baby up when he or she cries, or putting the baby down to sleep on his or her back? Remind them that parenting advice has changed a lot since they had their babies. Ensure them you are doing what's best for the baby.

Getting Back in Shape

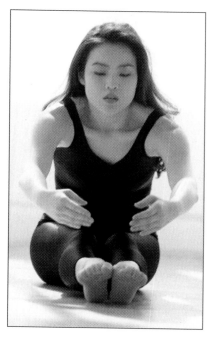

The demands of being a mother may have left you feeling too tired to exercise. The extra effort is worth it, though. Working out boosts your energy level and your sense of well-being. It also restores muscle strength and helps you get back in shape.

You can start working out as soon as you feel up to it. Talk to your doctor about when you can get started. If you had a cesarean delivery, a hard birth, or problems after delivery, it may take a little longer to feel ready for exercise. For safety's sake, follow the same guidelines you did when you were pregnant (see Chapter 5).

If you stayed fit during pregnancy, you'll have a head start. Even so, don't attempt hard workouts right away. If you didn't do much exercise before, take it slowly now. Start with easy exercises and work up to harder ones.

Walking is a very good way to ease back into fitness. Take a brisk walk a few times a week. This will help prepare you for more intense exercise when you feel up to it. Walking is a great activity. It's easy to do, and you don't need anything except comfortable shoes.

Swimming is another great postpartum exercise. There also are exercise classes designed just for new mothers. To find one, check with local health and fitness clubs, community centers, and hospitals.

Postpartum Exercises

Leg Slides

This simple exercise tones abdominal and leg muscles. If you had a cesarean birth, it doesn't put much strain on your incision. Try to do leg slides a few times a day.

- Lie flat on your back and bend your knees slightly.

- Inhale, and slide your right leg from a bent to a straight position.

- Exhale, and bend it back again.

- Be sure to keep both feet on the floor and keep them relaxed.

- Repeat with your left leg.

Postpartum Exercises (continued)

Head Lifts

Head lifts can progress to shoulder lifts and curl-ups. These all strengthen the abdominal muscles. When you can do 10 head lifts with ease, move on to shoulder lifts.

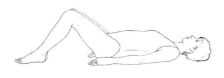

▶ Lie on your back with your arms along your sides.

▶ Keep your lower back flat on the floor.

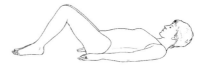

▶ Bend your knees so that your feet are flat on the floor.

▶ Inhale and relax your belly.

▶ Exhale slowly as you lift your head off the floor.

▶ Inhale as you lower your head again.

Shoulder Lifts

Start this exercise the same way you would head lifts. When you can do 10 shoulder lifts with ease, move on to curl-ups.

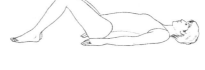

▶ Inhale and relax your belly.

▶ Exhale slowly and lift your head and shoulders off the floor. Reach with your arms so you don't use them for support. If this bothers your neck, place both hands behind your head.

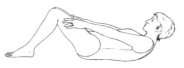

▶ Inhale as you lower your shoulders to the floor.

Curl-Ups

Start this exercise the same way you would head lifts.

▶ Inhale and relax your belly.

Postpartum Exercises (continued)

▶ Exhale. Reach with your arms, and slowly raise your torso until it's halfway between your knees and the floor (about a 45° angle). If you need more support for your neck and head, place your hands behind your head.

▶ Inhale as you lower your torso to the floor.

Kneeling Pelvic Tilt

Tilting your pelvis back toward your spine helps strengthen your abdominal muscles.

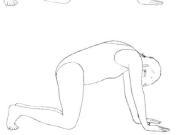

▶ Get on your hands and knees. Your back should be relaxed, not curved or arched.

▶ Inhale.

▶ Exhale and pull your buttocks forward, rotating the pubic bone upward.

▶ Hold for a count of three.

▶ Inhale and relax.

▶ Repeat five times. Add one or two repetitions a day if you can.

Kegel Exercises

Kegel exercises tone your pelvic-floor muscles. This, in turn, controls bladder leaks, helps the perineum heal, and tightens a vagina stretched from birth.

▶ Squeeze the muscles that you use to stop the flow of urine.

▶ Hold for up to 10 seconds, then release.

▶ Do this 10–20 times in a row at least three times a day.

No matter what sort of exercise you do, design a program that meets your needs. You may want to strengthen your heart and lungs, tone your muscles, lose weight, or do all three.

Also try to choose a program you'll keep doing. Staying fit over the long haul is more important than getting into shape right after birth. Your doctor can suggest forms of exercise that will help you meet your fitness goals.

Nutrition and Diet

It's common to lose as many as 20 pounds in the month after delivery. It may be tempting to follow up this weight loss with a crash diet so you can squeeze back into your old clothes. Don't—dieting can deny your body vital nutrients and delay healing after birth. If you are nursing, strict dieting will deprive your baby of the calories and nutrients he or she needs. (For details, see "Nutrition for Nursing Moms" in Chapter 10.)

Instead, try to be patient. Keep up the good eating habits you began in pregnancy. If you do, you'll be close to your normal weight within a few months. Combining healthy eating with exercise will help the process.

Going Back to Work

If, when, and how you go back to work after having a baby are personal choices. Paid maternity-leave policies vary from state to state and employer to employer. The federal Family and Medical Leave Act (FMLA) guarantees women up to 12 weeks of unpaid leave after giving birth. (For more on the FMLA, see "Your Workplace Rights" in Chapter 5.)

Beyond your recovery from birth, there are other factors to take into account. You have to think about how much money you make and how long your family can do without it. You have to look at the costs of and options for childcare, too. If you are breastfeeding, you should give yourself time to establish a good nursing relationship with your baby. You also may want to check into renting or buying a breast pump and learning how to use it.

(For details, see "Breastfeeding and Work" in Chapter 10.)

No matter what you choose to do about work, try to discuss it with your boss before the baby is born. Be careful to build in some leeway for yourself. You can't know how you'll feel about work until after your baby is born. Some women plan to scale back on work or even put their career on hold for a few years, for instance.

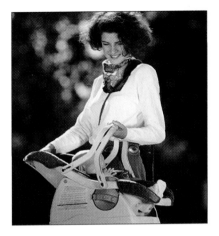

Then they find that they miss the excitement and self-esteem they get from their job. Other women plan to go back to work full-time shortly after giving birth. Once their baby arrives, though, they are less sure about being both a mother and a full-time worker.

Working mothers have a number of options these days. A growing number of employers let new mothers work part-time, work from home 1 or 2 days a week, job share, condense their work weeks, or work flexible hours. What's more, some companies offer on-site childcare. This is a real boon for new mothers— they can bring their babies to work with them and visit them during breaks and lunch hours.

There are three basic options to finding good childcare: your baby can be cared for in your home, in a caregiver's home, or in a childcare center. If you want to hire someone to care for your baby in your home, contact agencies that focus on childcare placements. Keep in mind that this type of care is very costly. To cut costs, some parents share a caregiver with another family. The caregiver in these "share-care" setups is paid to watch two babies in one family's home.

A less costly option is having a relative or a licensed provider care for your baby in their home. In most cases, these caregivers watch more than one child.

Childcare centers are yet another option. This type of setting often has a large number of children and a high staff turnover rate.

Finding Good Childcare

Follow this step-by-step guide to find the right care for your baby:

1. Gather the facts. Make a list of childcare providers, family childcare homes, and childcare centers in your area. Then find out:

   Where is the home or center located? _____

   Does the caregiver, home, or center care for infants? _____

   What hours are available? _____

   Is the home or center open year-round? _____

   What's the policy on sick children? _____

   What's the cost for care? _____

2. Check it out. If you are thinking about family home or center care, visit the site more than once. Make an appointment the first time. If you like what you see during this visit, drop in the next time. (If drop-in visits aren't allowed, keep looking.) Find out:

   Is the facility clean, safe, well-equipped, and child-friendly? _____

   Are there enough care providers (one adult per three to four infants, four to five toddlers, or six to nine preschoolers)? _____

   Are the caregivers attentive and loving? _____

   How is discipline handled? _____

   Do the children seem happy and well cared for? _____

   What's a normal day like? _____

   What's served at meal and snack times? _____

3. Set up an interview. Schedule a chat with a family childcare provider, nanny, or center director. Have your baby with you and note how the caregiver responds to him or her. Ask:

   What experience and training do they have? _____

   _____

   Have they cared for infants before? _____

   Why did they go into this line of work? _____

   How long do they plan to stay in it? _____

Finding Good Childcare (continued)

What do they like most—and least—about caring for children?

_____

What's their philosophy on caring for and disciplining children?

_____

For a caregiver, why did they leave their last job?   _____

For a center, what's the staff turnover rate?   _____

Do babies at a center have one main caregiver or do caregivers change often? _____

Has the care provider had training in first-aid and CPR? _____

Are they willing to give your child prescribed medications? _____

What plans are in place in case of a medical emergency? _____

If you are nursing, how do they feel about handling pumped breast milk? _____

Is the home or center licensed, or is the caregiver certified? _____

4. Check credentials. Never leave your baby with someone until you have checked out their background. Ask:

   If the home or center is licensed or registered or the caregiver certified, can you see the document? _____

   Is the facility in good standing with the agency that issued the license or registration?   _____

   Have there been any complaints? (Call to double-check.) _____

   If there are written policies on philosophy, procedures, or discipline, can you get copies?   _____

   Can you get references from other parents who have used the caregiver, home, or center? _____

5. Try it out. Once you have chosen a caregiver, do a few "practice" runs before you go back to work. This way, if anything strikes you as being "off," you still have time to keep looking. It also will help you and your baby get used to the setup before your maternity leave ends.

No matter which option you'd like to pursue, be sure to start your search early—while you are still pregnant, if you can. Ask around: your pediatrician, friends, neighbors, and coworkers are all good sources of information on childcare. Also check with parents' centers and your local childcare resource and referral agency (listed in the phone book).

Sex After Birth

After giving birth, you may find that you don't have much interest in sex. There are many reasons for this:

▸ *Fatigue.* Once you get your baby to sleep, all you or your partner may want to do is sleep, too.

▸ *Stress.* Coping with your baby's demands can leave you with little desire for sex.

▸ *Fear of pain.* Your breasts may be tender and your perineum may be sore. If you are breastfeeding, low estrogen levels may make your vagina dry. This, in turn, can make sex uncomfortable.

▸ *Lack of desire.* Hormone levels decrease after birth. As a result, so does your desire for sex.

▸ *Lack of opportunity.* Sex takes energy, time, and focus. When you are a new parent, these all tend to be in short supply.

Even if you want to have sex, wait until the healing process is complete to avoid hurting fragile tissues. It is fine to resume sex as soon as you feel comfortable. Most often, this takes at least 4 weeks. Make sure your partner understands this, too. When you feel ready to start having sex again:

▸ Try to spend time alone with your partner. Make talk about the baby or the household off-limits during these times. Instead, talk about yourself and each other.

▸ Get in the mood. Find a time for sex when you are not rushed. Wait until the baby is sound asleep or you can drop him or her off with a friend or a relative for a couple of hours.

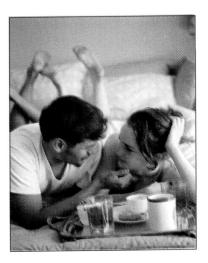

- Proceed slowly and gently. Start with a soothing massage. Try foreplay. Be sure to tell your partner what does—and doesn't—feel good.

- Use lubricant. If your vagina is less moist than normal, a water-soluble cream or jelly will help. If the problem persists, see your doctor.

- Try different positions. You may find that side-lying or kneeling on top of your partner gives you more control and freedom of movement, for instance. This can help you relax and aid arousal.

- Try something new. There's more than one way to give and receive sexual pleasure, after all. If sex isn't comfortable yet, try mutual masturbation or oral sex.

- Talk about it. If you have concerns about sexual problems, discuss them with your partner. This will help both of you avoid frustration and hurt feelings.

Family Planning

If you and your partner are ready to start having sex again, then don't forget one key thing: birth control. Even if you want your children to be close in age, it's best to wait 18–23 months before getting pregnant again. It is believed that babies conceived less than 6 months (or more than 10 years) after you give birth have a higher risk of preterm birth, low birth weight, and small size for time spent in the uterus. Babies born soon after their siblings may have these problems because the mother's body has not had time to replace nutritional stores. Postpartum stress also is a factor. It is unclear why the longer time between pregnancies may affect fetal health, though. Of course, each family has different needs and desires when it comes to child spacing. Discuss the issue with your partner and your doctor.

If you are not breastfeeding, you can be fertile within weeks of giving birth. If you are breastfeeding, it can be hard to tell when fertility returns. Keep in mind, too, that if you used fertility drugs to conceive your first baby, it doesn't mean you can't get pregnant without them.

To be on the safe side, choose a form of birth control before you have sex for the first time. Today, there's a wide array of birth control methods for both women and men. Each has pros and cons. Before choosing one, talk about it with your partner and your doctor. This way, you are more likely to choose birth control that best meets your needs. Some questions to ask:

▶ How well does the method work?

▶ How safe is it for your body (and, if you are nursing, for your baby)?

▶ How easy is it to use?

▶ How convenient is it (will you need to plan in advance or put sex on hold for a few minutes to use a certain method)?

▶ Will it prevent sexually transmitted diseases (STDs) as well as pregnancy?

▶ What are the side effects?

▶ How much does it cost?

▶ Is it permanent?

Any method of birth control can do a good job of preventing pregnancy if it's used the right way and used all the time. You may find, though, that one form of birth control suits your needs at a given time better than others.

That's why you shouldn't just start using your old birth control method after your baby is born. Certain types of birth control may interfere with breastfeeding. (For details on using birth control during breastfeeding, see "Breastfeeding and Sex" in Chapter 10.)

Birth control pills, hormone implants in your arm, hormone injections every 3 months, and the intrauterine device (IUD) are among the most effective methods. They also leave you the option of having more children later.

Used the right way, these methods give you constant protection from pregnancy. You don't have to do anything special when you want to have sex. Surgical sterilization also offers constant protection. You must be sure you don't want any more children, though.

Emergency Contraception

What if you and your partner have sex before you have settled on a birth control method? Or in the rush to make use of your baby's half-hour nap, you forget contraception one time? Talk to your doctor right away about emergency contraception. This is even more vital if your period has returned or you are not breastfeeding and you don't want to become pregnant.

Emergency contraception consists of a high dose of birth control pills taken within 72 hours of sex. It's followed by a second dose 12 hours later. This lowers the odds of getting pregnant by about 75 percent. Your doctor also can insert an IUD after unprotected sex to help prevent pregnancy.

These methods work by preventing ovulation, blocking fertilization, or keeping a fertilized egg from implanting in the uterus. There are two types of emergency contraceptive pills. One type is combined oral contraceptives—birth control pills that contain the hormones estrogen and progestin. The other type uses only one of the hormones—progestin. Your doctor may prescribe a combination of regular birth control pills, a prepared kit with a pregnancy test and four pills, or a package with two pills.

After taking emergency birth control pills, you may feel sick to your stomach for a day or two. Your belly also may feel bloated and your breasts may feel tender. Your next period may be earlier or later than you expect. If you don't get your period within 3 weeks, take a home pregnancy test.

Hormones

Hormonal birth control works by preventing ovulation. When there's no egg to fertilize, you can't get pregnant. You still have your period each month, though. There are three types of hormonal contraception:

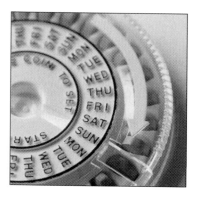

1. *Birth control pills.* Oral contraceptives are the most common method of hormonal birth control. Taken as directed, the pill is also one of the most effective forms of birth control. Combination pills contain manmade estrogen and progesterone, called progestin. If you are breastfeeding, estrogen can cut down on your milk supply. As a result, combination pills should not be used until milk flow is steady. This occurs about 3 months after delivery. Until then, use barrier methods such as condoms or a diaphragm with spermicide. Minipills contain progestin only. They are a better choice if you are breastfeeding because there is no estrogen to affect the milk supply. Its doses of progestins are even lower than those in low-dose birth control pills. Unlike other birth control pills, each pack consists of 28 tablets of active hormone. Minipills can be used by some women who cannot take estrogen.

2. *Implants.* After your upper arm is numbed with local anesthesia, your doctor makes a small cut. Next, he or she inserts six soft plastic tubes the size of match sticks under your skin. Implants are easy to use—after the tubes are in place, you don't need to do anything else to prevent pregnancy for the next 5 years. If you want to get pregnant or switch to another method before then, your doctor can remove the implants.

3. *Injections.* This is another very easy method to use. Each injection provides birth control for 3 months. You need four injections a year. As long as your injections are up-to-date, you don't have to do anything else to prevent pregnancy.

Intrauterine Device

The IUD is a small plastic device that contains copper or hormones. It's inserted into the uterus by a doctor. The copper or hormones in the IUD prevents an egg from being fertilized or prevents a fertilized egg from implanting in the uterus.

Both types of IUDs are T-shaped, but they work in different ways. The hormonal IUD releases a small amount of progesterone into the uterus. The copper IUD releases a small amount of copper in the uterus. A hormonal IUD must be replaced each year. A copper IUD can stay in place for up to 10 years. Both types of IUD can be removed if you want to get pregnant or switch to another form of birth control.

The IUD is simple to use. You don't need to do anything else to prevent pregnancy once it's in place. It's also very effective. However, the IUD may not be the best choice for women who have more than one sex partner.

Barrier Methods

Barrier methods include a spermicide, diaphragm, cervical cap, sponge, and male and female condom. They work by keeping sperm from getting to the egg.

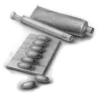

▶ Spermicides are chemicals that kill sperm. They include creams, jellies, foams, and vaginal inserts and suppositories. Before sex, they are placed in your vagina, close to the cervix.

▶ The diaphragm is a round rubber dome. It fits inside your vagina and covers your cervix. If you used a diaphragm before, you must be refitted after giving birth.

▶ The cervical cap is a small rubber cup. It fits over you cervix and stays in place with suction. If you used a cervical cap before, you must be refitted after delivering your baby.

▸ The male condom is a thin sheath made of latex (or, less often, animal membrane). It's worn over a man's penis. Latex condoms also help prevent STDs.

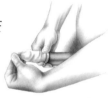

▸ The female condom is a plastic pouch that lines the vagina. It's held in place by a closed inner ring at the cervix and an open outer ring at the entrance of the vagina. Female condoms may help prevent STDs.

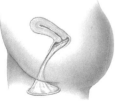

▸ The sponge is a doughnut-shaped device coated with spermicide. It is pushed up in the vagina to cover the cervix.

If you choose a barrier method, be sure to use it each time you have sex. To further reduce your chance of getting pregnant, use spermicide with a diaphragm, cervical cap, or condoms.

Natural Family Planning

Natural family planning also is called "periodic abstinence" or "the rhythm method." It involves not having sex during the days of the month that you are most fertile.

To prevent pregnancy, you must know when you ovulate. You can predict ovulation by watching for changes in your body temperature, watching for changes in your cervical mucus, or charting your menstrual cycle. Ovulation predictor kits also are available. For best results, it's a good idea to combine all three of these methods. Menstrual cycles often aren't regular after delivery and during breastfeeding. Thus, natural family planning may not work very well for new mothers.

Sterilization

You and your partner may think about sterilization if both of you are sure you want this baby to be your last. Sterilization is more than 99% effective, and, in most cases, it's permanent. Talk to your doctor about it well ahead of time if you think you want to

Sterilization

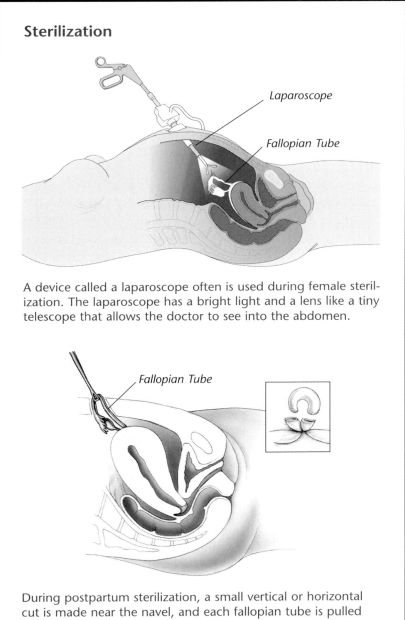

Laparoscope

Fallopian Tube

A device called a laparoscope often is used during female sterilization. The laparoscope has a bright light and a lens like a tiny telescope that allows the doctor to see into the abdomen.

Fallopian Tube

During postpartum sterilization, a small vertical or horizontal cut is made near the navel, and each fallopian tube is pulled through the incision. A section of the tube is closed off, and the section between the ties is removed.

be sterilized after delivering your baby. There may be time limits on when you can have it done.

Sterilization is done by surgery. General or local anesthesia is used. As with any surgery, sterilization has some risks. Problems occur in about 1 in 1,000 women who have the operation. Most of the time, these problems can be treated and corrected.

Female sterilization is called tubal ligation. It involves tying, cutting, banding, or clipping the fallopian tubes. This blocks sperm from reaching and fertilizing an egg. Tubal ligation won't affect your periods or your pleasure of sex.

Male sterilization is called *vasectomy*. It involves cutting or tying the vas deferens (tubes through which sperm travel). This means no sperm is released when a man ejaculates. Vasectomy won't affect your partner's ability to get erections or have orgasms.

Both types of sterilization can be done at any time. In most cases, you or your partner can go home the same day. Some

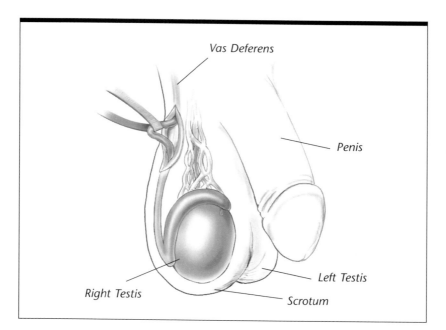

During a vasectomy, one or two small cuts are made in the skin of the scrotum. Each vas is pulled through the opening until it forms a loop. A small section is cut out of the loop and removed.

women choose to get sterilized right after their baby is born, while they are still in the hospital. The surgery is easier then because the uterus is still enlarged and pushes the fallopian tubes up in the abdomen. There, they can be grasped through a small cut near the navel, then tied or cut.

Talk to your doctor about it well ahead of time if you think you want to be sterilized after delivering your baby. There are time limits in some areas. You should be certain that you and your partner won't change your mind about having more children down the line. Although there is surgery to reverse sterilization, it doesn't always work. Also, the operation to reverse sterilization is major surgery. Most insurance plans won't cover it.

Your Follow-Up Visit

Arrange a visit to see your doctor 4–6 weeks after your baby's birth. (If you had a cesarean birth, the doctor may want to see you about 2 weeks after surgery to check the incision.) The goal of this checkup is to make sure that your body has recovered from pregnancy and birth and that you are not having any problems.

During the visit, the doctor will check your weight, blood pressure, breasts, and abdomen. He or she also will do a pelvic exam to make sure a tear or episiotomy has healed and that your vagina, cervix, and uterus have returned to their normal state.

Use this time to bring up any questions or concerns you have about the healing process, breastfeeding, birth control, weight loss, sex, or your emotions. Don't be shy—your doctor's heard it all before. So you don't forget anything, jot down any questions you have and bring them with you to this visit.

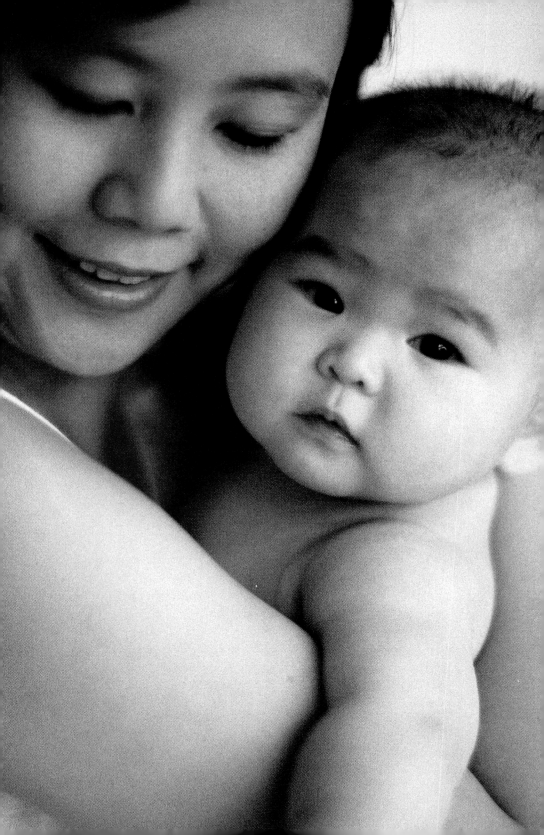

Special Care

Most of the time, pregnancy goes the way it should: you are healthy, the fetus grows normally, and the baby's birth is a happy and trouble-free event. Sometimes, though, pregnant women develop problems.

A mother or father may pass an inherited disorder to the baby, for instance. A fetus may not develop the way it should. A woman may have a health condition—or develop one during pregnancy—that puts her and her baby at risk. Complications can arise as a result of the pregnancy itself. Sadly, a pregnancy or a baby may be lost.

In some of these cases, close monitoring and treatment can help prevent problems or make them less severe. That's why planning your pregnancy, having a pre-pregnancy doctor's visit, and getting early and regular prenatal care is so vital to having a healthy baby and staying healthy yourself.

CHAPTER 13

Genetic Disorders and Birth Defects

Just about every mother-to-be worries about her baby having a problem. Most of the time, this worry is needless. Almost all children in the United States are born healthy. Out of 100 newborns, only 2 or 3 have major birth defects. Birth defects affect the baby's health, ability to function, or the way he or she looks. Many can be treated or corrected with medication or surgery.

What causes birth defects? Some are passed from parent to child. Just as a baby gets hair and eye color from his or her parents, he or she can inherit certain diseases or conditions. Other birth defects result from being exposed to harmful things during pregnancy. Getting certain infections, drinking alcohol in excess, or taking some medications, for instance, may result in birth defects. Birth defects also can be caused by being exposed to toxic substances such as mercury or lead (see Chapter 5 for details). Getting an infection such as rubella (German measles) during pregnancy may cause birth defects as well (see Chapter 16). Sometimes, a mixture of inheritance and exposure during pregnancy is the cause. In many cases, the reason for a defect isn't known.

Many birth defects can be seen right away. A defect that's present at birth—no matter when it is diagnosed—is called a ***congenital disorder***. A congenital disorder may or may not be inherited.

Many babies with birth defects are born to couples with no known risk factors. The risk of birth defects is higher when certain risk factors are present, though. During prenatal care, some tests are offered to some women with known risk factors. Tests may be offered to women at low risk of a problem. These tests, along with genetic counseling, will advise patients about their risk of a problem.

Choosing whether to have these tests is up to you. Some couples choose not to be tested for birth defects. Other couples find that testing and counseling can help them decide whether to become pregnant, end a pregnancy, or prepare for the birth of a baby with special needs.

Genes and Chromosomes

Genetics is the study of how traits are inherited. Traits are passed from parent to child through *genes* and *chromosomes*. Each cell in your body has pairs of genes and chromosomes that control your physical makeup.

Normally, a man's sperm and a woman's egg have 23 chromosomes each. All other cells in the body have 46. When an egg is fertilized by a sperm, the 23 chromosomes from the mother's egg and the 23 chromosomes from the father's sperm join to form the 46 chromosomes of the cell that will become the fetus.

One pair of these chromosomes—one each from the sperm and the egg—is called the sex chromosomes. There are two types of sex chromosomes: X chromosomes and Y chromosomes. A normal sperm has either an X or a Y chromosome. A normal egg always has an X chromosome.

The sex chromosome in the sperm determines the sex of the child. If a sperm with a Y chromosome joins with an egg, the fetus is male (XY). If a sperm with an X chromosome joins with an egg, the fetus is female (XX).

Each chromosome carries many genes. Genes also come in pairs. Half of a fetus's genes come from the mother. The other half comes from the father. Some traits are controlled by a single gene pair. Other traits—including skin color, hair color, and height—are the result of many pairs of genes working together.

DNA: The Key to the Genetic Code

Cells are the body's basic building blocks. Inside each cell is a **nucleus**. Inside each nucleus are chromosomes. All human cells have 46 chromosomes, except the eggs and sperm. These each have 23.

Chromosomes are made up of deoxyribonucleic acid (DNA) molecules. DNA molecules are double stranded. The two strands are shaped like a spiral staircase. The strands connect at what are called base pairs.

Each chromosome has between 50 million and 250 million base pairs, depending on its size. The human body has about 3 billion base pairs of DNA. Each DNA molecule contains the genetic code for the whole body.

A gene is a segment of DNA that's coded to pass along a certain trait. The body has about 50,000–100,000 genes. Each gene has a specific position on the chromosome. Each controls a specific function.

The human genome is the full set of genes. Together, these genes control all aspects of a person's growth, development, and function.

Scientists know the role of just a small number of genes. The Human Genome Project is an international effort to map the entire human genome. That is, they are trying to pinpoint each gene's place on a chromosome and the role it serves. By knowing the role and placement of each gene, scientists can better understand how it affects the body in both health and disease.

A gene is either dominant or recessive. If one gene in a pair is dominant, the trait it carries cancels out the trait carried by the recessive gene. For a recessive trait to appear, the gene that carries it must be inherited from both parents. For instance, the gene for blue eye color is recessive to the gene for brown eyes. If a fetus inherits a brown eye gene and a blue eye gene, he or she will have brown eyes. It requires two blue eye genes to result in blue eyes. Like eye color, genetic diseases also can be dominant or recessive.

Are You at Increased Risk?

When you have your pre-pregnancy checkup or start prenatal care, your doctor may give you a list of questions like the ones in the box. If you answer "yes" to any of them, you may be at increased risk for having a baby with a genetic disorder.

Genetic Counseling

If you're at risk for having a baby with a disorder, genetic counseling can help you and your partner choose whether to take tests to find out if you're carriers, whether to become pregnant, or whether to have prenatal testing to see if your fetus has a problem.

A genetic counselor is someone with special training in genetics. He or she can:

▶ Give you an idea of the risk you face

▶ Offer expert advice on the types of genetic disorders and how they affect babies born with them

▶ Help you weigh your options

▶ Discuss any concerns you have

▶ Calm undue fears

Your genetic counselor will ask you and your partner for a detailed family history. If a family member has a problem, the counselor may ask to see that person's medical records. He or she also may refer you or your partner for physical exams, blood tests, or prenatal tests. Using all the information he or she can gather, the counselor will try to figure out the risk of your baby having a problem and explain it to you.

Whether to have genetic testing is up to you and your partner. Some hopeful parents and parents-to-be would rather not know if they're at risk for a problem. Even so, finding out has benefits:

▶ If you have carrier testing before trying to conceive, the results can help you decide whether to become pregnant. If you learn that you have a strong chance of having a child with a genetic

Risk Factors for Genetic Disorders

Review the following list of risk factors and place a check after the "yes" responses.

___ Will you be age 35 or older when your baby is due?

___ If you or your partner are of Mediterranean or Asian descent, do either of you or anyone in your families have thalassemia?

___ Is there a family history of neural tube defects?

___ Have you ever had a child with a neural tube defect?

___ Is there a family history of congenital heart defects?

___ Is there a family history of Down syndrome?

___ Have you ever had a child with Down syndrome?

___ If you or your partner are of eastern European Jewish or French Canadian descent, is there a family history of Tay–Sachs?

___ If you or your partner are of eastern European Jewish descent, is there a family history of Canavan disease?

___ If you or your partner are African American, is there a family history of sickle cell disease or trait?

___ Is there a family history of hemophilia?

___ Is there a family history of muscular dystrophy?

___ Is there a family history of cystic fibrosis?

___ Is there a family history of Huntington disease?

___ Is anyone in your or your partner's family mental retarded?

___ If so, was that person tested for fragile X syndrome?

___ Do you, your partner, anyone in your families, or any of your children have any other genetic diseases, chromosomal disorders, or birth defects?

___ Do you have a metabolic disorder such as diabetes or phenylketonuria?

___ Have you had more than two miscarriages in a row?

___ Have you ever had a baby who was stillborn?

defect, you can explore other options for starting a family. You can adopt a child, for instance. You can be artificially inseminated with sperm from a donor. You can have a donated egg fertilized by your partner's sperm and implanted in your uterus.

▸ Carrier testing or genetic testing can give you information that will help other family members. Siblings and other relatives who may want to have children of their own someday can benefit from the knowledge that your family has the gene for a certain disorder.

▸ Testing can help you prepare for the birth of a child with special needs. You can learn about the disorder, line up special medical care for your baby, and seek out others for support.

▸ Genetic testing done during pregnancy can help you decide whether to continue your pregnancy. If you find out your baby has a severe problem, you have the chance to think about ending the pregnancy and trying again.

▸ Many parents with risk factors can have a baby who's just fine. Testing may spare you from spending the months before your child's birth in a state of fear, panic, and grief.

Genetic Disorders

There are many types of genetic disorders. Genetic defects fall into one of three categories:

1. *Inherited.* An inherited disorder is caused by a gene that's passed from parent to child. These disorders can be dominant, recessive, or X-linked.

2. *Chromosomal.* A chromosomal disorder is caused by a missing, damaged, or extra chromosome.

3. *Multifactorial.* A multifactorial disorder is caused by a mixture of factors. It often is not clear why the disorder occurred.

Prenatal tests may detect a genetic disorder in a fetus. Tests done before or during pregnancy may show if the mother or the father is a **carrier** for a certain genetic disorder.

In some cases, there are no risk factors for a disorder, so testing is offered to everyone. In other cases, a personal or family history may call for counseling and testing. Most birth defects occur when there is no history of problems in the family.

Dominant Disorders

Some genetic disorders are dominant. That means just one gene from either parent can cause them. If a parent has the gene, each of his or her children has a 1-in-2 chance of inheriting the disorder. Two dominant disorders are:

1. *Huntington disease.* Huntington disease is a nerve disorder that causes loss of control of movements and mental function. Most often, it's diagnosed in mid-life. Death often follows in about 15 years. Huntington disease affects about 1 in 100,000 people. If there's a family history, genetic testing can tell if you, your partner, or your baby have the gene and will later develop the disease.

2. **Polydactyly.** A baby with this disorder is born with extra fingers or toes. Polydactyly is fairly common. It's easily corrected with surgery.

Recessive Disorders

Some genetic disorders are recessive. That means a pair of genes, one from each parent, is needed to cause them.

Each person carries a few abnormal recessive genes. Most of the time, they don't cause a defect. The abnormal genes are canceled out by normal dominant genes. Even so, if you have a recessive gene for a certain disorder, you're a carrier. Although you may show no signs of the disorder yourself, you can still pass it on to your children.

If both you and your partner are carriers for the same recessive disorder, each of your children has a 1-in-4 chance of having the disorder. If one of you has the disorder and the other doesn't (and isn't a carrier), your children will be carriers.

Some recessive disorders are more common in certain ethnic groups. These disorders include:

▶ *Sickle cell disease.* In a person with this disorder, red blood cells have a crescent, or "sickle," shape rather than the normal doughnut shape. Because of their odd shape, these cells get caught in the blood vessels. This prevents oxygen from reaching the organs and tissues. This lack of oxygen, in turn, causes pain. The body destroys sickle cells faster than it can make normal cells to replace them. Anemia often results. Sickle cell disease occurs most often in African Americans. In the United States, about 1 in 625 African Americans has sickle cell disease. About 1 in 10 are carriers. For a couple to have a child with sickle cell disease, both parents must be carriers of the trait or have the disease.

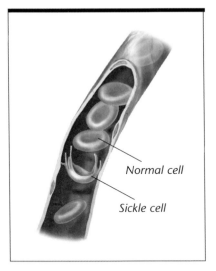

Normal cell

Sickle cell

The red blood cells of a person with sickle cell disease are shaped like a crescent (or a "sickle"). Normal red blood cells are shaped like a doughnut.

▶ *Tay–Sachs disease.* People with Tay–Sachs disease lack a chemical needed for normal brain function. Symptoms first occur at about 6 months of age. Tay–Sachs disease causes severe mental retardation, blindness, and seizures. Most people with the disease die before they are 7 years old. It occurs mostly in people of eastern European Jewish descent (Ashkenazi Jews). One in 3,600 Ashkenazi Jews is born with Tay–Sachs disease. It's also common among French Canadians. The chance of being a carrier is 1 in 30 for Ashkenazi Jews and French Canadians, and 1 in 300 for other people.

▶ *Cystic fibrosis.* This disorder appears in childhood—sometimes right after birth. The lungs produce thick, sticky mucus. This mucus clogs the airways and leads to lung infections. Thick mucus may affect the way the gut works. It mainly affects white people of northern European descent. In the United States, 1 in 2,500 white people have the disease. One in 25 are carriers. If you or your partner have a family history of cystic fibrosis, genetic testing will help you find out if you're carriers. Testing of the fetus also can tell you if the fetus has the disease.

▶ *Thalassemia.* This disorder causes anemia. It also can lead to liver and heart problems. One form, beta-thalassemia, is more likely to occur in people of Mediterranean descent. This includes people whose ethnic background is Italian or Greek. For them, the chance of being a carrier is about 1 in 250. Another form, alpha-thalassemia, tends to occur in people of Asian descent. Testing can tell you if you or your partner are carriers or if your fetus has the disorder.

X-Linked Disorders

Disorders that are caused by genes on the X chromosome are called "X-linked" or "sex-linked" disorders. In most X-linked disorders, the abnormal gene is recessive.

A woman may carry this gene but not have the disorder. That's because the normal gene on her other X chromosome cancels out the abnormal gene. In some X-linked recessive disorders, a woman may have a slight effect. A male child who inherits the X chromosome with the abnormal gene, however, may get the disorder. That's because he doesn't have another X chromosome with a normal gene to cancel that one out. Color blindness is a common X-linked trait.

If you're a carrier for an X-linked disorder and the father of the baby isn't, there's a 1-in-2 chance a son will have the disorder and a daughter will be a carrier. Very rarely, a daughter has an X-linked recessive disorder. In this case, her father has the disease and her mother's a carrier.

Genetic testing can show if you're a carrier of an X-linked disorder or if your fetus is affected. Common X-linked disorders include:

▶ *Hemophilia.* People with hemophilia lack a substance that helps blood clot. When they're injured, they risk bleeding to death. Hemophilia affects 1 in 10,000 males. Females can be carriers of the disease.

- *Duchenne muscular dystrophy.* Duchenne muscular dystrophy is the most common severe form of muscular dystrophy. This is a group of diseases that weaken the muscles. Duchenne muscular dystrophy affects almost only boys. It occurs at about age 2. As his muscles weaken, the child has trouble standing and walking. By age 12, he may be confined to a wheelchair. Most males with this disease die in early adulthood.

- *Family history of mental retardation.* Fragile X syndrome is the most common inherited cause of mental retardation. It affects 1 in 1,250 boys and 1 in 2,000 girls. Boys with the disorder have a long, triangular face and ears that stick out. Women with no problems may be carriers of the fragile X gene.

Chromosomal Disorders

Rarely, chromosomal problems are inherited. Most are caused by an error that occurs when the egg or sperm are forming. Extra, missing, or incomplete chromosomes often cause severe health problems. Most children with chromosomal disorders have physical defects and below-average intelligence.

The older you are, the greater your risk of having a child with a chromosomal disorder. If you're age 35, for instance, the chance is about 1 in 200. If you're age 40, it's about 1 in 60. Common chromosomal disorders include:

- *Down syndrome.* A person with Down syndrome has an extra chromosome—three number 21 chromosomes instead of two. This is called trisomy 21. Down syndrome causes mental retardation. It also can cause heart defects. People with Down syndrome have a flat face, slanting eyes, and low-set ears. About 1 in 800 babies is born with Down syndrome. The risk of having a baby with Down syndrome increases as you age. Still, it can happen to women of any age. In fact, 8 out of 10 women who have Down syndrome babies are younger than age 35. That's because most babies are born to younger women.

How Common Are Chromosomal Disorders?

Chromosomal disorders occur when there are too few or too many chromosomes. The table shows your risk of having a baby with Down syndrome or any chromosomal disorder. Your risk is based on your age.

The Risk of Having a Baby With a Chromosomal Disorder at Birth

Mother's Age	Risk of Down Syndrome	Risk of Any Chromosomal Disorder
20	1/1,667	1/526
25	1/1,250	1/476
30	1/952	1/385
35	1/378	1/192
40	1/106	1/66
41	1/82	1/53
42	1/63	1/42
43	1/49	1/33
44	1/38	1/26
45	1/30	1/21

Modified from Hook EB, Cross PK, Schreinemachers DM. Chromosomal abnormality rates at amniocentesis and in live-born infants. JAMA 1983;249:2034–2038 (ages 33–49), copyright 1983, American Medical Association; Hook EB. Rates of chromosome abnormalities at different maternal ages. Reprinted with permission from the American College of Obstetricians and Gynecologists (Obstetrics and Gynecology, 1981; 58, 282–285)

▶ *Klinefelter syndrome.* Klinefelter syndrome happens when a boy has an extra X chromosome—that is, two X chromosomes and one Y chromosome, for a total of 47 chromosomes. About 1 in 800 males has this disorder. It can—but doesn't always—cause infertility and lower intelligence.

▶ *Turner syndrome.* About 1 in 3,000 females has just one X chromosome. This is called Turner syndrome. These girls tend to be short and are almost always infertile. A woman carrying a fetus with Turner syndrome may have a miscarriage.

Multifactorial Disorders

Many disorders are thought to come from a mix of factors. The actual cause is unknown. This is called multifactorial inheritance. Some of these disorders can be detected during pregnancy. They often can be corrected with surgery. Following are common multifactorial disorders.

Congenital Heart Disease

Congenital heart disease is the most common major congenital disorder. It occurs in about 1 in 125 births. The outcome for babies with congenital heart disease depends on the type of heart defect they have and whether they also have other problems. Chromosomal disorders cause about 30–40% of cases of congenital heart disease. If a parent has a congenital heart defect, his or her children also are at greater risk for having a heart defect.

Congenital heart disease may be found during a routine ultrasound exam. Still, only about 1 in 10 cases is detected this way.

What if you know you're at high risk for having a baby with a congenital heart defect? Your doctor may suggest that you have a special ultrasound focused on the fetal heart. Routine ultrasound likely will not detect congenital heart problems.

Neural Tube Defects

Neural tube defects occur when the fetal brain, spinal cord, or their coverings don't form the way they should during the early stages of pregnancy. Most NTDs are "open." This means they're not covered by skin. The two major types of NTDs are:

1. **Spina bifida.** The effects of spina bifida depend on where the defect is located. When the defect is low in the spine, problems often are mild. If the defect is higher in the spine, it can cause leg paralysis, loss of feeling, lack of bladder and bowel control, hydrocephalus (extra spinal fluid in the brain), mental retardation, and even death. Spina bifida occurs in North America in 1–2 of 1,000 births.

2. **Anencephaly.** Anencephaly occurs when the brain and head don't form the way they should. Babies with this disorder often are stillborn or die soon after birth.

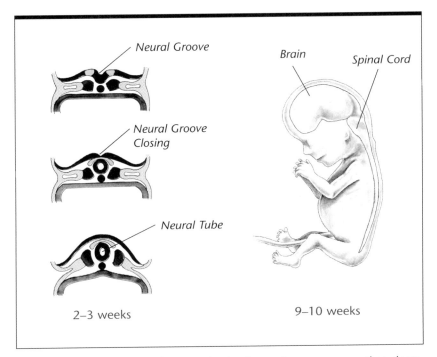

Neural Groove

Brain   Spinal Cord

Neural Groove
Closing

Neural Tube

2–3 weeks   9–10 weeks

In very early pregnancy, the neural tube forms from a groove that deep-
ens and normally closes (*left*). The brain and spinal cord of a fetus
develop later in pregnancy (*right*).

The cause of NTDs is unknown. About 9 in 10 babies with
such defects are born to parents with no family history of it.

To reduce the odds of having a baby with an NTD, a woman
should take 0.4 milligrams of folic acid a day before getting pregnant and during the first trimester. A woman at high risk for having a baby with an NTD should take 4 milligrams of folic acid a
day. (For details, see "Folic Acid" in Chapter 6.)

Cleft Lip and Cleft Palate

Cleft lip is a gap in the upper lip. It's sometimes called a "hare-
lip." *Cleft palate* is a hole in the roof of the mouth. Cleft lip and
palate are among the most common congenital defects. It occurs
in about 1 in 1,000 births. Most cases are multifactorial. Cleft lip
also can be caused by a chromosomal disorder or inherited as a

dominant trait. An ultrasound sometimes can detect the problem during pregnancy. After birth, surgery can correct it.

Clubfoot

With *clubfoot*, a baby is born with one or both feet twisted at the ankle. It occurs in about 1 in 1,000 births. If the problem is slight, special exercises often will correct it. For more severe cases, a baby may need to wear splints or casts for at least a year or have surgery.

Pyloric Stenosis

In pyloric stenosis, the opening between the stomach and the intestine is blocked. It can cause vomiting that doesn't go away, constipation, and failure to gain weight. It often is diagnosed between the second week and second month after birth. Most children with pyloric stenosis are boys. The defect is easily treated with surgery.

Other Defects

Certain defects are sometimes (but not always) linked to a chromosome problem. These defects don't tend to be inherited. With abdominal wall defects, for instance, the skin doesn't finish forming over the abdomen. This leaves it open. Prenatal testing sometimes detects this problem. There are two major types of abdominal wall defects:

1. *Omphalocele.* In this type of defect, the muscle and skin that cover the wall of the abdomen is missing. As a result, the organs in the abdomen are covered by only a membrane. The amount of missing tissue varies from very little to most of the abdominal wall. Omphalocele occurs in about 1 in 5,000 births. A baby with this defect may have other defects as well. The outcome depends on whether there are problems.

2. *Gastroschisis.* In this disorder, part of the bowel sticks out through a hole in the abdominal wall. Unlike omphalocele, the defect isn't covered by a membrane. Most often, it's not linked with other defects. Gastroschisis occurs in about 1 in 8,000 births. Surgery often corrects the problem.

Genetic Tests

Some genetic tests are offered to all pregnant women. Others may be offered if your medical history, family history, or physical exam raise questions about your baby's health. Genetic tests can't find all problems. In fact, in most cases, these tests focus on a certain genetic problem. They do not look for all genetic problems that could occur. They're also not 100% accurate. Your fetus could have a birth defect even if testing doesn't show a problem. Also, if a positive test result raises a red flag, your baby likely will be healthy. Your genetic counselor can explain what the test results mean. He or she can also tell you what the chance is that the result isn't right.

There are two main types of genetic tests:

1. *Screening tests.* These tests are done as a matter of routine, even when a woman has no symptoms or known risk factors. Some screening tests are blood tests. A blood sample is taken from you and studied for certain things that can signal an increased risk for certain birth defects. It won't tell you if your baby has a defect, though. A positive screening test suggests that you may want to think about having diagnostic tests to check your baby's health. Screening tests include alpha-fetoprotein (AFP), multiple marker screening (MMS), and ultrasound.

2. *Diagnostic tests.* If a screening test or other factors raise concerns about your baby, these tests often can show whether the fetus has certain birth defects. If a woman is already at an increased risk of having a baby with a disorder, she may be offered the diagnostic test first. Diagnostic tests include amniocentesis, chorionic villus sampling (CVS), and ultrasound.

Maternal Serum Screening Tests

Maternal serum screening tests are used to find out if you have a higher-than-normal risk of having a baby with certain birth defects. These tests measure the level of certain substances in your blood. These levels may be higher or lower than normal if your fetus has open neural tube defects, Down syndrome, or abdominal wall defects. If the results raise concerns, screening tests are followed up with other tests. The two most common screening tests are AFP and MMS.

The Alpha-Fetoprotein Test

Alpha-fetoprotein is a substance made by the fetus. A small amount of AFP crosses the placenta and enters your blood.

This test is done between 16 and 18 weeks of pregnancy. A small amount of blood is taken from a vein in your arm and tested in a lab. Results come back in about a week. A high level of AFP can signal a risk of neural tube defects and certain other defects. A low level, though, can signal a risk of Down syndrome.

These tests may be alarming when the results are abnormal. Keep in mind, in most cases the baby is healthy even if there is an abnormal blood test result. These tests are used only to tell your doctor which women should be offered a diagnostic test.

A high AFP level can simply mean you are further along in pregnancy than you thought. It also can mean you're carrying more than one baby. A low level can mean the fetus is younger than you thought.

The Multiple Marker Screening Test

The multiple marker screening test measures the levels of estriol and human chorionic gonadotropin (hCG), as well as AFP, in your blood. Estriol is a hormone made by the placenta and the fetal liver, and hCG is a hormone made by the placenta. The multiple marker screening test can be done at the same time, using the same blood sample, as the AFP test. Most often, the results come back in about a week.

The MMS test is thought to be a better check for Down syndrome than AFP alone. If a fetus has Down syndrome, hCG levels often are higher than normal. Estriol and AFP levels often are lower than normal.

If the levels of these three markers are in the high-risk range, your doctor will offer you further testing. This might include ultrasound or amniocentesis. In almost all cases, a follow-up test shows that the baby is fine.

Much research is being done in this area. Soon, the test may be able to detect more chemicals.

Ultrasound

If the blood test showed an abnormal result, an ultrasound can help find out the reason. This test uses sound waves to create a picture of the fetus growing inside you. It can show:

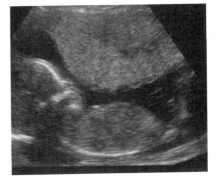

▶ Some information about the fetal anatomy

▶ The age of the fetus

▶ If you're carrying more than one fetus

▶ How well the fetus is growing

▶ The location of the placenta

▶ The fetal heart rate

About half the time, ultrasound explains why AFP levels are high. If your pregnancy is further along than you thought, for instance, it can alter screening results. The presence of twins also can affect AFP results. If ultrasound doesn't detect the reason, you may be offered amniocentesis.

Ultrasound also is used to follow up abnormal MMS results. Ultrasound can be used to check for signs of Down syndrome. It's not so good at ruling the disorder out, though. Because of this, amniocentesis may be an option for you. (See Chapter 17 for more information about ultrasound.)

Amniocentesis

Most often, amniocentesis is done at 16–18 weeks of pregnancy. To perform the procedure, a doctor uses ultrasound to guide a thin needle through your abdomen and uterus. A small sample of amniotic fluid is withdrawn and sent to a lab.

In the lab, cells that have been shed from the baby are grown in a special culture. This can take up to 3 weeks.

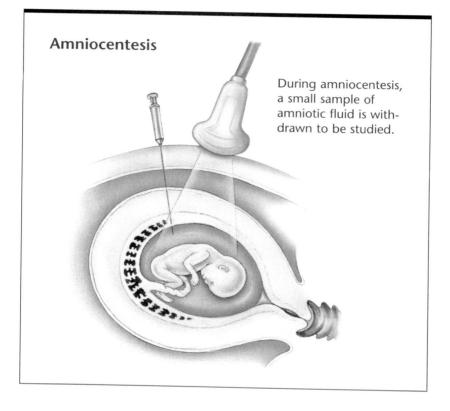

Amniocentesis

During amniocentesis, a small sample of amniotic fluid is withdrawn to be studied.

Next, the chromosomes in these cells are studied under a microscope. This shows if there's an extra chromosome (as in Down syndrome). It also can show if there are other chromosomal defects.

For a woman whose fetus is thought to be at risk for a single gene disorder—like cystic fibrosis or muscular dystrophy—the fetal cells can be studied to see if the fetus will have these conditions. However, such testing is only done on women whose genetic history suggests a risk for the single gene disorder.

Amniocentesis shows whether the fetus is male or female. It can help figure the risks of some genetic disorders. Also, testing the AFP level in the amniotic fluid can help determine if the fetus has an open neural tube defect.

Complications from amniocentesis are rare. Side effects may include cramping, vaginal bleeding, and leaking of amniotic fluid.

Very rarely, the fetus is injured. There is a slight chance of miscarriage as a result of amniocentesis.

Chorionic Villus Sampling

Chorionic villus sampling detects some of the same chromosomal problems as amniocentesis. It can be performed earlier, though—often at 10–12 weeks of pregnancy. Chorionic villus sampling is newer than amniocentesis. Fewer doctors are trained to perform CVS than are trained in amniocentesis. As a result, it isn't offered in all areas. You might need to travel to a center where it is performed.

To perform CVS, a doctor uses ultrasound to guide either a small tube through your vagina and cervix or a thin needle

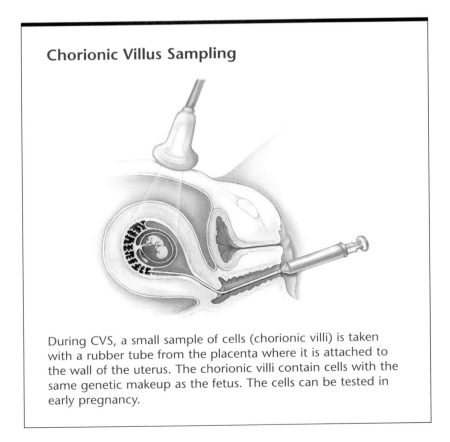

Chorionic Villus Sampling

During CVS, a small sample of cells (chorionic villi) is taken with a rubber tube from the placenta where it is attached to the wall of the uterus. The chorionic villi contain cells with the same genetic makeup as the fetus. The cells can be tested in early pregnancy.

Amniotic Fluid

Your baby grows nestled safely inside the amniotic sac. This sac is formed by two membranes: the amnion and the chorion. Inside the sac, a liquid called amniotic fluid collects to support and protect the fetus.

Amniotic fluid starts forming around the tiny embryo a few weeks after conception. At first, it's made up mostly of fluid from your body. Because the fetus swallows some of this fluid, new fluid is needed all the time.

As early as 11 weeks, the baby's kidneys start to put out weak urine. After 20 weeks, this urine makes up most of the amniotic fluid.

The fluid also has cells that have been shed from the skin of the fetus. These cells have all of the baby's genetic material. That's why amniotic fluid is sometimes used for prenatal testing.

Amniotic fluid helps your growing baby in many ways:

▸ It cushions the fetus if you fall or have an accident.

▸ The fluid puts pressure on the walls of your uterus. This gives the fetus room to grow.

▸ It provides a safe, warm place for the fetus to exercise muscles and practice the movements he or she will need after birth.

▸ The fetus breathes in and swallows amniotic fluid. This helps develop the baby's ability to breathe and swallow.

▸ This fluid stops the growth of some kinds of bacteria. This protects the fetus from infection.

through your abdomen and uterine wall. He or she then takes a small sample of chorionic villi from the placenta. Chorionic villi (the plural of villus) are tiny, fingerlike projections of tissue. Villi come from the same fertilized egg as the fetus. This means they have the same genetic makeup. The villi are sent to a lab, where they're grown in a culture. This can take up to 3 weeks. Chromosomes from the villi then are studied under a microscope to check for chromosomal or other certain genetic defects.

Chorionic villus sampling carries some risks. There's a small chance, for instance, that the test will cause miscarriage.

The Next Steps

As hard as it may be, try not to panic or give up hope if a screening test signals that further tests may be needed. To be sure, the days and weeks that lapse between having an alarming screening test result and finding out the results of other tests are among the worst in many couple's lives.

If there really is a problem, talk about the facts and your feelings with your partner, your family, your doctor, your genetic counselor, and others with whom you can share your thoughts. You may have to make some hard choices in a short time. There's no "right" choice in these cases. Your personal or religious values, your finances, the amount of support you have, and your baby's outlook will all come into play. The choice that's right for one couple may not be right for another.

Some couples choose to continue the pregnancy. If this is your choice, use the months before the birth to prepare yourself and your family. Line up special care from medical experts. Arrange to deliver at a hospital with facilities and specialists to care for your baby. Read as much as you can about your baby's condition. Join support groups for parents of children with the condition.

Other couples choose to end the pregnancy when a major problem is found. If this is your choice, it can be hard to come to terms with your loss and move on. The support of your loved ones is vital. You also must allow yourself time to grieve. You may want to seek counseling. (See Chapter 18 for advice on dealing with loss.)

Keep in mind, too, that a baby with major health problems can be a valued part of your family and your life. With help from your doctor and your loved ones, you can start to plan for your child's future. That way, he or she will have the best care right from the start and the best chance to lead a full and happy life.

CHAPTER 14

Medical Problems in Pregnancy

Pregnancy puts a lot of new demands on a woman's body. It can alter the course of a health problem that a woman already has. Some conditions can affect the pregnancy itself. It's best if any health problem is under control before a woman becomes pregnant. (See "Before You Become Pregnant" in Chapter 1.) This increases the chance that her baby will be born healthy.

Doctors keep close tabs on the health of women with medical problems that can affect their pregnancy—or vice versa. These women may need to have extra tests, see the doctor more often, or have special treatment. They may need to monitor their condition from home and check in often with the doctor. They may need to stay in the hospital while they are pregnant.

Women with medical problems can—and do—have healthy babies. It takes special care and extra effort, though. Doctors may work as a team of experts to make sure that both mother and baby receive the special care they need for the condition.

High Blood Pressure

Each time the heart beats, it pumps blood rich in oxygen into vessels called arteries. The arteries carry the blood to all parts of the body. After your organs and tissues take what they need from the blood, veins bring it back to the heart. There, it's refilled with oxygen. Then the whole process starts again.

Blood pressure is the pressure in the arteries that pushes the blood throughout the body. When the pressure becomes too high, it is known as hypertension, or high blood pressure. Women with long-term blood pressure problems before they became pregnant have what is called chronic hypertension.

Pregnancy also can cause high blood pressure in women who have never had it before. Blood pressure that goes up during pregnancy may be a sign of **pregnancy-induced hypertension.** This type of high blood pressure occurs only during pregnancy.

Small arteries, called arterioles, also affect blood pressure. These blood vessels are lined with a layer of muscle. When the blood pressure is normal, this muscle is relaxed and the arterioles dilate (open) so that

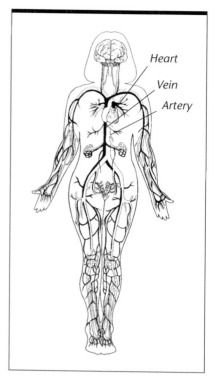

The heart pumps blood rich in oxygen through the arteries (light blood vessels) to the body. Veins (dark blood vessels) carry blood back to the heart.

blood can flow easily through them. If a signal is sent to increase the blood pressure, the muscle layer tightens and the arterioles become narrow. This makes it harder for the blood to flow. The pressure then rises in the arteries. Imagine that an arteriole is the nozzle on a hose. When the nozzle is open, the water can escape, so the pressure in the hose is normal. When it is closed, the water is trapped. The pressure in the hose rises, but less water comes out.

Both chronic and pregnancy-induced hypertension affect mothers-to-be and their babies in different ways. One effect may be that the fetus does not receive enough oxygen and nutrients to

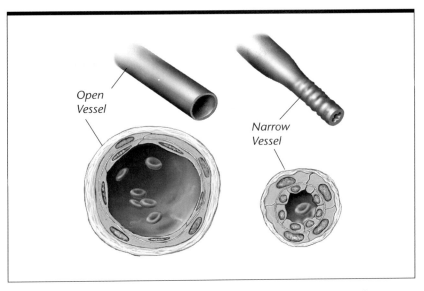

When your blood pressure is normal, blood vessels are open so that blood can flow easily through them. When your pressure is high, though, the vessels are narrow. This makes it harder for the blood to flow.

grow. Organs in the mother's body also may receive less blood than normal. The effects depend on how severe the problem is and how well it's managed. With pregnancy-induced hypertension, a woman's blood pressure returns to normal soon after delivery. With chronic hypertension, it stays high even after the baby is born.

Measuring Blood Pressure

During each visit to the doctor, your blood pressure is checked. This is done with a stethoscope and a device called a sphygmomanometer. The sphygmomanometer is made of a pressure gauge and an inflatable cuff that wraps around the upper arm.

A blood pressure reading has two numbers. Each is separated by a slash: 110/80, for instance. (You may hear this as "110 over 80.")

The first number is the pressure in the arteries when the heart contracts. This is called the *systolic blood pressure.* The second number is the pressure in the arteries when the heart relaxes. This is the *diastolic blood pressure.*

Blood pressure changes during the course of the day. It increases when you exert yourself or get excited, for instance. Most often, it decreases when you are resting. These short-term changes are normal. It's only when blood pressure stays high for some time that it may signal a problem.

When women have a high reading, it may be double-checked with a second reading. This helps prevent normal ups and downs in blood pressure from being confused with a problem. "Normal" blood pressure may be the average of a few readings that are taken while resting.

Blood pressure varies from person to person. In women who aren't pregnant, readings of 130/80 or less are normal. For women who are pregnant, a reading of 140/90 or higher is cause for concern. Blood pressure drops a bit during the middle part of pregnancy. It inches back up as the due date nears.

Your doctor checks your blood pressure before you get pregnant or in early pregnancy. This tells him or her what your normal level is. The doctor also will take a blood pressure reading at each prenatal visit. This way, he or she can spot an increase early.

Chronic High Blood Pressure

Diet, lifestyle, and heredity all play a role in causing chronic high blood pressure. If it isn't treated, it increases the risk of a heart attack or a stroke.

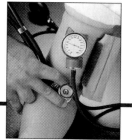

Your Blood Pressure Reading

110	systolic	pressure in arteries when heart contracts
____ =	____ =	
80	diastolic	pressure in arteries when heart relaxes

High blood pressure also poses a risk for problems during pregnancy. Babies may be born too small, for instance. The placenta may tear loose from the uterine wall before the baby is born. This is called abruptio placentae. For these reasons, it's vital for women to bring high blood pressure down before they get pregnant. They can do this by:

▶ Watching what they eat

▶ Losing weight, if needed

▶ Exercising

▶ Cutting down on alcohol and cigarettes

▶ Lowering stress

▶ Taking blood pressure medication if it is prescribed

Women with high blood pressure should be sure to go to all prenatal visits. That way, the doctor can check for blood pressure changes and other symptoms that may signal a problem. The doctor may switch medication to a safer type during pregnancy.

Pregnancy-Induced Hypertension

Pregnancy-induced hypertension may lead to preeclampsia, *eclampsia*, or toxemia. Most often, it occurs after the 20th week of pregnancy. Pregnancy-induced hypertension affects about 7 out of 100 pregnant women. No one knows for sure what causes it.

Signs of high blood pressure during pregnancy include sudden weight gain, swelling of the hands and face, and protein in the urine. At each prenatal visit, the doctor may check for swelling and ask for a urine sample.

Women with chronic high blood pressure are more likely to get pregnancy-induced hypertension. In most cases, though, women with pregnancy-induced hypertension have never had high blood pressure. Others at increased risk include women who:

▶ Are pregnant for the first time

▶ Are African American

▶ Are older than age 40

▶ Are carrying more than one fetus

▶ Have diabetes or kidney disease

▶ Have blood vessel problems (other than varicose veins)

▶ Have a family history of pregnancy-induced hypertension

In most cases, pregnancy-induced hypertension doesn't come back in later pregnancies. Women with chronic hypertension, blood vessel problems, or kidney disease are more likely to have pregnancy-induced hypertension again, though.

Pregnancy-induced hypertension can range from mild to severe. It can slowly worsen or slowly improve. It also can get worse very quickly. The degree of risk to mother and baby depends on how severe the problem is and when it starts.

Pregnancy-induced hypertension is harmful because it can reduce the blood flow through the vessels in the uterus. This may deprive the baby of oxygen and nutrients. As a result, the fetus may not grow as much as it should.

If pregnancy-induced hypertension isn't controlled, it also can damage the mother's heart, liver, kidneys, and brain. Preeclampsia may occur. In severe cases, it can lead to seizures—a severe contraction of the muscles. If that happens, the disease is called eclampsia. In rare cases, this can be fatal.

Warning Signs and Symptoms of Pregnancy-Induced Hypertension

Call your doctor right away if you have:

▶ Headaches that are constant or severe

▶ Swelling (edema) in the face or hands

▶ Pain in the upper right part of your abdomen

▶ Blurred vision or spots in front of your eyes

▶ Sudden weight gain—1 pound a day or more

As long as pregnancy-induced hypertension is mild, rest may be advised. This should help lower blood pressure or bring it back to normal. Women also may be told to lie on their side. This improves blood flow to the uterus and kidneys. Tests such as ultrasound or electronic fetal monitoring may be used to make sure the baby is healthy and growing well.

If rest doesn't help, women may be checked into the hospital. There, doctors will try to bring their blood pressure into a safe range.

Sometimes pregnancy-induced hypertension can't be controlled, even in a hospital. If the condition is severe or progresses to eclampsia, the baby may need to be delivered right away.

It's best to postpone delivery until the baby is fully grown. That's because a preterm baby may have problems, such as trouble breathing because his or her lungs aren't fully formed. Waiting isn't always possible, though. In some cases, staying in the uterus is more of a risk than being born too early.

Diabetes

Diabetes occurs when the body has trouble making or using insulin. Insulin is a hormone that converts glucose in food into energy. Glucose is a sugar that is the body's main source of fuel. If there isn't enough insulin, or if the insulin doesn't convert enough glucose into fuel, the level of glucose in the blood becomes too high. Good control of the levels of blood glucose lowers the risks to the mother and fetus.

Some women have diabetes before they become pregnant. Others develop the disease during pregnancy. In either case, insulin may be needed to control glucose levels.

Gestational Diabetes

When a woman develops diabetes during pregnancy, it's called gestational diabetes. It results from hormones made by the placenta. These hormones can alter the way insulin works.

Taking It Easy

One of the most common treatments for certain problems in pregnancy is a simple one: rest. It's rare to need total bed rest during pregnancy. Some women, though, are asked to limit their activity. Following are tips to help women cope when they have been asked to restrict their activity:

▶ Find out just what your doctor means by "bed rest." Can you spend any time on your feet? If so, how much? Do you need to stay in a certain position, such as on your side or propped up? (Don't lie flat on your back in the last half of pregnancy.) Can you use the bathroom, or must you use a bed pan? Can you do some work from bed? What other activities can you do?

▶ Make arrangements. You may need to go on leave from your job, arrange childcare, or check into disability pay.

▶ Call in extra help. Depending on what you can and can't do, you might have to line up full-time childcare and find someone to fix meals, clean house, run errands, and so on.

▶ Set up your room so things are in easy reach. This way, you won't have to get out of bed to answer the phone or hunt for the TV remote control, books and magazines, prescription medications, paper and pen, toiletries, and hobbies such as crossword puzzles.

▶ Stick to a daily routine. Wake up at the same time each day. Plan activities. This will help you feel more in control.

▶ Eat right. Don't gorge on junk food because you are bored. Be sure to eat fruits and vegetables and drink lots of fluids. Lack of activity can bring on constipation. A healthy diet will help prevent it.

Glucose levels often return to normal after delivery. A woman who has gestational diabetes has a higher risk of developing diabetes later.

Nearly half of the women who develop gestational diabetes have no known risk factors. But certain things put a woman at risk:

▶ Being older than age 30

▶ Being obese (See BMI chart in Chapter 1)

Taking It Easy (continued)

▶ Exercise. If your doctor says it is OK, flex your muscles while you lie in bed. It will help you relax and avoid stiffness. Ask the doctor if it's safe to try deep breathing, pelvic tilts, leg lifts, neck circles, and Kegel exercises. If you can't exercise, take some deep breaths every 20 minutes and wiggle your fingers and toes. This helps your blood circulate.

▶ Let your family come to you. If you can't join your partner at the dinner table, for instance, have a cozy "picnic" in bed. If you have an older child, plan quiet activities that you can do together on the bed. Reading story books, cutting out shapes, and doing puzzles will help you spend quality time with your children.

▶ Shop from home. You can't hit the mall to outfit your baby's nursery, but you can stock up on the items your little one will need. Send friends and family out with lists of items to pick up for you. Leaf through catalogs and place your orders by phone. If you have a computer, you can even buy baby gear on the Internet.

▶ Get some support. There are groups that put women who are confined to bed in touch with others who have had to do the same thing. Check with your doctor or local hospitals to find a support group near you.

▶ Accept your situation rather than fight it. Allow your partner, family, and friends to take care of you. Don't feel guilty about the things you can't do. Instead, focus on what you can do to help your baby.

▶ Keep your eyes on the prize. Staying in bed for days, weeks, or even months is not easy. Think of the sacrifices you are making as an act of love for the child you are carrying.

▶ Having a family history of diabetes

▶ Being a member of an ethnic group with a high rate of the disease

Gestational diabetes often causes no symptoms. To be on the safe side, the doctor may ask you for a urine sample at each prenatal visit. The urine then is tested for the presence of glucose.

The doctor may test for diabetes in other ways. This simple test is called a glucose screening. It's often given at 24–28 weeks of pregnancy. During the test, the patient drinks a special sugar mixture. An hour later, a blood sample is drawn from her arm and sent to a lab. There, a technician measures the level of glucose in the blood.

If the glucose screening test shows the level is high, the patient is given a glucose tolerance test. This test is similar to a glucose screening. However, it lasts longer—about 3 hours—and requires four blood samples. The test is taken on an empty stomach.

Women with mild gestational diabetes may be able to control their blood glucose levels with a special diet and exercise. If the problem is more severe, they will need to take insulin. They will need to test the level of glucose in their blood each day, too. They must watch their diet and insulin dose closely to keep blood glucose levels in check.

If diabetes isn't controlled, the extra sugar in the blood raises the odds of *macrosomia*. Babies with macrosomia are overly large. They weigh 10 pounds or more. They may be too big to fit safely through the birth canal.

Overly large babies often have health problems. They include:

▸ Low glucose levels

▸ Low blood calcium and magnesium levels

▸ Too many red blood cells

▸ Jaundice

▸ Breathing problems

To see how the baby is doing, the doctor may order special tests. Ultrasound may be used to assess the baby's weight. Amniocentesis can show if the baby's lungs are mature enough to handle an early delivery.

A few months after birth, the doctor may order another glucose tolerance test. This will confirm whether the patient still has diabetes.

If the disease subsides, steps can be taken to stay healthy. Overweight women, for instance, can follow a balanced program of diet and exercise. This may lower the odds of problems in future pregnancies. It also may help reduce the risk of getting diabetes later in life.

Diabetes Before Pregnancy

About 1 woman in 100 has diabetes before she gets pregnant. At one time, the disease posed a major health threat to both mother and baby during pregnancy. Today, though, doctors know much more about how to control diabetes. As a result, pregnancy is safer than ever for most women with diabetes. The risks involved are now almost as low as those for any woman without the disease.

For a woman who has diabetes, it's best that the disease be brought under control *before* she is pregnant. During her pregnancy, a woman and her doctor should monitor her health closely and keep blood glucose levels in check. With planning, control, and expert care, the chances she will stay healthy and have a healthy baby are very good.

Diabetes can't be cured. It can only be controlled. Women who have chronic diabetes should get early care to help lower the risks related to the disease:

▸ *Miscarriage.* Women with diabetes have a higher risk of pregnancy loss. The risk is even greater for women whose condition isn't under control.

▸ *Birth defects.* Heart defects, kidney defects, and spinal problems are more common in babies whose mothers have diabetes. This is even more true if the disease isn't well managed.

▸ *Pregnancy-induced hypertension.* Pregnancy-induced hypertension can slow the baby's growth in the uterus or require an early delivery.

▸ *Hydramnios* (too much amniotic fluid). Hydramnios may make it hard for the mother to breathe. It also can lead to preterm labor and birth.

▶ *Macrosomia.* An overly large baby can make it hard to give birth vaginally. If the doctor suspects that a woman's baby has grown too large, he or she will talk about options for delivery. Whether she has a vaginal birth or cesarean birth depends on a number of factors.

▶ *Stillbirth.* Although stillbirth is rare, mothers with diabetes are more likely to lose their babies than women without the disease.

▶ **Respiratory distress syndrome (RDS).** Respiratory distress syndrome can occur when the baby's lungs aren't fully developed. This can affect his or her breathing after birth.

Controlling Diabetes

A woman who has diabetes should do a number of things to keep her glucose levels under control.

▶ Watch her diet. The amount of calories she needs depends on how much she weighs. Even if diabetes is well-controlled, she may need to follow a new diet during pregnancy. She might have to adjust her diet from time to time, too. This will help lower glucose levels or better meet the growing baby's needs. Most often, the diet consists of special meals and snacks spread over the course of the day. A bedtime snack helps keep blood glucose at the right level during the night.

▶ Exercise. Exercise lowers the amount of insulin the body needs to keep blood glucose at normal levels. The kind and amount of exercise needed depends on the woman's health and fitness level and how far along the pregnancy is.

▶ Take insulin if it is prescribed. Insulin shots or pills will help blood glucose stay at a normal level. It doesn't cross the placenta, so it doesn't affect the fetus directly. How much insulin is needed and how often depend on a number of factors. Many women take insulin at least twice a day during pregnancy. It's likely that insulin needs will increase during pregnancy and level off near the end. This means the dosage will have to be adjusted from time to time.

▶ Keep tabs on blood glucose levels. To find out how much insulin is needed, a woman with diabetes must monitor blood glucose levels at home each day. In fact, blood glucose levels may need to be checked a few times a day. There are many ways to do this. Two common methods are using a blood glucose meter or colored strips. For either, a simple device is used to get a small drop of blood. Most often, this blood comes from the tip of the finger. Then, the blood is put in a meter that measures the blood glucose level. It also may be put on a strip of special paper. Next, the color on the paper is compared with the colors on a chart. This will help pinpoint the blood glucose level.

Special Care

Women who have diabetes need special medical care during pregnancy. They may:

▶ See the doctor more often

▶ See a doctor who has special training in diabetes care

▶ Work with a dietitian to develop a meal plan

▶ Stay in the hospital if treatment at home isn't working

Certain tests also may be needed during pregnancy. These tests will help spot any problems that arise. Then steps can be taken to correct or reduce these problems.

One such test measures hemoglobin A_{1C}. This is a substance in the blood. When the level increases, it means glucose levels have been poorly controlled for a number of weeks.

Women with diabetes may need tests such as ultrasound, amniocentesis, and fetal monitoring, too. This allows the doctor to track fetal growth and tell how the baby is doing. These tests are even more important if the baby needs to be delivered early.

Most women are able to have a vaginal birth when it's time for the baby to be born. In years past, nearly all mothers with diabetes had cesarean births. That was because the stress of labor and delivery could worsen some of the problems linked with diabetes. These days, though, special tests and monitoring during pregnancy can help prevent many of these problems.

Heart Disease

Many women think of heart disease as something that happens only to older people. Heart disease also can affect about 1% of pregnant women.

Some women have rheumatic heart disease that can affect them during childbearing. Rheumatic heart disease is caused by an infection called rheumatic fever. This infection can occur in childhood and can damage the heart valves. Modern medicine has made both rheumatic fever and the heart problems linked with it rare in this country.

A woman with congenital heart disease is born with a defect in her heart. The heart might have a hole between two of the four chambers, for instance. Half of all women with heart disease during pregnancy have congenital defects. The risk of problems during pregnancy depends on the type of defect and how severe it is.

Ideally, heart disease is diagnosed before a woman gets pregnant. Then doctors can take the steps needed to correct the condition.

Women who have heart disease should talk to the doctor before trying to conceive. Some patients may be referred to a cardiologist who is an expert in heart disease. The cardiologist can provide details on the impact heart disease can have on pregnancy and on how pregnancy may affect the heart.

Sometimes doctors with different types of training will team up to manage a patient's care. They may prescribe certain medications, extra rest, and limits on activities. Pregnancy makes the heart work harder. The amount of blood this organ pumps out increases by as much as 40% during pregnancy. Taking it easy will help offset the extra demands on the heart.

Some women with heart disease have an artificial heart valve and take pills to thin the blood. They may be switched to other medication while they are pregnant. They also will need *antibiotics* during delivery. Women with congenital heart defects also will need antibiotics during delivery.

Labor and delivery put added stress on the heart, too. During labor, contractions increase the heart's workload. Even so, vaginal delivery is safer than cesarean birth in most cases. More problems may result from surgery than from vaginal delivery. The pain and anxiety that sometimes go along with labor also can take a toll on the heart. Pain medication will help reduce this problem. The doctor may suggest the use of forceps or vacuum extraction to decrease the amount of pushing and shorten labor time.

Heart disease can raise the risk of early delivery or a small baby. Also, babies of women who have congenital heart disease have a 4–5% chance of having the disease as well. It may not be severe, though. In some cases, ultrasound can spot heart defects before birth.

Lung Disorders

During pregnancy, the growing uterus alters the shape of the chest cavity. This, in turn, changes breathing patterns. It's normal to feel short of breath during the later part of pregnancy. (For hints on dealing with this, see "Shortness of Breath" in Chapter 7.) Some lung disorders, though, can cause some problems:

▶ *Asthma.* This lung disease causes wheezing and trouble with breathing. The condition can deprive the mother and fetus of oxygen if it's not treated. Most asthma medicine is safe to use during pregnancy. Women should not stop using their inhaler or taking prescribed pills when they get pregnant. They should first talk to the doctor about these medications. Women with severe asthma more than likely will keep having attacks while they are pregnant. Regular medical care is vital. This way, the doctor can keep tabs on the baby's health and help the mother control her asthma.

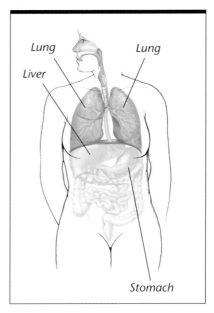

Lung

Lung

Liver

Stomach

‣ *Pneumonia.* This lung infection may be more severe in pregnancy than it is at other times. It can cause both mother and baby to get less oxygen. Women who think they may have pneumonia should see the doctor right away. He or she may order a chest X-ray to confirm the condition. This type of X-ray isn't thought to be harmful during pregnancy. A woman should tell both the doctor and the X-ray technician that she's pregnant. To be on the safe side, a lead apron will be draped over the belly to shield the fetus from radiation.

A women who has pneumonia needs to take antibiotics. She may have to stay in the hospital until the infection clears up.

Kidney Disease

If the kidneys are scarred from a prior illness or don't function the way they should, it could affect pregnancy. The risks of kidney disease in pregnancy include miscarriage, hypertension, preterm birth, and stillbirth. Some forms of kidney disease can be passed to the baby. An ultrasound exam may be done to check for them. With good medical care, risks can be lowered.

Kidney disease often can be diagnosed from the patient's medical history, physical exam, and blood and urine tests. Protein in the urine can signal kidney disease, for instance. This is another reason why the doctor may ask for a urine sample at each prenatal visit.

Seizure Disorders

Epilepsy and certain other disorders cause seizures (convulsions). A seizure can consist of a few muscle twitches, or it can be a major attack that causes a blackout and loss of bladder or bowel control.

Most women with seizure disorders have healthy babies. Even so, these women deliver babies with birth defects two to three times more often than normal. Cleft lip, cleft palate, and heart defects are the most common problems in babies born to women with seizure disorders. No one is certain just why these problems occur. Some of the medications used to treat the condition may be the cause. Also, the disease itself can be a factor.

During pregnancy, women should not stop taking their medication for a seizure disorder without talking to the doctor first. In some cases, seizures may be more harmful than the medication used to control or prevent them.

The amount of medication needed often changes during pregnancy. The doctor will monitor drug levels and adjust the dosage as needed. With good control of drug levels, there should be little change in the number or strength of seizures.

Medications that treat seizure disorders can use up stores of folic acid. This is a vital nutrient during pregnancy. Taking folic acid supplements will lower the risk of having a baby with a neural tube defect (see "Genetic Disorders and Birth Defects" in Chapter 13). These defects are linked with not getting enough folic acid.

Autoimmune Disorders

Autoimmune disorders are a group of diseases in which the immune system goes awry. Instead of protecting the body from disease, the immune system attacks the body's own tissues. As a result, organs such as the thyroid or other parts of the body can be injured.

Many autoimmune diseases have symptoms that overlap with other illnesses. This makes them hard to detect. Most of these disorders are chronic. Often, they have no cure because the cause isn't always known. Symptoms may go away for a time, then flare up with little warning and no clear reason. For women who suffer from an autoimmune disorder, its effect on pregnancy depends on the type of disorder and how severe it is. Their doctor may work with a specialist to plan care during pregnancy.

Systemic Lupus Erythematosus

Systemic lupus erythematosus (SLE) is a disease that can affect the whole body, including the skin, joints, kidneys, and nervous system. Some women with SLE may have a rash on their face. Others develop a more severe condition that causes their kidneys to fail and affects their nervous system, heart, and blood.

Systemic lupus erythematosus tends to strike women during their childbearing years. It doesn't seem to affect a woman's ability to get pregnant. It does raise the risk of miscarriage, preterm birth, and stillbirth, though. Systemic lupus erythematosus also can slow the fetal heart rate.

In about one third of women, SLE gets worse during pregnancy. Symptoms can flare up after delivery, too. A woman with SLE whose kidneys aren't affected and who goes 6 months without symptoms before getting pregnant is less likely to have problems during pregnancy.

Systemic lupus erythematosus is treated with medications called *corticosteroids*. During pregnancy, only about 10% of this medicine reaches the fetus.

Aspirin or medication like aspirin also can be taken to control joint pain. Most often, the doctor will keep the dosage low to prevent side effects such as fetal bleeding.

Rheumatoid Arthritis

Rheumatoid arthritis often is thought of as a disease of the joints. It causes pain, soreness, heat, and swelling in the small- and medium-sized joints. Many women also have stiffness in the morning and a general feeling of fatigue and discomfort.

Rheumatoid arthritis can flare up and then lessen for a time, or it can get worse and damage the joints. The disease also can affect the blood. This can lead to severe anemia. It can affect the heart and lungs, too.

During pregnancy, rheumatoid arthritis often is treated with aspirinlike medications. Sometimes other drugs are used as well. Many women find that their symptoms lessen during pregnancy. Some have a relapse between 6 weeks and 6 months after giving birth, though.

Antiphospholipid Antibody Syndrome

Women with antiphospholipid antibody syndrome have high levels of a certain antibody in their blood. Antibodies are proteins that protect the body against disease.

Antiphospholipid antibody syndrome can cause blood clots and bleeding problems. Injuries may bleed longer than normal, for instance. During pregnancy, the disorder can cause miscarriage. It also can slow fetal growth or cause fetal death. Antiphospholipid antibody syndrome often is treated with anticoagulant therapy (blood thinners).

Thyroid Disease

The thyroid is a gland in the neck that controls key body functions. Certain disorders cause the thyroid to release too much or too little thyroid hormone. Either can harm a mother or her fetus during pregnancy.

Hypothyroidism means the thyroid isn't as active as it should be. This condition is treated with thyroid hormone pills.

Hyperthyroidism means the thyroid is too active. This condition is treated with medications that help reduce the amount of thyroid hormone the body makes.

Women who have a thyroid problem that's well controlled shouldn't have any special problems during pregnancy. To ensure the best treatment, the doctor will order blood tests to pinpoint the best medication dosage.

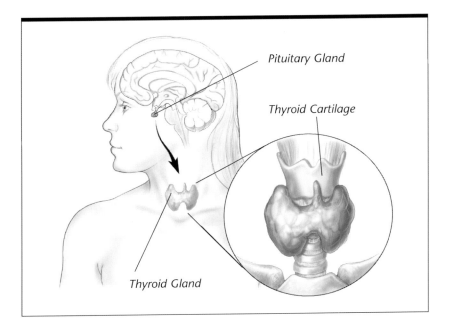

Pituitary Gland

Thyroid Cartilage

Thyroid Gland

Physical Disability

For women who are physically disabled, pregnancy and being a parent pose special challenges. That doesn't mean they can't—or shouldn't—become mothers.

It's a good idea for women with disabilities and their partners to meet with the doctor before getting pregnant. This will help reduce the odds of medical problems during pregnancy.

Talking to the doctor ahead of time also will help in preparing for pregnancy and being a parent. Your doctor can suggest community resources that will benefit the family.

Special care will be needed after pregnancy begins, too. The doctor may work closely with the primary care physician or other specialists, for instance. He or she also may suggest occupational or physical therapy to help women better cope with the stresses pregnancy puts on the body.

Before the baby arrives, special equipment may have to be installed or modified at home to help in caring for the baby. Leaving the hospital may require postpartum home care for mother and baby as well.

Mental Illness

Mental illness may have a genetic factor. Women with a mental illness may want to see a genetic counselor before they become pregnant. Women with a history of mental illness should tell their doctor about their condition and medical history. The doctor also needs to know if medications are used to control such a disorder. This will help ensure the needed care is given for a healthy pregnancy.

Women with a mental illness should not stop taking medication that has been prescribed unless their doctor and mental health provider say it is OK. In many cases, keeping a mental condition under control outweighs any possible risks from the drugs used to treat it.

Mental illness can affect pregnancy in a number of ways. As many as 1 in 6 pregnant women have mental health problems, including:

- Mood disorders, such as severe depression and bipolar disorder

- Schizophrenia

- Anxiety disorders, such as obsessive–compulsive disorder and phobia

- Personality disorders

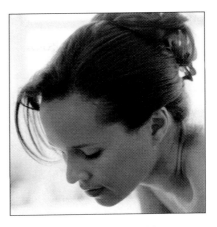

A woman who has a mental illness that is not treated may do things that could harm her baby. She may have trouble eating well, getting enough rest, or taking care of herself in other ways. She also may be less likely to get regular prenatal care.

Many women take prescription medications to treat mental or emotional disorders. In some cases, these medications can harm a growing fetus. For other medications, the effect on the fetus simply isn't known. In still other cases, a medication is thought to be safe during pregnancy—or at least safer than the effects of going without it.

Even if the baby's health isn't an issue, being pregnant can cause mental illness to worsen. For others, it causes emotional problems to occur again. Why? Even if a woman wants to become a mother, pregnancy often is a very stressful time. For a woman prone to anxiety, for instance, pregnancy brings with it all sorts of new things to worry about—going through labor and delivery, the baby's health, or family finances. This, in turn, can worsen a mental or emotional problem.

During pregnancy, the doctor should be told right away if a patient's mental state is a danger. He or she can arrange for counseling or community agencies to provide social or mental health services. It's vital for both mother and baby that these services be used if they are needed.

Mental health care is vital after the baby's born, too. Although it's rare, some women have a problem after delivery. Women with mental health problems are 20 times more likely to be admitted to a hospital for a psychiatric illness in the month after giving birth than they are in the 2 years that lead up to it. They also are more likely to have postpartum depression.

The first weeks after a newborn arrives can be stressful for any woman. The more help mothers have during these early weeks, the more comfortable they'll feel as they adjust to being a mother. They should ask for support from their partner and loved ones and seek counseling if they need it. Community services can help as well.

What Women Can Do

Women who have a chronic illness should see a doctor before getting pregnant. It's best to get the disease under control first. This will lower the risks as well as raise the odds of staying healthy during pregnancy and having a healthy baby.

Pre-pregnancy and prenatal care is vital even when the condition is well-controlled. Because some of these conditions can be passed to the baby, genetic counseling may be a good idea. Keep in mind that the treatment routine worked out with a primary care doctor or specialist may need to change during pregnancy. Medications may need to change. Sometimes it should be taken more or less often, the dosage needs to be changed, or a safer medication needs to be used during pregnancy.

If women are just learning that they have an illness, it can come as a shock. On top of learning about pregnancy and birth, they must learn how to care for a medical condition. A doctor can help women adjust and work out a treatment plan.

CHAPTER 15

Complications of Pregnancy

Although pregnancy and childbirth are natural events, problems can arise. They may be minor or major. Some problems require prompt treatment or special care to do the best for the mother and her baby. Some women have certain risk factors that increase their chances of problems. In even the most healthy and fit women, though, things can go wrong with no warning.

If you have a high-risk pregnancy, your doctor and health care team will watch your progress closely. They will adjust your prenatal care as needed and give you special care through labor and delivery. If you suspect or find any problems, such as the ones described here, contact your doctor.

Infection

An infection can be passed from the mother to the fetus during pregnancy or to the baby as it is born. Both the mother and the baby have a natural defense to many infections and can fight them when they occur, but some agents can cross the placenta and infect the fetus in the uterus (see Chapter 16).

Only a small number of babies get infected during or after birth. Hospitals have policies aimed at stopping the spread of infection. The hospital staff will check your baby for signs of infection. They can advise you on ways to decrease the risk, such as washing your hands often, using good hygiene when you feed the baby, caring for the umbilical cord properly, and staying away from people with infections.

Vaginal Bleeding

Vaginal bleeding in pregnancy has many causes. When bleeding occurs, its cause must be found. To do this, your doctor or nurse may ask you questions, examine you, or do special tests. In many cases, the bleeding stops and the baby is carried to term with no problems.

Sometimes bleeding is a serious problem. Your health and that of your fetus may depend on prompt treatment. You should report any bleeding to your doctor or nurse. He or she can decide the proper course of action based on the symptoms, signs, and stage of pregnancy.

Early Pregnancy

At the start of pregnancy, some women may have light bleeding (spotting or staining). It happens when the fertilized egg becomes attached to the lining of the uterus. Some women may confuse this bleeding with a menstrual period. When there is doubt, lab tests can confirm you are pregnant.

Warning Signs in Early Pregnancy

Call your doctor if you have:

- Spotting or bleeding with or without pain
- Heavy or constant bleeding with abdominal pain or cramping
- A gush of fluid from your vagina but no pain or bleeding (you may need an exam to see if your membranes have broken)

If you have heavy bleeding and think you have passed fetal tissue, place it in a clean jar and take it to the doctor to be checked. Your doctor will want to examine you to see if your cervix has dilated.

During early pregnancy, there is a chance of a miscarriage. This means the pregnancy ends before the fetus can survive outside the uterus. Miscarriage occurs in about 15–20% of all pregnancies, often during the first 3 months. Bleeding is the most common sign that a miscarriage may occur. Another sign is cramping pain in the lower abdomen. This pain often comes and goes. The pain often is stronger than menstrual cramps.

Many women who have bleeding have little or no cramping. In more than half of the women who bleed in early pregnancy, the bleeding stops and the pregnancy goes on to term. At other times, the bleeding and cramping become more heavy and strong, ending in miscarriage.

A miscarriage often occurs without known cause. Some women may have more than one miscarriage. If she has three in a row, she may have a problem that causes her to miscarry. She will need more tests to see if there is a problem and if it can be treated. The woman may be advised to see a doctor with special skills in this area.

When bleeding occurs in early pregnancy, you may be given a pelvic exam and a repeat pregnancy test. Ultrasound, which creates pictures of the internal organs and the fetus from sound waves, may be used to decide if:

▪ The pregnancy is ectopic (located outside the uterus).

▪ Miscarriage has occurred or is about to occur.

▪ You have a normal pregnancy with some bleeding.

Often when miscarriage occurs early in pregnancy, tissue is left in the uterus. If this happens, the bleeding may not stop. In such cases, the tissue is removed by a surgical technique called *dilation and curettage (D&C)*. The cervix is widened (dilation). Then the tissue is gently scraped (curettage) or suctioned from the lining of the uterus.

The cause of some miscarriages is not known. Miscarriage may be the body's way of dealing with a pregnancy that may not be growing as it should. A miscarriage doesn't always mean that a woman can't become pregnant again. Nor does it always mean

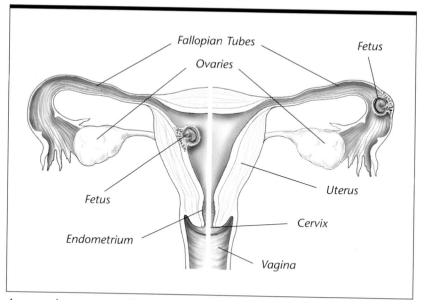

A normal pregnancy (*left*) occurs in the uterus. An ectopic pregnancy (*right*) may occur in the fallopian tube.

that something is wrong with her health. There is no evidence that emotional stress or physical or sexual activity causes miscarriage.

Late Pregnancy

The cause of bleeding during the second half of pregnancy may be something minor. If the cervix becomes inflamed, for instance, it can cause bleeding.

Some bleeding can be severe, though. It may pose a threat to the woman or the fetus. Contact your doctor or nurse right away if you have any bleeding in late pregnancy. You may need to go to the hospital for special care.

Heavy vaginal bleeding often suggests a problem with the placenta. The most common problems are abruptio placentae and placenta previa. With abruptio placentae, the placenta comes loose from the wall of the uterus before or during birth. This often causes vaginal bleeding and constant, severe pain in the abdomen. The fetus may get less oxygen, which could be harmful.

Dilation and Curettage

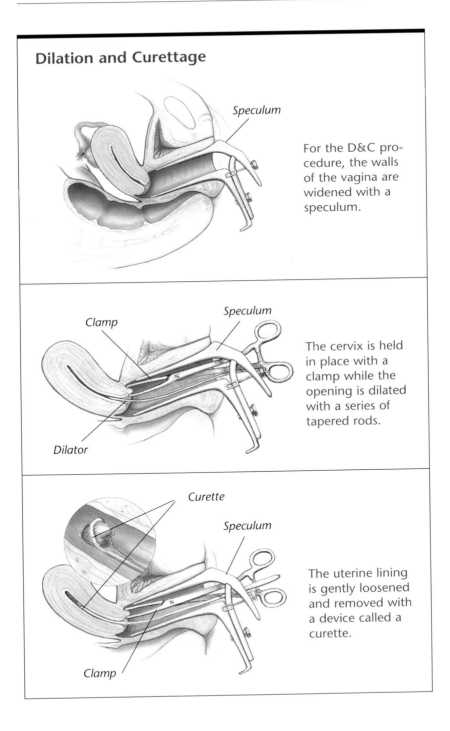

Speculum

For the D&C pro-
cedure, the walls
of the vagina are
widened with a
speculum.

Clamp

Speculum

Dilator

The cervix is held
in place with a
clamp while the
opening is dilated
with a series of
tapered rods.

Curette

Speculum

Clamp

The uterine lining
is gently loosened
and removed with
a device called a
curette.

Placental Problems

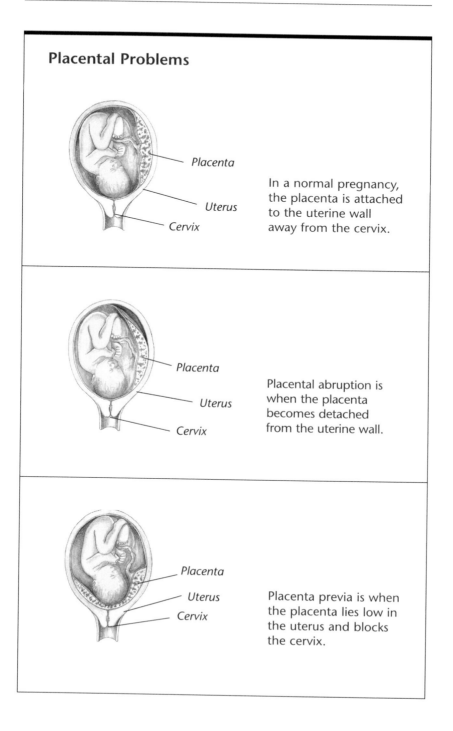

Placenta

Uterus

Cervix

In a normal pregnancy, the placenta is attached to the uterine wall away from the cervix.

Placenta

Uterus

Cervix

Placental abruption is when the placenta becomes detached from the uterine wall.

Placenta

Uterus

Cervix

Placenta previa is when the placenta lies low in the uterus and blocks the cervix.

With placenta previa, the placenta lies low in the uterus and covers part or all of the cervix. This blocks the baby's exit from the uterus. When the cervix starts to open in women who have placenta previa, they bleed. This requires prompt care.

If you have bleeding in late pregnancy, your doctor may suggest you have an ultrasound exam. Sometimes, you may need to stay in the hospital for a few weeks. Both abruptio placentae and placenta previa may be severe enough to require that the baby be born early. In this case, the baby likely will be delivered by cesarean birth.

Blood Group Incompatibility

Each person's blood is one of four major types: A, B, AB, or O. Blood types are determined by the types of *antigens* on the blood cells. Antigens are proteins on the surface of blood cells that can cause a response from the immune system.

Type A blood has only A antigens, type B has only B antigens, type AB has both A and B antigens, and type O has neither A nor B antigens. There are other antigens that can make blood types even more specific. One of the most common is the Rh factor.

As part of your prenatal care, you will have blood tests to find out your blood type. If your blood lacks the Rh antigen, it is called Rh negative. If it has the antigen, it is called Rh positive. More than 85% of people in the world are Rh positive.

When the mother is Rh negative and the father is Rh positive, the fetus can inherit the Rh factor from the father. This makes the fetus Rh positive, too. Problems can arise when the fetus's blood has the Rh factor and the mother's blood does not.

If a small amount of the fetus's blood mixes with the mother's blood, which often happens, the mother's body may respond as if it were allergic to the fetus. It may make antibodies to the Rh antigens in the fetus's blood. This means the mother has become sensitized. Her antibodies then can attack the fetus's blood. The antibodies will break down its red blood cells and cause anemia. This can lead to severe illness or even death in the fetus or newborn.

Sensitization and Rh Immune Globulin

Sensitization can occur any time fetal blood mixes with the mother's blood. This can happen during pregnancy or after an abortion, miscarriage, ectopic pregnancy, or amniocentesis. After any of these events, an Rh-negative woman often is given RhIg to prevent sensitization. Its effects seem to last only about 12 weeks. Thus, it is given again any time blood from the fetus and mother might mix.

A small number of Rh-negative women become sensitized during the last 3 months of pregnancy. To prevent this, they may be given RhIg near 28 weeks. When an Rh-negative woman gives birth to an Rh-positive baby, she will be given a dose of RhIg soon after delivery. This is the case even if she received a dose at 28 weeks. The dose of RhIg will remove the risk to the fetus during her next pregnancy. Repeat doses of RhIg are given each time the woman gives birth to an Rh-positive child.

It is safe for pregnant women to receive RhIg. The only known side effects are soreness from the injection or a slight fever. There is no risk of infection with human immunodeficiency virus (HIV) with RhIg.

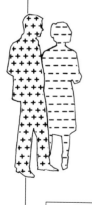

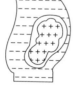

1st pregnancy: An Rh-negative woman may have an Rh-positive fetus.

- Rh-negative
+ Rh-positive
⊕ Antibodies

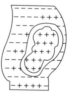

Cells from Rh-positive fetus enter the mother's bloodstream. Woman may become sensitized—antibodies form to fight Rh-positive cells.

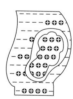

2nd pregnancy: in the next Rh-positive pregnancy, antibodies attack fetal blood cells.

The first pregnancy poses little risk. It takes time for the mother's antibodies to build up after being exposed to the antigens. Once they are formed, though, antibodies do not go away. The best course is to keep the mother from being sensitized and forming antibodies in the first place.

If you are Rh negative and blood tests show that you have not become sensitized, your doctor will prescribe *Rh immune globulin (RhIg)* shots. This blood product prevents the mother from forming antibodies. It will be given during pregnancy, at about 28 weeks. It also is given again right after the birth of your first baby (if your baby is Rh positive) to prevent harm to your next child. You also will need to be given RhIg if you had a miscarriage and certain procedures during pregnancy.

If you have become sensitized already, your fetus is at risk. As the weeks of your pregnancy go by, your doctor will check the levels of antibodies in your blood. If they become high, tests may be done to check the health of your fetus.

The fetus may be anemic. If so, the fetus will need a blood transfusion. After 18 weeks of pregnancy, the transfusion can be given while the fetus is still in the uterus. If the fetus is old enough, early birth may be an option. The baby most likely will be treated in a special-care nursery.

Breech

It is normal for a baby to be in any position until 34 weeks of pregnancy. To get ready for their entrance into the world, most babies move a few weeks before birth so their heads are down near the birth canal. If this does not happen, the baby's buttocks, or buttocks and feet, will be in place to come out first during birth. This is called breech presentation. It occurs in about 1 of 25 full-term births.

The causes of breech presentation are not fully known. But it is more common when:

▶ You have had more than one pregnancy

▶ You have more than one fetus in the uterus

▸ You have a preterm delivery

▸ Your uterus has too much or too little amniotic fluid

▸ Your uterus is an abnormal shape or has growths, such as *fibroids*, that are not normal

▸ You have placenta previa

There are three main types of breech presentation:

1. *Frank breech.* The fetus's buttocks are aimed toward the birth canal and the legs stick straight up in front of the body. The feet are near the head.

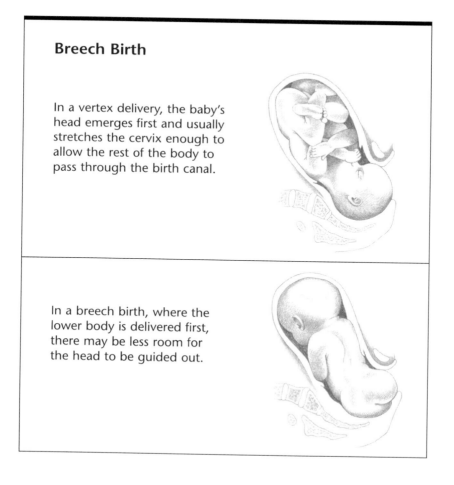

Breech Birth

In a vertex delivery, the baby's head emerges first and usually stretches the cervix enough to allow the rest of the body to pass through the birth canal.

In a breech birth, where the lower body is delivered first, there may be less room for the head to be guided out.

2. *Complete breech.* The buttocks are down, with the legs folded at the knees and the feet near the buttocks.

3. *Footling breech.* One or both of the fetus's feet are pointing down and will come out first.

Most breech babies are born healthy. They do have a higher risk for certain problems than babies born head first. Birth defects are slightly more common in breech babies. A birth defect may be why they have not moved into the right position before birth. Your doctor may advise cesarean or vaginal birth after checking a number of factors, such as the stage of your pregnancy, the size of the baby and your pelvis, and the type of breech position.

Sometimes, the baby can be moved within the uterus by a method called *external version.* It does not involve surgery. The baby is turned by hand into the head-down position. The doctor places his or her hands at certain key points on your lower abdomen. He or she then gently pushes the baby, as if the baby were doing a somersault in slow motion.

You may be given medication first to relax your uterus. An ultrasound exam may be done before the doctor turns the fetus. This allows the doctor to better check the status and placement of the baby, the location of the placenta, and the amount of amniotic fluid in the uterus. Ultrasound also is used to view the fetus during the turning.

Before, during, and after external version, your baby's heartbeat will be checked closely. If any problems arise, efforts to turn the baby will be stopped right away. The best time for trying external version is as you approach term.

Multiple Pregnancy

Multiple pregnancy is when a woman is carrying more than one fetus. In the most common kind of multiple pregnancy, the uterus contains two fetuses (twins). Twins are born once in about every 41 births in the United States. Twins occur in one of two ways. Either two separate eggs are fertilized, causing *fraternal twins*, or a single egg divides into two fetuses, known as *identical twins*.

?

How Are Twins Formed?

You may wonder why sometimes twins look so much alike and other times don't seem to look alike at all. It has to do with how twins are formed.

Most twins are fraternal. Each grows from a separate egg and sperm. As a rule, the ovaries release one egg each month to be fertilized. Sometimes two or more eggs are released. Fraternal twins each have their own placenta and amniotic sac. (Sometimes these twins will be described as dizygotic, meaning two zygotes or two fertilized eggs.) Because each twin grows from the union of a different egg and a different sperm, these twins look no more alike than any brother and sister do. The twins can be both boys, both girls, or one of each.

Sometimes, for unknown reasons, one fertilized egg splits early in pregnancy and grows into two or more fetuses. Two fetuses formed this way are identical (or monozygotic) twins. They share a placenta. Often each has its own amniotic sac. Because they share the same genetic material at the start, they are the same sex and have the same blood type, hair color, and eye color. These twins can look so much alike that even their mothers may not be able to tell them apart.

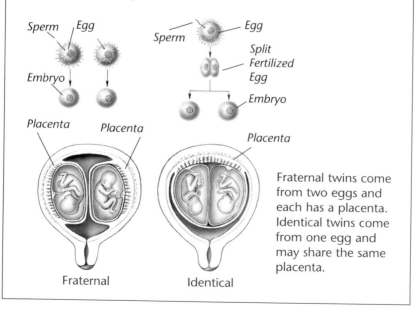

Fraternal twins come from two eggs and each has a placenta. Identical twins come from one egg and may share the same placenta.

Identical twins are somewhat rare. They occur less than once in every 100 births.

Even more rare is when three or more fetuses result from a single pregnancy. The risk of problems during these pregnancies is greater than that in pregnancies with twins. Triplets (three fetuses) occur naturally in only 1 of 10,000 births. Three or more fetuses can be formed by more than one egg being fertilized, a single fertilized egg splitting, or both methods combined.

African-American women are more likely to have multiple pregnancies than white women. Asian women are the least likely to have multiple pregnancies. Some families are more likely than others to have fraternal twins.

Multiple pregnancies have become more common. They now make up about 3% of all pregnancies. One of the reasons for this is that more women are using methods to help them get pregnant. The methods cause more eggs to be released, and more eggs are implanted in the uterus. Some women take fertility drugs to help them ovulate. The drugs can cause more than one egg to be released from the ovaries at once.

Most multiple pregnancies are found before delivery. One may be suspected if:

▸ Fraternal twins tend to run in your family.

▸ Your uterus grows more quickly or is larger than expected.

▸ More than one heartbeat can be heard.

▸ You have been taking fertility drugs.

▸ You have extreme bouts of nausea and vomiting in the first trimester.

▸ You feel more fetal movement than you did in any pregnancies you had before.

▸ You are older than age 35.

If your doctor suspects a multiple pregnancy, an ultrasound exam will be done to confirm it. Sometimes twins are revealed when an ultrasound exam is done for other reasons during pregnancy.

Multiple pregnancy can make your pregnancy more uncomfortable. The uterus becomes much larger. It now must make room for more than one fetus. Multiple pregnancy also brings a higher risk of problems. For instance, the mother is more likely to get high blood pressure or anemia. She also is more likely to go into preterm labor (see "Preterm Birth").

In almost half of multiple pregnancies, the fetuses are small for the stage of pregnancy. Twins also tend to differ in size.

If you are carrying more than one fetus, you may need special care during pregnancy, labor, and delivery. One or both of the twins may need to be born by cesarean birth. If both are head first, they are more likely to be born vaginally. The heart rates of both twins will be monitored during labor. A pediatrician or neonatologist—a doctor who is an expert in the care of newborns—will examine the babies.

Preterm Birth

Preterm labor (labor that starts before the end of the 37th week) can lead to preterm birth. About 1 of every 10 babies born in the United States is born preterm. The earlier the baby is born, the greater the risk of a problem. Preterm birth accounts for three fourths of newborn deaths that are not related to birth defects. Preterm birth may result from preterm labor or problems with the mother or the baby.

Labor starts with regular contractions of the uterus. The cervix thins out (effaces) and opens up (dilates) so the baby can enter the birth canal. Sometimes babies are born before they have had a chance to finish developing. Growth in the last part of pregnancy is vital to the baby's health. Preterm babies (also called premature babies or "preemies") may have problems right away that need special care in the hospital. Long-term problems include learning and behavioral problems and trouble with vision, hearing, and breathing.

Preterm labor can happen in any woman. However, some of the following factors have been linked to preterm birth:

▶ Past pregnancies with preterm labor or birth

▶ Special problems in this pregnancy

—Multiple pregnancy
—Defects in the uterus such as incompetent cervix or fibroids
—Abdominal surgery during pregnancy
—Infection in the mother
—Bleeding in mid-pregnancy
—Weight less than 100 pounds
—Placenta previa
—Premature rupture of membranes ("water breaks" too soon)
—High blood pressure
—Chronic illness in the mother
—Too much fluid in the amniotic sac
—Birth defects in the fetus

Signs of Preterm Labor

If preterm labor is found early, birth often can be postponed. This gives your baby extra time to grow and mature. Even a few more days may mean a more healthy baby. See the box for signs of preterm labor.

Preterm Labor Warning Signs

Call your doctor or nurse right away if you notice:

▶ Vaginal discharge

—Change in type (watery, mucus, or bloody)
—Increase in amount

▶ Pelvic or lower abdominal pressure

▶ Constant, low, dull backache

▶ Mild abdominal cramps, with or without diarrhea

▶ Regular or frequent contractions or uterine tightening, often painless

▶ Ruptured membranes (your water breaks)

Sometimes the signs that preterm labor may be starting are fairly easy to detect. For instance, if the membranes rupture, you may feel a trickle or gush of fluid from the vagina. Other times, the signs are mild and may be harder to detect.

You can monitor yourself. Lie down and gently feel the entire surface of your lower abdomen with your fingertips. Feel for a firm tightening over the surface of your uterus. Often this tightening is not painful. If you feel these contractions, count them. Call your doctor or nurse—they will instruct you on what to do next. You may be in preterm labor. You may need to be seen right away to check whether your cervix has begun to change. This is the only way to know whether you are truly in preterm labor.

Fetal monitoring may be used to record the heartbeat of the fetus and contractions of your uterus. Ultrasound may be used to estimate the size and age of the baby. Ultrasound also will locate the fetus in the uterus. You may be watched for a time and then examined again to see whether your cervix has changed.

Sometimes you may think labor has begun but the membranes have not ruptured and the cervix has not dilated. If this happens between weeks 24 and 35 of pregnancy, the doctor may measure the amount of a substance called fibronectin in the vaginal discharge. A normal amount of fibronectin can rule out preterm birth within the next 2 weeks for women at risk. Other new tests are being studied.

If preterm birth seems likely, your doctor will need to decide if the baby's lungs are mature enough to function outside the uterus. Amniocentesis may be used to check your baby's lungs. If the lungs are not mature, they are not coated with enough of a substance called surfactant. Without this coating, the baby may get respiratory distress syndrome. This means the baby has trouble breathing. It is the most common cause of death in preterm babies.

If it looks as though you may have the baby early, you may be given a medication called a corticosteroid. It will increase the amount of surfactant in the amniotic fluid. This helps the baby's lungs mature, reduces bleeding problems, and increases the baby's chance to live. Studies suggest that corticosteroids are most likely to work when preterm labor begins between 24 and 34 weeks of pregnancy.

Preventing Preterm Birth

If labor is detected at its earliest stages and there is no sign that you and the fetus are in danger from infection, bleeding, or other problems, your doctor may try to stop labor. This will allow the fetus more time to grow and mature. You may be asked to:

▸ Limit physical activity and increase rest.

▸ Take extra fluids by mouth or through a tube inserted in a vein.

▸ Take medications that can stop or suppress uterine contractions.

Many medications can be used to stop or slow preterm labor. These medications are called tocolytics. It is not always clear which, if any, of these medications should be used. As with all medications, tocolytics can have side effects. Each woman responds in her own way. Side effects can include:

▸ Fast pulse

▸ Chest pressure or pain

▸ Feeling dizzy

▸ Headache

▸ Feeling of warmth

▸ Feeling shaky or nervous

If you are not truly in preterm labor or if labor is stopped, you may be able to go home. Some women may need to stay in the hospital for a while. This depends on the findings of the exam and other factors.

Your Preterm Baby

Sometimes preterm labor may be too advanced to be stopped. In some cases, the baby is better off being born—even if it is early.

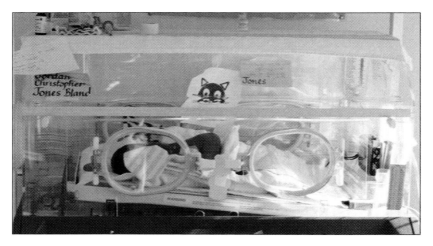

Some preterm babies are kept in an incubator in the hospital to keep them safe and warm.

Reasons can include infection, high blood pressure, bleeding, or signs that the fetus is having problems.

Preterm babies are more likely to be born by cesarean birth. Preterm labor and delivery involve risks that require special care. You or your baby may be moved to a hospital that can provide this expert care.

Preterm babies look different from term babies. They may be red and skinny because they have little fat under their skin and their blood vessels are close to the surface. The earlier a baby is born, the less developed it is. This can lead to breathing problems (such as respiratory distress syndrome), feeding problems, or increased risk of infection.

Early Rupture of Membranes

A common sign that labor has begun is when "your water breaks"—a rupture of the membranes that hold the amniotic fluid. In most cases, rupture of the membranes is followed by other signs of labor. Sometimes the membranes break before labor begins. This is called *premature rupture of membranes.* If it occurs before the baby is ready to be born (before 37 weeks), this is called preterm premature rupture of membranes.

Your doctor will want to confirm that your membranes have ruptured. Sometimes you may have a discharge for other reasons. Diagnosis of rupture of the membranes depends on your medical history, physical exam, and lab tests. It is confirmed when there is a pool of amniotic fluid in the vagina. Other tests, such as ultrasound, can be done when the diagnosis is not clear.

Although some fluid is lost when the membranes rupture, the fetus will produce more fluid. This may cause more leaking from the uterus.

Premature Rupture of Membranes

One of every 10 women has premature rupture of membranes. The reasons are not clear. Some causes may be infection or bleeding.

With premature rupture of membranes, four problems can occur:

1. The amniotic fluid, the fetus, or the mother could become infected.

2. The umbilical cord could be compressed because the fluid is not there to protect it. The fetus may not get the nutrients it needs.

3. The umbilical cord could become prolapsed.

4. Abruptio placentae could occur.

The mother will be watched closely for these problems. In a few cases, the doctor will decide to induce labor.

Certain conditions may require extra special care if premature rupture of membranes occurs. For instance, because of the threat of infection, women with group B streptococci (GBS) disease should be managed with care. They can transmit the infection to the baby during labor and delivery. Medication is given during this process if:

▸ At least 18 hours have passed since the membranes ruptured.

▸ The pregnancy is less than 37 weeks.

▸ The mother's temperature is more than 100.4°F.

▸ The membranes rupture at less than 37 weeks (preterm premature rupture of membranes).

▸ The mother has delivered a baby before with group B streptococci disease.

The medication used most often is penicillin G or ampicillin. Clindamycin or erythromycin also can be used.

Preterm Premature Rupture of Membranes

In most cases of preterm premature rupture of membranes, efforts are made to delay birth until the baby is likely to be healthy. The major problems are preterm birth and infections.

Rest, fluids, and medications may be used to manage preterm premature rupture of membranes (see "Preventing Preterm Birth"). You may be given antibiotics or corticosteroids (see "Preterm Birth"). Antibiotics can prolong pregnancy, reduce infection and bleeding in the newborn, and reduce the risk of respiratory distress syndrome.

Postdate Pregnancy

Most women (80%) give birth between 38 and 42 weeks of pregnancy. These pregnancies are called term. Only 5% of babies arrive on the exact due date. Up to 10% of normal pregnancies are not born by 42 weeks. These are called postdate pregnancies.

Knowing the gestational age of the fetus is key in knowing if your pregnancy is postdate. It can be hard, though, to pinpoint the age of the fetus. You may be unsure of your menstrual cycle history. This makes it harder to predict your exact due date. For this reason, more than one method may be used to cross-check the age of the fetus (see "What's Your Due Date?" in Chapter 4). The due date should be set early in pregnancy. It is less exact when it is set later.

If pregnancy goes past 42 weeks, the fetus could face some problems. These risks occur in only a small number of postdate pregnancies. More than 90% of babies born between 42 and 44 weeks have no problems as a result of the longer pregnancy.

As pregnancy moves past 42 weeks, a fetus has a higher risk of:

▸ *Dysmaturity syndrome.* The baby is malnourished and born with a long and lean body, an alert look on the face, lots of hair, long fingernails, and thin wrinkled skin.

▸ *Macrosomia.* The fetus grows larger than normal, which can pose problems during birth.

▸ *Meconium aspiration.* The fetus inhales meconium (greenish waste that is emptied from the fetus's bowels into the amniotic fluid). Often, a baby born with meconium staining does just fine.

It is vital to know if the baby is at risk so action can be taken. As a fetus passes full term, the placenta may stop working the way it should. This means the baby may not get as much oxygen and nutrients and may not grow as fast. The baby also may make less urine. This can reduce the volume of amniotic fluid in the sac. If the amount of amniotic fluid decreases, fetal movements or uterine contractions can pinch the umbilical cord.

A number of tests can be used to check the well-being of the baby. Tests often are started between 40 and 42 weeks of pregnancy. Some tests are done in the doctor's office. Others are done in the hospital. Tests that may be used include electronic fetal monitoring and ultrasound.

If the baby seems to be active and healthy and the amniotic fluid volume appears normal, the mother and baby may be monitored at set times until labor starts on its own. Many women wonder why the doctor doesn't simply bring on labor at 42 weeks. First, there is a chance that the due date is off. Estimates can be wrong. Often, neither the mother nor her doctor can be sure that the fetus is fully mature and ready to be born. Second, in some women, the cervix is not ready for labor to start.

If the cervix is not ready, a number of agents can be used as a first step to induce labor. These are called "cervical-ripening" agents. (For more details, see "Helping Labor Along" in Chapter 8.) They may be used to help dilate the cervix.

Your baby may need to be born if it seems to be at risk. Your doctor may induce labor by giving the drug oxytocin. This drug causes uterine contractions.

If problems arise, the baby may be born by cesarean birth. After birth, a postdate baby may need special care.

Close Care

If your pregnancy involves certain complications, your doctor will monitor your health until you give birth. In most cases, you will deliver a healthy child. You should follow your doctor's advice and take steps to keep yourself healthy.

CHAPTER 16

Infections During Pregnancy

Infections are caused by tiny organisms that invade the body and then spread. The body draws on its immune system to fight back and try to kill the invaders. While this fight is going on, you may have symptoms of the infection, such as a rash, pain, fever, and swelling. You also form antibodies in your blood. These are special proteins that form to combat infection when it strikes.

Antibodies are a key part of the immune system. You are not aware of antibodies when they form, but tests can show if they are present. If you have antibodies to a disease, you have been exposed to that disease. In many cases, once antibodies to a disease are made, you have become immune to the disease and will not get it in the future.

Infections can range from a mild cold or flulike illness to life-threatening disease. Certain infections can harm the fetus if the mother is exposed to them during pregnancy. Although a cold or flu often is not harmful to the mother or fetus, over-the-counter medications to treat it may cause harm. You should call your doctor or nurse if you have symptoms of an infection.

Sometimes you can have an infection but not have any symptoms. Sometimes the symptoms don't occur right away. Without these clues, you can have an infection and not know it. The earlier an infection is found and treated, the less likely you or your baby will have long-term health problems as a result.

Some infections can be prevented if you receive vaccines. Certain types of vaccines are not safe during pregnancy, though. A vaccine contains either a small amount of the same organism that causes the infection or a small amount of an organism like it. The amount is just enough to cause antibodies to form and make you immune, but not enough to make you ill.

The best way to protect yourself from infections to which you are not immune is to avoid being exposed to them before and during pregnancy. If you think you have been exposed to an infection, tell your doctor or nurse right away. Sometimes steps can be taken to avoid problems and lower the risk to your baby.

Sexually Transmitted Diseases

Sexually transmitted diseases (STDs) are infections that are passed from person to person during sex. All STDs can lead to serious problems. Some STDs are even more harmful during pregnancy. For instance, if you have an STD, you are more likely to have preterm labor and an inflammation called *endometritis.*

If you think you may have an STD, get tested and treated right away. Your partner also should be treated. Neither of you should have sex until you have finished treatment.

Chlamydia, Gonorrhea, and Pelvic Inflammatory Disease

Chlamydia and gonorrhea are the most common STDs in the United States. They are caused by bacteria that are passed from person to person during sex. The infections are alike in many ways, and often occur at the same time. They infect the same sites in a woman's reproductive tract. In many cases, the cervix, rectum, and urethra (the opening through which urine is passed) are infected.

The most common symptoms in men with chlamydia or gonorrhea are a drip from the penis and painful urination. Many women have no symptoms. They may learn they have chlamydia or gonorrhea only when their sexual partners are found to have the disease or if they are tested during pregnancy.

TABLE 1. How Sexually Transmitted Diseases Can Affect You and Your Baby

Disease	Symptoms in Women	Effects On:	
		Mother	Fetus/Baby
AIDS*	May have no symptoms; appetite or weight loss, fatigue, swollen lymph nodes, night sweats, fever or chills, persistent diarrhea or cough	Immune system damage leading to infections (such as pneumonia) or cancers, death	Immune system damage leading to death in as early as 3 years in some infants
Chlamydia	May have no symptoms; vaginal discharge, painful or frequent urination, pelvic pain	Endometritis or postpartum infection, preterm labor, pelvic inflammatory disease, ectopic pregnancy	Eye infection, pneumonia
Genital Herpes	Flu-like symptoms (fever, chills, muscle aches, etc); small, painful, fluid-filled blisters on genitals or buttocks	Recurrent outbreaks	Severe skin infection, nervous system damage, blindness, mental retardation, death
Genital Warts	Possible genital itching, irritation, or bleeding; warts may appear as small, cauliflower-shaped clusters	Warts grow in size and number; may have abnormal Pap test	Warts on the vocal cords in early adolescence (rare)
Gonorrhea	Most women have no symptoms; vaginal discharge, minor genital irritation, pain, and fever	Pelvic inflammatory disease, arthritis	Eye infection if left untreated
Syphilis	A painless open sore called a chancre; later rash, sluggishness, or slight fever	Damage to heart, blood vessels, and nervous system; blindness, insanity, death	Miscarriage, stillbirth, syphilis in liveborn infant, birth defects

*AIDS stands for acquired immunodeficiency syndrome.

Sometimes a pelvic exam is not enough to diagnose the problem, and other tests need to be done. If you have these diseases, you can be treated with antibiotics, even during pregnancy.

Pregnant women who are infected have an increased chance of having their membranes break early and having the baby before it is fully mature. Some women may even have a miscarriage.

Chlamydia and gonorrhea can infect the fetus while passing through the vagina during birth. They can cause eye infection and other problems. A newborn's eyes are an easy target for gonorrhea. To prevent damage, the eyes of all newborns are treated at birth whether or not the mother has gonorrhea.

Chlamydia and gonorrhea can cause pelvic inflammatory disease. This is a severe infection that spreads from the vagina and cervix through the pelvic area. It may attack the uterus, fallopian tubes, and ovaries.

Herpes Simplex Virus

Genital herpes is an infection caused by herpes simplex virus. Symptoms are sores and blisters on or around the sex organs. Herpes also can affect the tongue, mouth, gums, lips, eyes, fingers, and other parts of the body. Other symptoms include swollen glands, fever, chills, muscle aches, fatigue, and nausea. Sometimes there are no symptoms.

The infection is spread by direct contact with a person who has active sores. In some cases, the virus can be passed to others even when the sores have healed.

Some people have only one outbreak of genital herpes. Others have many bouts during their lifetime. In rare cases, babies can become infected with the herpes virus during birth. This can cause severe skin infection, damage to the nervous system, blindness, mental retardation, or death. Infected infants are treated with medication (acyclovir, for instance).

If you have ever had genital herpes or have had sex with someone who has, tell your doctor or nurse. He or she will want to see if you have open lesions. If you have no herpes sores, the baby can be born vaginally. If there are signs of active infection when you are in labor, you may need to have your baby by

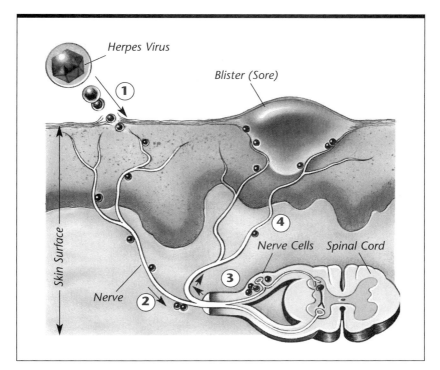

The herpes virus passes through your skin (*1*). It travels through your body (*2*) and settles at nerve cells near your spine (*3*). When something triggers a new bout of herpes, the virus leaves its resting place and travels along the nerve, back to the surface of the skin (*4*).

cesarean birth. Cesarean birth lessens the chance that the baby will come in contact with the virus in the vagina. If the membranes have ruptured a number of hours before birth, the baby still may become infected.

Human Papillomavirus

Human papillomavirus (HPV) is a virus that causes genital warts. These warts are sometimes called condyloma acuminata. Warts in the genital area are easily passed from person to person during sex. This includes oral and anal sex.

You can have HPV even without having genital warts, and you may not be found to have HPV until years after you've been exposed. Sometimes a Pap test will show signs of HPV infection. Some types of HPV infection are linked with higher rates of cervical cancer.

There is a very slight risk that babies born to mothers with HPV can get the infection. Sometimes it is not found in these babies until adolescence. At that time it affects the larynx (voice box). This is not a reason for cesarean delivery, though.

Genital warts may go away on their own. If there are a lot of them or they are large, your doctor may suggest minor surgery to remove them. This treatment is safe to have during pregnancy in most cases. In some cases, your doctor may suggest you wait until after the baby is born to begin treatment. Your condition will be watched closely during your pregnancy.

Warts can go grow in number and size during pregnancy. Rarely, warts can grow so large they block the birth canal or make it very narrow. If this occurs, cesarean birth is needed.

Trichomoniasis

Trichomoniasis is an STD that affects the vagina. Women may have no symptoms, or they may have a vaginal discharge, burning, and irritation. There may be more problems with premature rupture of membranes and preterm delivery in women who are infected.

Pregnant women can be treated with an antibiotic that is safe to use during pregnancy. This will relieve symptoms, increase the chances of curing it, and make it less likely that the infection will be passed to others.

Syphilis

Syphilis, a disease that has been known for hundreds of years, can be a severe STD. It is caused by organisms called spirochetes. Syphilis occurs in stages. It is more easily spread in some stages than in others. If not treated, syphilis may affect your eyes, heart, nervous system, and blood vessels. It can cause brain damage, blindness, paralysis, and death. If syphilis is found and treated early, it may cause less damage.

Syphilis can be passed from a pregnant woman's bloodstream to her fetus. This may cause miscarriage, stillbirth, or premature rupture of membranes. If the infant lives, it may be born with syphilis. Infants born with syphilis may have problems of the nervous system, skin, eyes, bones, liver, lungs, or spleen.

Syphilis can be hard to detect in women. The sore that marks the site of infection—called a chancre—may be in the vagina where it cannot be seen. For most heterosexual men, the chancre appears on the penis, but it may be anywhere around the genital area.

In its early stages, when a chancre is present, syphilis may be diagnosed by scraping tissue from the chancre. A blood test may or may not find the disease in its very early stages. The chancre will go away even without treatment, but the disease remains. After the chancre goes away, the only sure way to diagnose syphilis is a blood test.

Treating an infected pregnant woman with antibiotics will halt further damage to her fetus, but it will not reverse any harm already done. If a woman is treated during the first 3–4 months of pregnancy, most likely the infant will not have any long-term damage. Treating an infected infant after birth will prevent more damage in many cases.

Human Immunodeficiency Virus Infection and Acquired Immunodeficiency Syndrome

Human immunodeficiency virus (HIV) enters the bloodstream by way of body fluids—mainly blood or semen—from an infected person. The main ways that HIV is passed to others are by sexual contact and by injecting drugs. In rare cases, blood transfusions can transmit the disease. Since 1985, though, the blood supply in the United States is tested. Infected blood is not used. Breast milk from a woman with HIV also can pass the virus.

Once in the body, HIV invades and destroys CD4 cells that are part of the immune system—the body's natural defense against disease. This leaves the body open to infections that can cause death. When a person infected with HIV gets one of these infections or has a very low level of CD4 cells, he or she is said to have *acquired immunodeficiency syndrome* (AIDS). A person with HIV or AIDS is also more likely to have or get other STDs.

When a person is infected with HIV, he or she carries the infection for life. Initial symptoms are like the flu, with weight loss, fatigue, and fever. They come on slowly. It may take more than 5 years for symptoms to appear. There is no cure for HIV or AIDS, but treatment can prolong life.

Testing

HIV and AIDS can be passed from mother to fetus. Because with treatment the chance of the fetus being infected is greatly reduced, all pregnant women will be told that they will be tested for the disease. Results will be discussed with you. If you have concerns about the test, talk to your doctor.

A test called the enzyme-linked immunosorbent assay (ELISA) is used to detect HIV. It will show if your blood contains HIV antibodies. This is a sign that you have been infected. Positive results then are confirmed by a second ELISA and by Western

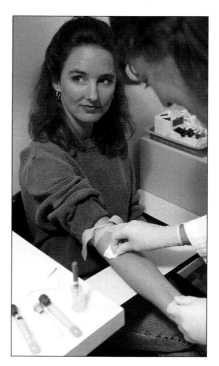

blot, another test used as a double check. If both tests are positive, HIV infection is diagnosed. This does not mean that you have AIDS. It means that you have been infected with HIV and that you run a high risk of passing it to others. Very rarely, the tests will give a false-positive result. A false-positive result means the test shows you have been infected when you haven't been. Another test can be done.

Other factors can cause test results that are not correct. After you are exposed to the virus, weeks or months must pass before enough antibodies show up in your blood to produce a positive test result. This means that if you were exposed to the virus only a week before being tested, the test would show a negative result. A negative test can't tell you if you are now infected. It shows only that you didn't have antibodies when the test was done. A negative test also doesn't mean that you can't get AIDS in the future.

To protect yourself from infection or, if you're infected, from infecting others:

▸ Use latex condoms during sex.

▸ Avoid other risky behavior, such as:

—Injecting drugs
—Having sex with more than one partner
—Having sex with a partner who may use drugs or have other sexual partners

Treatment

If a pregnant woman is infected, she can transmit the virus to her fetus. The virus can attack the fetus as early as week 8 of pregnancy. It also can occur during labor and delivery. Without treatment, about 1 in 4 pregnant women who are infected with HIV pass the virus to their fetus.

For women who are treated with medication between weeks 14 and 40, the risk of passing the virus to the fetus is greatly reduced. For best results, the medication should be taken during pregnancy, labor, and delivery, and the infant should take the drug during the first 6 weeks of life. Treatment with certain medications also helps prevent other common problems in the mother, such as infection, preterm labor, and giving birth to a very small baby.

After birth, a mother should take special care not to pass the infection to the baby in other ways. She should not breastfeed her baby. She should be careful not to cause contact of her body fluids with the baby's mucus membranes (the mouth, eyes, nose, and bottom). It is important for the mother to continue her treatment and not infect others. The best way to do this is to practice safe sex or not have sex.

Bacterial Vaginosis

An imbalance of the bacteria growing in the vagina can cause the infection *bacterial vaginosis*. It is the most common cause of a vaginal discharge. The discharge has a fishy odor. Bacterial vaginosis is not an STD.

Some women may have a greater risk of preterm birth, premature rupture of membranes, and endometritis if they have this infection. Women with the infection may need treatment.

Bladder and Kidney Infections

Bladder infections (also called urinary tract infections) are common in pregnancy. Severe infections can cause problems for both mother and fetus. Some bladder infections can be found only by tests. Because there may be no symptoms to let you know that you are infected, you will be tested as part of your routine care. Some symptoms linked with a bladder infection, such as pain when you urinate, can be caused by other problems such as infection of the vagina or vulva.

Cystitis is a lower-tract (bladder) infection. Cystitis is treated with antibiotics. Its symptoms may include:

▪ Increased need to urinate

▪ Burning and pain when you urinate

▪ Pain in the lower abdomen

▪ Blood in the urine

Pyelonephritis is an upper-tract (kidney) infection. This can occur if bladder infections are not treated or are not cured by treatment. Thus, medication prescribed for a bladder infection should be finished, even if symptoms go away. Symptoms are chills, fever, rapid heart rate, and nausea or vomiting. It can lead to premature labor or severe infection. You may be hospitalized and may need antibiotics. It may take a while before you get well.

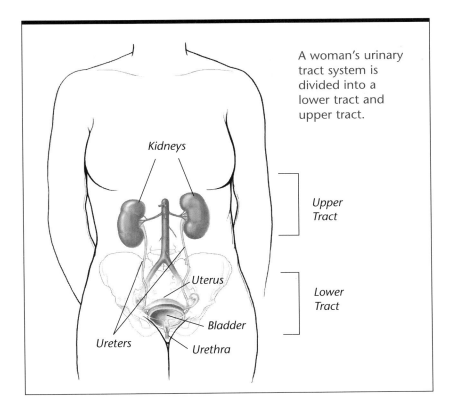

Kidneys

A woman's urinary tract system is divided into a lower tract and upper tract.

Upper Tract

Lower Tract

Uterus

Bladder

Ureters

Urethra

Childhood Diseases

Although certain infections are thought of as childhood diseases, they also can occur in adults. Some can cause serious problems in pregnant women.

If you've had these diseases as a child, you are not likely to get them again. You are immune because you have antibodies that protect you against them. There are vaccines for many of these diseases. If you haven't had these diseases yet, it's a good idea to be vaccinated against them before your next pregnancy. In a few cases, vaccination is safe during pregnancy.

Because many children have not been vaccinated, these diseases have become widespread. If you are exposed to these diseases during this pregnancy, your doctor may be able to treat you or your fetus to prevent the fetus from getting sick.

Chickenpox

Chickenpox is caused by varicella–zoster virus. Adults who get chickenpox often get sicker than children do. Pregnant women with this infection may get pneumonia at the same time.

If you have not had chickenpox, you should be vaccinated at least 1 month before you become pregnant. Once you are pregnant, you should not be vaccinated because the vaccine is made with live virus.

It takes about 14 days from the time you are exposed to chickenpox to get symptoms of the illness. Symptoms include fever and fluid-filled bumps that itch. Chickenpox can be passed on to others even before the rash appears.

If you get chickenpox early in pregnancy, the chance of harm to the fetus is low. However, if you get it a week or more before giving birth, the fetus can catch the infection in your uterus and be born with it. Sometimes the antibodies you form while you are sick pass through the placenta into the fetus's blood. This helps protect it from serious illness. The baby may be born with chickenpox, but likely will recover fully. If you get chickenpox less than a week before delivery, though, there is not enough time for antibodies to form and protect the baby. In such cases, babies are more likely to get very sick.

Because chickenpox is so easy to catch, pregnant women who are not immune to it should stay away from people who have the disease. Extra caution is needed near the time of birth.

You can be tested if you can't remember if you've had the disease or not. If a pregnant woman has contact with an infected person, a medication called varicella–zoster immune globulin may keep her from getting seriously ill if it is given within 4 days of being exposed.

Fifth Disease

Fifth disease was given its name because it was the fifth to be found among a group of diseases that cause fever and skin rash in children. It is caused by a virus called parvovirus B19. This common childhood illness often is mild but is easily passed to others.

Vaccines

Vaccines help prevent diseases caused by infection. Like all medicines, vaccines should be used during pregnancy only when it is needed and safe. It is best for a woman to have all her vaccinations before she becomes pregnant (see Chapter 1). If a vaccination is needed during pregnancy, waiting until the fourth month is best.

Some vaccines are not given to pregnant women as a rule, but are safe to be used if you are likely to come in contact with the infections:

- Hepatitis A
- Hepatitis B
- Pneumonia caused by Pneumococcus
- Rabies
- Influenza (Women who are at high risk or are in their second or third trimester during flu season, October through February, should be vaccinated.)
- Polio
- Diphtheria
- Tetanus

Certain vaccines contain a live virus and should be avoided during pregnancy:

- Lyme disease
- Measles
- Mumps
- Rubella
- Varicella (chickenpox)

Being exposed to measles, rubella, mumps, and chickenpox should be avoided during pregnancy. Women should be vaccinated against measles, rubella, and mumps at least 3 months before they become pregnant. They should be vaccinated against chickenpox at least 1 month before becoming pregnant. If you are pregnant but not yet vaccinated, you should ask your doctor when you should be. Vaccination is safe for both you and your baby while you are breastfeeding.

Its main symptom is a rash that often starts on the cheeks and is later found on the backs of the arms and legs. In rare cases it causes joint pain and affects the nervous system. About half of all adults have antibodies to fifth disease because they have been exposed to it.

Women who have close contact with children are at higher risk of getting infected than are women whose contact is more casual. Teachers in a school with an epidemic of the disease or mothers who have an infected child at home are at high risk.

During pregnancy, infection with parvovirus B19 may be a concern. If you get fifth disease in the first 3–4 months of pregnancy, you have a slightly higher risk of miscarriage (about 1–2% higher than normal). When infection occurs later in pregnancy, it can cause anemia in the fetus and may require treatment. During the course of the disease, the fetus must be closely watched by ultrasound.

Rubella

There are a number of types of measles. Each is caused by a different virus. Most types do not cause problems during pregnancy. The type that can be harmful is caused by rubella virus. It is known as German measles.

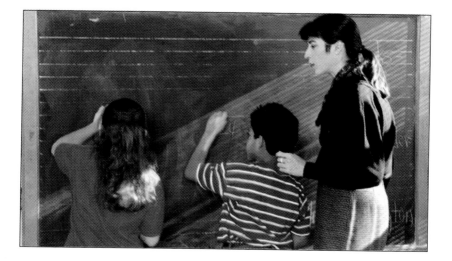

In 1969, a vaccine for rubella was found. Since then, preschool and young school-aged children have been vaccinated routinely. About 75–80 of every 100 women are immune to rubella by the time they reach childbearing age. This is because they have been exposed to rubella, have had the disease, or have been vaccinated. You can be infected with the rubella virus without knowing it. Once infected with rubella virus, you are immune for life.

It's a good thing that most people are immune to rubella—the virus can cause birth defects and long-term problems in babies exposed to the virus while their mothers were pregnant. The risk depends on the stage of pregnancy at the time that the mother was infected. If she was infected during the first month, her baby has a 1-in-2 chance of being affected. By the third month, the risk is lowered to about 1 in 10. The most common problems include cataracts (an eye problem that can cause blindness), heart defects, and deafness. If these problems occur, it is called congenital rubella syndrome. Other problems, such as diabetes, can occur later in life.

As a routine part of prenatal care, each pregnant woman is tested for antibodies to show if she is immune to rubella. If there are signs that a woman is not immune but may have been exposed to rubella or if she develops symptoms, she will be tested again. Symptoms include fever, rash, and swollen lymph glands.

It is best to get the rubella vaccine before you are pregnant. This is because rubella can have a severe impact on the fetus and nothing can be done during pregnancy to protect the fetus.

Women who have never had the disease or the vaccine can be vaccinated just after delivery. They should get the vaccine before they become pregnant again. Although the vaccine does not cause congenital rubella syndrome, the virus it contains may be passed to the fetus. Therefore, it is best to wait 3 months after getting the vaccine before you try to become pregnant. If you get the vaccine early in your pregnancy, though, the risk that your baby will have a problem is very low.

Mumps

Mumps is a disease also caused by a virus. Less than 1 case in 10 occurs in people older than age 15 years. Mumps causes fever and swollen glands under the jaw. It does not spread as easily as measles or chickenpox. Thus, mumps is not common during pregnancy. If you do get mumps during pregnancy, your symptoms are likely to be no worse than if you were infected any other time. Problems may occur with your fetus, though.

When a woman gets mumps in the first 12 weeks of pregnancy, it doubles her risk of having a miscarriage. Mumps also may cause preterm labor. Because this infection is so rare during pregnancy, it is not clear whether it is linked to birth defects.

The vaccine against mumps that is given to children has greatly reduced the number of pregnant women who are exposed to the disease. Having mumps as a child also protects against getting mumps later. If you are pregnant and not immune to mumps, it would be a good idea to get vaccinated after you give birth. There is a very small chance that the vaccine could hurt the fetus if given during pregnancy. Thus, it is not given to pregnant women.

Cytomegalovirus

Cytomegalovirus (CMV) infection is the most common virus transmitted during pregnancy. Cytomegalovirus is hard to detect because people who have it often do not have symptoms. People with symptoms have a fever, swollen lymph glands, and a sore throat. They also feel tired. Rarely does CMV cause serious illness in an adult. Although about 6–7 of every 10 people have been infected with CMV at one time or another, almost all of them never had symptoms.

Cytomegalovirus infection poses a problem during pregnancy and the period after birth because it can be passed to the baby through the placenta, the vagina, or breast milk. Unlike other viral infections, CMV can come back even if a person has been infected before and has formed antibodies. The risk of the fetus getting infected is greatest during the first bout of infection in the mother. Few women are first infected with CMV while they are pregnant. If they are, the chance of the fetus getting infected is fairly high. Studies have shown that among mothers with first-time CMV infections during pregnancy, about half of their fetuses are infected with CMV. Only 1 in 10 has signs of disease. Those who do have symptoms at birth have a higher risk of dying or having severe illness or handicaps. Some problems linked to CMV infection include:

- Jaundice (yellow skin and eyes caused when the liver doesn't work as it should)

- Microcephaly (having a very small head and being mentally retarded)

- Deafness

- Eye problems

Cytomegalovirus infection has no treatment. Because it rarely causes symptoms when a pregnant woman is infected, screening or routine testing is not useful. Those at highest risk are health care and lab workers, mothers of small children in childcare, and childcare providers. The best way to keep from getting CMV is to avoid contact with infected people and to wash your hands often.

Group B Streptococci

Group B streptococci (GBS) bacteria are fairly common in pregnant women. They are often found in the vagina and rectum. These bacteria differ from the streptococcus bacteria that cause strep throat. You can carry GBS in your body without symptoms. Group B streptococci can infect your bladder, kidneys, or uterus and cause pain and inflammation. These infections often are not serious and can be treated with antibiotics. When GBS is present but does not cause infection, the person is "colonized."

If GBS bacteria are passed from a woman to her baby, the baby may become infected. This happens to only a few babies. Babies who do become infected may have early or late infections.

Early infections occur within the first 7 days after birth. Most occur within the first 6 hours. Most newborns with early infection got it from their mother during labor and delivery. Early infection can cause inflammation of the baby's blood, lungs, brain, or spinal cord. This can cause severe problems. Infections in some babies may result in death.

> **!**
>
> ## Risk Factors for Group B Streptococci Infection
>
> Women with these risk factors are more likely to have babies with group B streptococci (GBS) infection:
>
>) Preterm labor (labor that begins before 37 weeks of pregnancy)
>
>) Preterm premature rupture of membranes (breaking of the amniotic sac before 37 weeks of pregnancy)
>
>) Prolonged rupture of membranes (18 hours or more since the amniotic sac broke)
>
>) Prior child with GBS infection
>
>) Fever during labor
>
>) Presence of GBS in urine

Late infections occur after the first 7 days of life. About half of late infections are passed from the mother to the baby during birth. The other half result from other sources of infection, such as contact with other people who are GBS carriers or with the mother after birth. Late infections also can cause harm. The most common problem is meningitis, an inflammation of the membranes of the brain or spinal cord. Meningitis can have long-term effects on the baby's nervous system. Babies with late infections are less likely to die than those with early infections.

Testing

Some doctors test for GBS during pregnancy as a routine. Some tests can detect GBS, but they are not perfect. One way to test for GBS is through cultures. For cultures, samples are taken from the vagina, perineum, and rectum and grown in a special substance. A urine sample also may be used for cultures. It may take up to 2 days to get the results.

Cultures are only somewhat useful because of the nature of GBS. A woman may be positive (colonized) at some times and not at others. This means test results may be negative (not colonized) at the time the sample was taken, but positive at another time during pregnancy. Also, at any given time, one place in the body (such as the vagina) may be negative, while another (such as the rectum) may be positive. Thus, the test cannot always detect women who will be colonized at the time of delivery.

Treatment

The best way to prevent early-onset GBS infection in the baby is to treat the woman with antibiotics during labor. Treating the pregnant woman before labor cannot be relied on to prevent infection in the baby. If she is treated during pregnancy, a woman can become positive again after treatment, before her baby is born. If she becomes positive, she can pass GBS to her baby.

A woman in labor may be treated even if she was not tested during pregnancy. Certain risk factors increase the chance that the baby of a mother with GBS will become infected. Treatment is most effective in these women.

Hepatitis

Hepatitis is a viral infection that affects the liver. The four common kinds of hepatitis are types A, B, C, and D. Hepatitis B (HBV) is the biggest concern during pregnancy because it can cause harm. It can be transmitted by blood, kissing, or sex.

People with HBV may not feel sick or show any signs of the disease. Some people who are infected can be chronic carriers, though. This means they keep the virus in their bodies all their lives and can pass it to other people. Some people who get infected with HBV have liver problems, such as cirrhosis (hardening) of the liver or liver cancer. Some people have a higher risk of HBV infection. You may be more likely to get the disease if you:

▸ Inject drugs and share needles

▸ Have multiple sexual partners

▸ Work in a health-related job that exposes you to blood or blood products

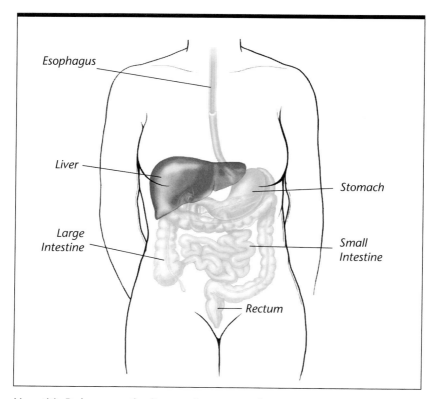

Esophagus

Liver

Large
Intestine

Stomach

Small
Intestine

Rectum

Hepatitis B damages the liver and can cause harm during pregnancy. All pregnant women should be tested for this infection.

▶ Live with someone infected with HBV

▶ Received blood products (for example, for a clotting disorder)

About 8 of every 10 infants born to women with chronic HBV get infected, often during birth. Most of these infants also become chronic HBV carriers and are at risk for the long-term problems of HBV infection.

Any teen or adult with a higher risk of getting the disease should be vaccinated. All infants should get the vaccine, too. Most of the time, the vaccine is given in three doses. The first two doses are given 1 month apart, and the third is given 6 months later.

Using condoms during sex and stopping any activity that results in contact with another person's blood can prevent hepatitis B.

All pregnant women should be tested for HBV infection. The infection can be hard to find without testing because its symptoms—nausea and vomiting—often occur in pregnancy. If you think you have been exposed, you will be given a vaccine to prevent the illness. If you might be infected already, you also will be given a drug called hepatitis B immune globulin. It can make the illness less severe. Rest, diet, and liquids also may be prescribed. With both vaccination and medical treatment, chances of passing the infection to the baby during birth are reduced to about 5%.

If you have chronic hepatitis B infection, it can be passed easily to others who are in daily contact with you. Your baby should be given hepatitis B immune globulin and one dose of vaccine within 12 hours of birth. Your baby should receive two more doses of vaccine within 6 months. With this treatment, chances of your baby getting the infection even

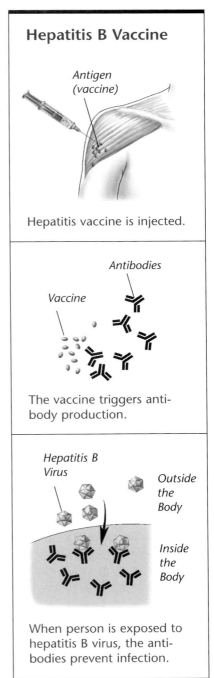

Hepatitis B Vaccine

Antigen
(vaccine)

Hepatitis vaccine is injected.

Antibodies

Vaccine

The vaccine triggers antibody production.

Hepatitis B
Virus

Outside
the
Body

Inside
the
Body

When person is exposed to hepatitis B virus, the antibodies prevent infection.

if you have it are only 1 in 20. Also, if your baby is given the vaccine, it is safe to breastfeed.

Hepatitis C is a disease that occurs more often than before. Hepatitis C does not spread as easily as hepatitis B. It is very rare that it is passed to your baby by breastfeeding. There is no vaccine to prevent infection with hepatitis C.

Listeriosis

Listeriosis is an illness caused by bacteria found in certain foods. The foods most likely to have the bacteria are unpasteurized milk, soft cheese, raw vegetables, and shellfish. Symptoms occur several weeks after you are exposed to the bacteria. They can include fever, chills, muscle aches, and back pain. However, there may be no symptoms.

When a pregnant woman is infected, the disease can cause serious problems for the fetus, including miscarriage. Babies born to mothers who were infected while pregnant can have trouble breathing, low body temperature, and other problems. Some babies who seem healthy at birth can get symptoms weeks later, such as fever or feeding problems. Some studies suggest that pregnant women are more likely to get the disease than most other people.

Because the symptoms of listeriosis are like the flu, it's not always found. If you have a fever or flulike illness, samples from your vagina, cervix, and blood can be checked. If the bacteria are found, you and your fetus can be treated with antibiotics. If there is a chance that a newborn is infected, he or she also can be tested and treated.

To prevent listeriosis, wash all fresh fruits and vegetables before using them. While you are pregnant, don't eat:

‣ Unpasteurized soft cheeses

‣ Undercooked meat, poultry, fish, or eggs

‣ Cold meat

‣ Raw animal foods such as unpasteurized milk or raw meat, eggs, fish, or shellfish

Lyme Disease

Lyme disease is caused by a bite from an infected tick. When the tick bites, it injects a germ into the body that causes disease. The first sign of Lyme disease is a sore that may look like a bull's-eye. This sore may go away, but the infection re-

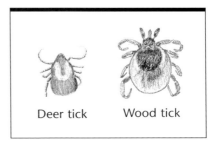

Deer tick   Wood tick

mains. It spreads to the joints, causing arthritis. It also can cause muscle pain. Antibiotics often will cure the infection. If it is not treated, it can attack the heart and nervous system.

Keep in mind that ticks can carry diseases other than Lyme disease. It is wise for pregnant women to avoid densely wooded areas. Wear long-sleeved shirts and long pants tucked into your socks in areas where ticks can be found. If you find a tick that has been on you for more than 24 hours, see your doctor. A vaccine is available that may help prevent infection in women who are at high risk for Lyme disease.

Toxoplasmosis

The parasite that causes *toxoplasmosis* lives in any animal that lives outdoors. Humans can get infected by eating raw or under-cooked meat or unwashed vegetables. Infection also is caused by coming into contact with animal feces. The most common way it occurs in the United States is by working in the garden. Rarely, it occurs from changing a cat's litter box, especially if the cat roams outdoors. Toxoplasmosis causes only mild illness in adults. Often, those exposed have no symptoms.

About one third of the public has been exposed to toxoplas-mosis. Once you have been exposed, you form antibodies and become immune to the disease. Toxoplasmosis is rare, but you should take steps to prevent it.

Toxoplasmosis creates a problem in pregnancy only when the mother is first infected while she is pregnant. Of women infected with toxoplasmosis during pregnancy, about one third pass the infection to the fetus. Only one third of infected fetuses will show signs of the disease, though. The chances of the fetus getting infected are highest in the last 12 weeks of pregnancy. The problems are more severe when the infection occurs in the first 12 weeks.

If the mother gets infected, the lymph glands in her neck may swell. She may have fever, fatigue, a sore throat, and a rash. She may not have symptoms at all. Her baby may be born early or too small. The baby also may have fever, jaundice, eye problems, or other severe long-term problems. Both the mother and fetus can be treated with antibiotics in some cases. Infected babies are treated soon after birth to prevent long-term problems.

The best way to protect against toxoplasmosis is to avoid being exposed to it. Be sure meat is well cooked, and avoid contact with the cat litter box. Pregnant women should wear waterproof gloves or avoid gardening in areas where there are feces. Always wash your hands with soap and water after touching soil, cats, or uncooked meat or vegetables. Once feces become infectious, they stay that way for a long time.

Tuberculosis

Tuberculosis (TB) is a disease that affects the lungs. It can spread to other parts of the body such as the brain, kidneys, or bones. It was becoming a rare disease in the United States, but the number of people with TB has started to increase again. The disease is caused by bacteria that are carried through the air, often when an infected person coughs or sneezes. A person slowly becomes sick and may have no symptoms at first. Over time, TB can cause fever, weight loss, night sweats, a dry cough, and chest pain. Even before symptoms occur, TB can be found by a simple skin test. It can be treated with a mixture of drugs that must be taken for a number of months.

Women can be treated for tuberculosis during pregnancy. When a mother has TB, the fetus can get infected through her blood or by breathing in the bacteria at birth. The baby also can get infected by contact with the mother after birth. For this reason, infants born to mothers with TB are treated to protect them from getting the disease. Women with TB should talk to their doctor to see if they can breastfeed. The baby may need to be kept away from you for a while.

Keeping Well

The best way to prevent infections during pregnancy is to make sure your vaccines are up-to-date before you become pregnant. Know the symptoms of infections so you can act on them if they occur. Try to avoid being exposed to an infection.

If you get an infection during pregnancy, it may be treated to prevent further harm to you or your baby. In some cases, there is no treatment for the disease or it is not safe to have during pregnancy. Your baby may need treatment after it is born to treat the illness.

CHAPTER 17

Testing for Fetal Well-Being

Many techniques are used to check the well-being of your fetus. Those described in this chapter often are used in the second half of pregnancy. They will be used only if there is a need to check the health of the fetus—they will not be used on all pregnant women. These tests may be done to confirm other test results or to provide further information. The results may assure you and your doctor all is going well.

These tests cannot cure a problem, nor can they ensure a healthy baby. What they can do is alert your doctor that you may need special care.

The results of routine tests or risk factors will reveal if more tests are needed to diagnose a problem. These tests may include amniocentesis or chorionic villus sampling. They are detailed in Chapter 13.

Kick Counts

You may be asked to keep track of your fetus's movements. These are called kick counts. A number of methods are used. A common one is to record the length of time it takes for the fetus to make 10 movements. You can pick any time of day to count movements, but a good time is after dinner, when the fetus is likely to be most active. Each fetus has its own level of activity, and most have a sleep cycle of 20–40 minutes. If you have been asked to note your baby's kick counts, your doctor or nurse will tell you what to do and when to call them.

Ultrasound

Ultrasound creates pictures or sounds of the baby from sound waves. It is used today in all major hospitals and in many doctors' offices. This device has many uses in the routine health care of women, but it is even more useful during pregnancy and childbirth. No harmful effects to either the mother or the baby have been found in more than 30 years of using ultrasound.

Ultrasound is energy in the form of sound waves produced by a small crystal. The sound waves move at a frequency too high to be heard by the human ear. A device called a *transducer* directs the sound waves into a certain area of the body.

There are two types of transducers:

1. A handheld transducer that is moved along the abdomen

2. A vaginal transducer that is placed in the vagina

The handheld transducer is moved across the skin. The sound waves bounce off tissues inside the body, like echoes. They are changed into pictures of the internal organs and the fetus. The

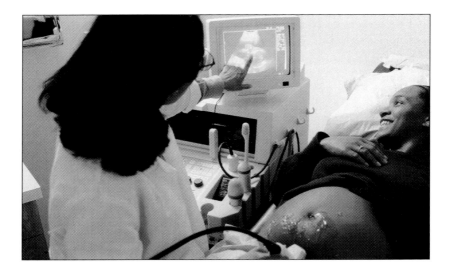

pictures appear on a screen that looks like a TV. Real-time ultrasound quickly combines still pictures one after another to show movement. This is somewhat like the single frames that make a motion picture.

The vaginal transducer can be inserted in the vagina to help view the pelvic organs. Ultrasound with a vaginal probe may feel like the exam you have for a Pap test. This exam is being done more often to detect certain disorders, such as placenta previa.

Ultrasound often is used to help find a problem or check a known condition. It is a useful diagnostic tool that gives information other tests do not. In a way, ultrasound is a type of physical exam of a fetus. Ultrasound cannot detect all abnormalities. It can provide useful information about the fetus's health and well-being, such as:

‣ Age of the fetus

‣ Rate of growth of the fetus

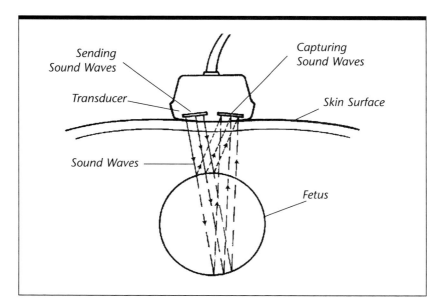

With ultrasound, energy in the form of sound waves is reflected off the fetus. The reflected sound waves are changed into pictures of the fetus that you and your doctor can see on a TV-type screen.

▸ Placement of the placenta

▸ Fetal position, movement, breathing, and heart rate

▸ Amount of amniotic fluid in the uterus

▸ Number of fetuses

▸ Some birth defects

Ultrasound is not designed to take pictures of the fetus for mementos. Ultrasound should not be done only to try to detect the baby's sex, although the images sometimes show if the fetus is male or female.

To prepare for an ultrasound exam, wear clothes that allow your abdomen to be exposed easily. A top and a skirt or slacks work best. You may be asked to wear a hospital gown. You may need a full bladder for exams done early in pregnancy.

A doctor or another team member trained in doing ultrasound exams will conduct the test. As you lie on the table with your abdomen exposed from the lower part of the ribs to the hips, a gel is applied to the abdomen. This improves contact of the transducer with the skin surface. The transducer then is moved along

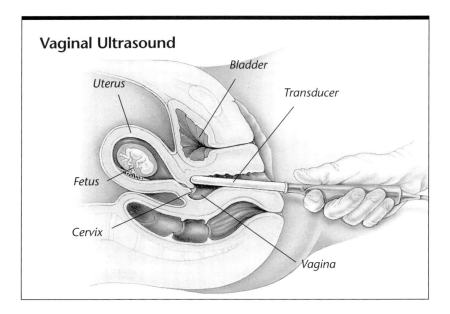

Vaginal Ultrasound

Bladder

Uterus

Transducer

Fetus

Cervix

Vagina

the abdomen. The sound waves sent out from the transducer enter the body and reflect back when they make contact with the internal organs and the fetus.

A new test, called Doppler velocimetry, uses a form of ultrasound to look at the uterus to check blood flow. It sometimes is used with other tests. It is not available in all areas.

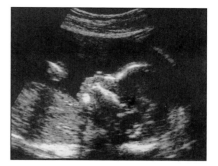

Ultrasound of a fetus in the mother's uterus.

Fetal Heart Rate Monitoring

Ultrasound can be used not only to make images, but also to listen to the fetal heartbeat. When used this way, it is called fetal heart rate monitoring. There are two methods of fetal heart rate monitoring. One method—called auscultation—involves listening to your baby's heartbeat at certain times. The other method—electronic fetal monitoring—uses equipment to record the heart rate on an ongoing basis. At the same time, the contractions of the uterus are measured. This can be done by feeling the abdomen or by using electronic equipment.

Auscultation

There are two ways of listening to the baby's heartbeat with auscultation:

1. A special device like a stethoscope—called a fetoscope—is placed in the ears of your doctor or nurse. The open end is pressed on your abdomen. The fetoscope allows your baby's heartbeat to be heard clearly.

2. A Doppler ultrasound is a small, handheld device that is pressed against your abdomen. It uses sound waves that reflect from your baby to create a signal of the heartbeat that can be heard.

Electronic Fetal Monitoring

For electronic fetal monitoring, a small device transmits sound waves (Doppler ultrasound). It is pressed against the mother's abdomen or is attached with belts. When the fetal heartbeats are reflected, they make sounds you can hear. These signals also are shown on a graph. Monitoring the fetal heart gives helpful information before labor. It also can show how the fetus is coping with labor (see "Monitoring" in Chapter 8).

There are two ways to monitor the fetal heart rate before labor starts—the nonstress test and the contraction stress test. Both of these tests measure the fetal heart rate in response to some form of stimuli. These tests can assure you if the results are normal. If the results are not normal, it is not certain there is a problem. You may need to have the test again.

Nonstress Test

The nonstress test measures the fetal heart rate in response to the fetus's own movements. Often the fetal heart rate quickens when the fetus moves, just as your heart beats faster when you exercise. Changes in the fetal heart rate are believed to be a sign of good health. During the nonstress test, you lie on a bed or examining table with a belt around your abdomen. The belt is attached to transducers, and the fetal heart rate is measured by Doppler ultrasound. You push a button each time you feel the baby move. This causes a mark to be made on a paper that is recording the fetal heart rate. (The nonstress test also can be done with a device that senses fetal movement.) The length of the test ranges from 10–40 minutes.

If the fetus does not move for a while during the nonstress test, it may be asleep. A device like a buzzer may be used to produce sound and vibration to wake the fetus and cause it to move. This test is called **vibroacoustic stimulation**. The doctor also may suggest you have something to eat or drink.

Contraction Stress Test

The contraction stress test measures how the fetal heart rate reacts to the uterus when it contracts. When the uterus contracts,

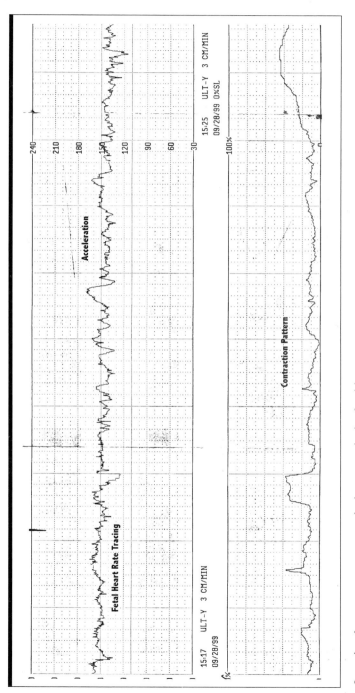

Sample of a nonstress test graph that records the fetal heart rate.

the blood flow to the placenta decreases for a brief time. Normally, contractions do not affect the fetal heart rate. If there is something wrong with the placenta or the baby is showing signs of having a problem, the contraction can decrease the oxygen flow and cause the fetal heart rate to drop. The contraction stress test often is used if the nonstress test shows no change in the fetal heart rate when the fetus moves.

To make the woman's uterus contract mildly, she is given a drug called oxytocin. (In a small number of cases the woman's uterus may contract on its own, especially if the test is done late in pregnancy.) The response of the fetal heart rate to the contractions then is measured by Doppler ultrasound. For results to be obtained, three contractions must take place over about 10 minutes, and each must last about 40 seconds. The test can take up to 2 hours. An abnormal response means that further testing or treatment is needed.

Biophysical Profile

The biophysical profile is a nonstress test combined with ultrasound. The biophysical profile examines the fetal heart rate, muscle tone, body movement, and the amount of amniotic fluid (the liquid around the fetus inside the uterus). It also checks breathing movements. Although the fetus does not truly breathe air, it does make chest wall movements with muscles used for breathing after birth. The fetus gets oxygen directly through the placenta. The test takes about 30 minutes.

Each of these items is given a score, and a total is obtained. A score of 8–10 is normal. If the score is below that range, you may need to have the test redone the next day. As with electronic fetal monitoring, the biophysical profile does not cause any harm to the fetus. It can be done again as needed to check the progress of your pregnancy. The score will help decide whether you need special care or whether your baby should be born sooner than planned.

Test Results

Testing during the second half of pregnancy can assure you and your doctor that all is going well with you and your baby. If there is a problem, tests may be able to find it early. Keep in mind tests cannot always find a problem, or the results may say there is a problem when there isn't one. Results of your tests may mean that you and your baby will need special care before and during pregnancy. This may seem scary, but it may help keep you and your baby as healthy as possible—and give your baby the best start in life.

CHAPTER 18

Grieving

It's normal to hope that your pregnancy will go smoothly and you'll have a baby that's perfect in every way. Most of the time, babies are born healthy. Once in a while, though, things go wrong and a baby may die. If you lose a baby, you may feel shock, anger, sorrow, and pain. If your baby has a severe physical or mental problem, you also may have feelings of grief. These feelings are normal and will lessen with time. There are ways to work through the normal grieving process to help you and your loved ones cope with the loss.

Cause of Loss

The loss of a baby can occur during pregnancy or after birth. Miscarriage is one of the most common causes of fetal loss. A miscarriage is the loss of a pregnancy before the fetus is able to live on its own outside the mother's uterus. It occurs in at least one fifth of all pregnancies. Miscarriages occur most often in early pregnancy.

A pregnancy also can be lost in later stages. A baby can be delivered that shows no signs of life. This is called stillbirth.

A fetus also may be lost if there is an ectopic pregnancy. Ectopic pregnancy occurs when the fertilized egg grows outside the uterus (in the fallopian tube in most cases). About 1 pregnancy in 50 is ectopic. Often this problem is diagnosed in the first 8 weeks of pregnancy, even before a woman realizes she is pregnant. She may have pains, cramps, or vaginal bleeding that signal the problem. A woman must have treatment right away to remove it.

Sometimes newborns die after birth. They may have a defect or were born too early. Babies may die in their sleep for no clear reason. This is called sudden infant death syndrome (SIDS). About 3 of 1,000 babies between the ages of 1 month and 4 months die from SIDS. Although no one knows what causes SIDS, it appears to be linked with long pauses in the baby's breathing. This is known as apnea. It is believed that the best way to prevent SIDS is to lay babies on their backs or sides to sleep and to avoid covering them with blankets. Although the loss of a baby can happen for many different reasons, mothers and fathers feel grief.

The Grieving Process

Most women get emotionally attached to their babies long before the actual birth. This process is called bonding. The bond grows stronger throughout pregnancy. As the weeks and months of your pregnancy go by, you may imagine how the baby will look and

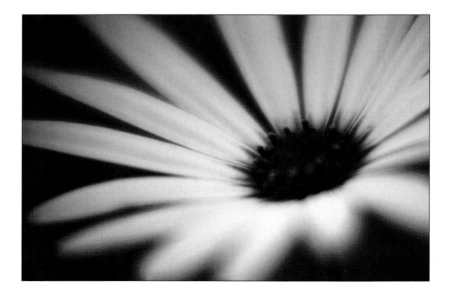

what he or she will be like. Around 16–20 weeks of pregnancy, when you first feel your baby move, the bond may become much more intense. The father also develops a strong tie to his unborn child. He may have many of the same feelings you do.

Losing your baby can bring intense sadness and shock. In almost all cases, you did not expect it to happen. The loss of a baby at any stage—during pregnancy or after birth—is tragic. Your feelings can be the same as when any person you love dies.

Grief is a normal, natural response to the loss of your baby. Working through grief and mourning your loss are healing processes that help you adapt and move ahead with your life.

The Stages of Grief

Grieving includes a wide range of feelings. Just as each pregnancy is unique, ways to react to losses of pregnancy are unique, too. How intense your feelings are does not always relate to the time in pregnancy when the loss occurs. A miscarriage can bring the same sorrow as a stillbirth, for instance.

Each family member mourns in his or her own way. The process you follow may be affected by your experiences with death, the culture you were raised in, your role in the family, and what you think others expect of you.

Grieving is a hard and tiring process. It can last 2 years or more. Often, the feelings of loss never go away completely.

Grieving happens in stages. These stages can overlap and repeat. They have a common pattern in many people, but do not always follow the same course.

▶ *Shock, numbness, and disbelief.* When faced with news of their baby's death, parents often think "This is not really happening" or "This can't be true." You may deny that the loss has occurred. You may have trouble grasping the news. You may feel nothing at all. Even though you and your partner may be together physically, you may each feel a very private sense of being alone or empty.

▶ *Searching and yearning.* These feelings tend to overlap with your initial shock and get stronger over time. You may start looking for a reason for your baby's death—who or what caused it to die? It is common during this stage to feel very guilty. You may think that somehow you brought about your baby's death and blame yourself for things you did or did not do. You may have dreams about the baby and yearn for what might have been. You may even think you are going crazy.

▸ *Anger or rage.* "What did I do to deserve this?" and "How could this happen to me?" are common feelings after losing a baby. You may direct your anger at your partner, the doctor or nurse, the hospital staff, or even other women whose babies were born healthy. If you feel angry toward your partner—or if he feels angry toward you—it may be hard for you to comfort each other. In this stage of grief you may find yourself questioning your religious beliefs. It's good to accept your anger, express it, and try to get it out of your system. Anger is not healthy when you try to deny it.

▸ *Depression and loneliness.* In this stage, the reality sinks in that you have lost your baby. You may feel tired and run down, sad, out of sorts, and helpless. You may have trouble getting back into your normal routine. The support from friends and family that you received during the early weeks of your loss may be gone, even though you still need comfort and kindness. Your relationships with people may be strained because others do not understand your feelings. Slowly you start to get back on your feet and work through your loss.

▸ *Acceptance.* In this final stage of grieving, you come to terms with what has happened. Your baby's death no longer rules your thoughts. You start to have renewed energy. Although you will never forget your baby, you begin to think of him or her less often and with less pain. You pick up your normal daily routine and social life. You laugh with friends and make plans for the future. You may feel ready to start planning your next pregnancy.

Other Signs of Grieving

As you grieve, you may have other feelings or symptoms that are natural and normal. These are more likely to occur in the first months after your loss and may include:

▸ Aches and pains in the breasts and arms

▸ A tight feeling in the chest and throat

▸ Heart flutters

▸ Headaches

▸ Trouble sleeping

▸ Nightmares

▸ Loss of appetite

▸ Tiredness and easy fatigue

▸ Loss of memory and trouble concentrating

▸ Pictures of the baby in your mind

Grieving mothers often feel as if their bodies have failed them. At first you may want to ignore your health or how you look. These feelings may be worse if your body is sore or slow to heal from the baby's birth. Although you may not be concerned about your own health, you need to take special care of yourself. If at any time you have concerns about what's going on in your body or mind, talk to someone who makes you feel comfortable and will listen.

You and Your Partner

Your relationship with your partner may suffer from the stress of the loss of a child. You may have trouble getting your thoughts and feelings across to each other. One or both of you may feel hostile toward the other. You may find it hard to have sex again or do other things together that you used to enjoy. This is normal. Try to be patient with each other. Let each other know what your

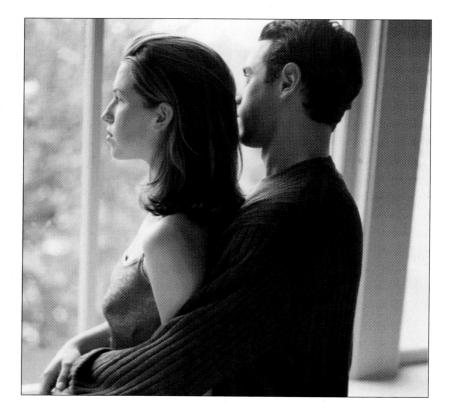

needs are and what you are feeling. Take time to be tender, caring, and close. Make an extra effort to be open and honest.

Throughout the grieving process, your partner may not respond in the same way as you do. Your partner may feel different things at different times. Your partner may not be ready to talk about the loss when you are. Each person should be allowed to grieve in his or her own way. Try to understand and respond to your partner's needs as well as your own.

Making Decisions

When you lose a baby, you must face certain decisions—even if you don't feel like facing anything. You also may choose to take certain actions, such as naming the baby or holding a memorial service, that help you through the healing process.

Saying Goodbye

One of the most important decisions you will make is whether to see your baby when it is born. Although this may sound scary or morbid at first, other bereaved parents suggest that seeing your baby will be very helpful to you. It can help you realize your loss more fully and may make it easier to let go of him or her. It also creates a personal memory of your baby that you can carry with you.

Even if your baby has features that are not normal, you should think about seeing him or her. A nurse can wrap your baby in a blanket so that you can see as much or as little as you want. Most parents find that the truth is far kinder and gentler than what they had imagined.

Choosing a Name

Naming the baby helps give him or her an identity. A name allows you, your friends, and your family to refer to a specific child, not just "the baby you lost." You may want to use the name you first chose or use another one.

Mementos

Many parents treasure mementos of their baby. You may want to ask the nurse to give you a lock of hair, a handprint or footprint, an ID bracelet, or a crib card from your baby.

Photos also can help create a memory of your baby. Even if you don't think you will want pictures of your baby, think about having them taken anyway so that you will have them if you change your mind later.

Autopsy

Your doctor may ask to do an autopsy—an exam of your baby's organs—to help find the cause of death. Although the doctor may not be able to tell the exact reason why your baby died, an autopsy may help answer questions about what happened. The information the autopsy provides may be useful for your family in planning future pregnancies.

Many parents express relief at knowing the cause of death. Others are relieved to know that no special problems were found. An autopsy does not delay burial and does not prevent having an open casket.

Funeral or Memorial Service

You may choose to have a religious or memorial service. For many parents, it is a great comfort to have family and friends acknowledge the life and death of their baby and to show their sorrow at a special service.

You will need to decide what to do with your baby's body. You may wish to contact a funeral home for burial or cremation. Some parents find comfort in having a grave site they can visit. Some hospitals can take care of your baby's remains, if this is what you prefer. In most cases they will have the body cremated.

Going Home

It's hard to leave the hospital with empty arms and face an empty nursery. Once you arrive home, it also may be hard to deal with family and friends. Most people will not be aware of the impact your loss has on you or how best to support you as you grieve. Although they do not mean to hurt you, people often cannot understand the pain involved in losing a baby.

They care for you and want to comfort you. However, they may say things that cause you pain, such as "You're young, you can try again," "Be grateful for your other children," "Some things happen for the best," "Be brave," or "You'll get over it." Some people may avoid you. They may avoid talking about the baby because they feel awkward.

During this time you should put your own needs first. Let people know what you want from them and how you are feeling. You don't need to force yourself to be brave just to please others.

To ease the pain of telling other people what has happened, you can send out announcements of the baby's birth and death. People you know casually who see that you are no longer pregnant may not be aware of your loss. They may ask questions. Prepare a simple sentence you can use in response.

If you have other children at home, tell them that the baby has died. Trying to shield children from death doesn't work. They can sense your sadness, anger, and fear. When telling young children about what happened to the baby, avoid placing blame. Make sure they understand that the baby's

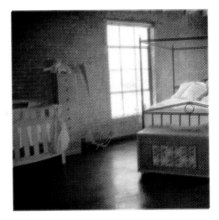

death is not their fault. Children often feel angry and jealous toward a new baby. The news of the baby's death may make them wonder if their thoughts and feelings somehow caused it.

Children sometimes fear that they or their parents also may be in danger of dying. You need to assure them that nothing they did caused the baby's death and that there is no danger to them. Children's response to death varies. It depends on their ages and personalities. Let them know you can see they are upset over the baby's death and that you feel the same way. Be sure to include your children in any funeral or memorial service.

Once you've returned home, take off the time you had planned after the baby's birth if you can. Going back to the pressures of work and seeing coworkers can be hard if you are not up for it. Sometimes you have no choice but to go back to your job or resume a full life right away.

Don't be surprised if feelings of grief come back on your due date or on anniversaries of your baby's birth or death. This is called an "anniversary reaction" or "shadow grief." You may dread these days and suffer through them, while family and friends seem to have forgotten. It helps to be aware of these feelings and to let others know how you feel. Often, parents find that doing something special to mark the date—such as making a visit to the grave site or giving money in the baby's name—is helpful.

Seeking Support

As you go through grieving, you will feel defenseless at times. The pain of your baby's death can remind you of hurts from the past, such as other losses and deaths, infertility, or family problems. Often these old hurts can return and get in the way of the healing process.

Find a network of people who can support you right after the baby's death and in the months that follow. Know you are not alone. A number of people have the knowledge and skills to help you. Your doctor or nurse may be able to direct you to support systems in your community. These can include childbirth educators, self-help groups, social workers, and clergy. Some of these

Support Systems

Getting in touch with one of the resources listed here may help you cope with your loss. These organizations offer support, friendship, and understanding.

The Compassionate Friends
PO Box 3696
Oak Brook, IL 60522-3696
Phone: 630-990-0010
Web site: www.compassionatefriends.org

SHARE: Pregnancy and Infant Loss Support, Inc.
c/o St. Joseph's Health Center
300 First Capital Drive
St. Charles, MO 63301-2893
Phone: 1-800-821-6819
Web site: www.nationalshareoffice.org

SIDS Alliance
1314 Bedford Avenue #210
Baltimore, MD 21208
Phone: 1-800-221-7437
Web site: www.sidsalliance.org

resources may be more helpful than others. You will need to find the one that fits your needs.

Many grieving parents find it helpful to get involved with groups of parents who have gone through the same loss. Members of such support groups respect your feelings, understand your stresses and fears, and have a good sense of the kindness you need.

Professional counseling also can help to relieve your pain, guilt, and depression. Talking with a trained counselor can help you understand and accept what has happened. You may wish to get counseling for yourself only, for you and your partner, or for your entire family. Some reasons for seeking help may be:

▶ Getting "stuck" in one phase of the grief process so that you cannot work through certain problems.

▶ Having severe physical or emotional problems that keep you from functioning. These include feeling not able to return to work, losing interest in your health and looks, having trouble sleeping, or staying in bed all day.

Another Pregnancy?

Before thinking about getting pregnant again, allow time for you and your partner to work through your feelings. After losing a baby, some couples feel a need to have another baby right away. They think it will fill the empty feeling or take away the pain. A new baby cannot replace the baby that was lost. If you have another baby too soon after your loss, you may find it hard to think of the new child as a separate and special person.

Should you choose to have another pregnancy, keep in mind that the chances of losing another baby are very small in most cases. Even so, you may be anxious and worried during your next pregnancy. Talk with your doctor or nurse about the reason for the baby's death. Find out the chances that it will happen again and what you can do to reduce these risks. Your doctor may suggest certain tests before or during your pregnancy to find problems as early as possible.

The Future

The hurt will never vanish completely, but it will not always be the main focus in your life and thoughts. At some point you will be able to talk and think about the baby more easily and with less pain. One day you'll find yourself doing more of the things you used to do—like enjoy favorite activities, renew friendships, and look forward to the future.

Pregnancy Diary

My Health Care Team

Doctors' names: _____

_____

Doctors' addresses: _____

_____

Telephone/answering service:

Day: _____Night: _____

Hospital: _____Email: _____

Nursing staff: _____Receptionist: _____

Pediatricians' names: _____

_____

Pediatricians' addresses: _____

_____

Telephone/answering service:

Day: _____Night: _____

Hospital: _____Email: _____

Nursing staff: _____Receptionist: _____

My Childbirth Education

Educator:_____

Educator's address: _____

_____

Beginning date: _____Ending date: _____

Telephone: _____

Email: _____

First Signs

I first heard my baby's heartbeat: _____

_____

I first felt my baby move: _____

_____

Medications

Medications Taken	Dose	Date Started	Date Ended

Vital Statistics

My pre-pregnant weight:_____lbs.   Last menstrual period: _____

My blood type: _____   Rh factor:_____

Rubella status: _____

Special Tests

Date	Procedure	Findings

Prenatal Visits

Visit	Date	Weeks	Weight	Blood Pressure	Uterus Height (cm)	Questions/ Comments
1st						
2nd						
3rd						
4th						
5th						
6th						
7th						
8th						
9th						
10th						
11th						
12th						
13th						

Labor and Delivery

My due date: _____My labor began: _____

The date my baby was born: _____

Time of delivery: _____

Delivered by: _____

My baby's weight: _____My baby's length: _____

Hospital where my baby was born: _____

Medical Record

Mother:_____Baby: _____
                     (no.)   (no.)

Postpartum Visits

Mother:

Date:_____Weight: _____Blood pressure: _____

Family planning: _____

Comments: _____

_____

_____

_____

Baby:

Date:_____Weight: _____Length: _____

Special care: _____

Baby's feeding: _____

Comments: _____

_____

_____

_____

My Baby's Growth Charts

When you take your baby for a checkup, he or she will be weighed and measured. Your baby's steady growth in height and weight is one of the best signs that he or she is healthy. Track your baby's growth by filling in the length and weight at each age in the charts on the following pages.

Length for Age—Boys

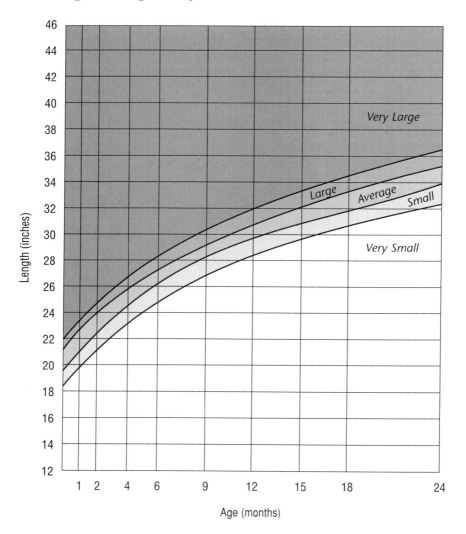

Length (inches)

Age (months)

Length for Age—Girls

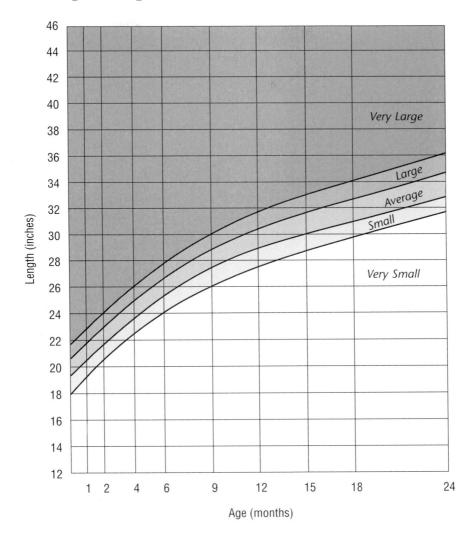

Age (months)

Weight for Age—Boys

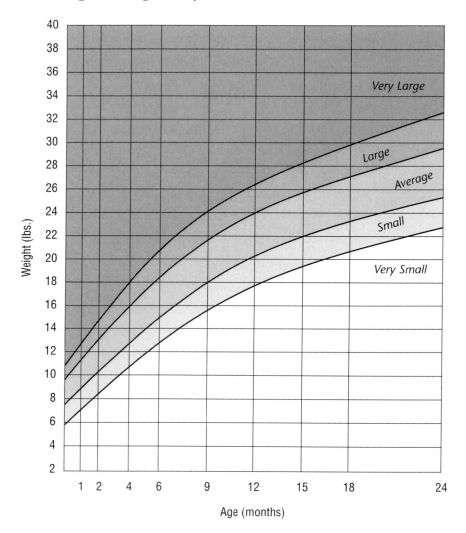

Weight for Age—Girls

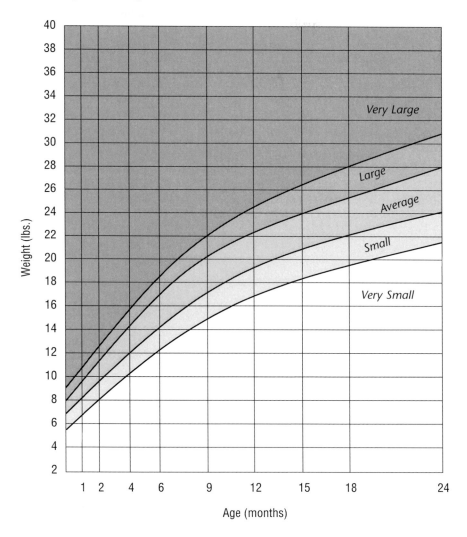

Adapted from *My Health Diary*, 1992, by the U.S. Department of Health and Human Services, Health Resources and Services Administration, Washington, DC

Resources

Pregnancy and Childbirth

C/SEC (Cesarean Sections: Education and Concern)
22 Forest Road
Framingham, MA 01701
508-877-8266

Confinement Line
PO Box 1609
Springfield, VA 22151
703-941-7183

Doulas of North America (DONA)
1100 23rd Avenue, East
Seattle, WA 98112
206-324-5440
www.dona.com

Healthy Mothers, Healthy Babies (HMHB)
121 North Washington Street
Suite 300
Alexandria, VA 22314
703-836-6110

High-Risk Moms, Inc.
PO Box 389165
Chicago, IL 60638-9165
630-515-5453

National Center for Education in Maternal and Child Health
2000 15th Street, North
Suite 701
Arlington, VA 22201-2617
703-524-7802
www.ncemch.org

National Maternal and Child Health Clearinghouse
2070 Chain Bridge Road
Suite 450
Vienna, VA 22182-2536
888-434-4MCH
www.ncemch.org

Childbirth Classes

International Childbirth Education Association (ICEA)
PO Box 20048
Minneapolis, MN 55420-0048
612-854-8660
www.icea.org

Lamaze International
1200 19th Street, No. 300
Washington, DC 20036-2422
800-368-4404
www.lamaze-childbirth.com

Breastfeeding

**International Lactation
Consultant Association**
4101 Lake Boone Trail, Suite 201
Raleigh, NC 27607
919-787-5181
www.ilca.org

**La Leche League International
(LLLI)**
1400 Meacham
Schaumburg, IL 60173
800-LA-LECHE
www.lalecheleague.org

Grieving and Loss

The Compassionate Friends
PO Box 3696
Oak Brook, IL 60522-3696
630-990-0010
www.compassionatefriends.org

**SHARE: Pregnancy and Infant
Loss Support**
St. Joseph's Health Center
300 1st Capitol Drive
St. Charles, MO 63301
800-821-6819
www.nationalshareoffice.com

SIDS Alliance
1314 Bedford Avenue #210
Baltimore, MD 21208
800-221-7437

Multiple Pregnancy

**National Organization of
Mothers of Twins Clubs**
PO Box 23188
Albuquerque, NM 87192-1188
800-243-2276
www.nomotc.org

Triplet Connection
PO Box 99571
Stockton, CA 95209
209-474-0885
www.inreach.com/triplets

Postpartum

Depression After Delivery (DAD)
PO Box 278
Belle Mead, NJ 08502-0278
800-944-4773

**March of Dimes Birth Defects
Foundation**
1275 Mamaroneck Avenue
White Plains, NY 10605
914-428-7100
www.modimes.org

Glossary

Abruptio Placentae: A condition in which the placenta has begun to separate from the inner wall of the uterus before the baby is born.

Acquired Immunodeficiency Syndrome (AIDS): A group of signs and symptoms, usually of severe infections, occurring in a person whose immune system has been damaged by infection with human immuno-deficiency virus (HIV).

Alpha-Fetoprotein (AFP): A protein produced by a growing fetus; it is present in amniotic fluid and, in smaller amounts, in the mother's blood.

Amniocentesis: A procedure in which a small amount of amniotic fluid is taken from the sac surrounding the fetus and tested.

Amniotic Fluid: Water in the sac surrounding the fetus in the mother's uterus.

Amniotic Sac: Fluid-filled sac in the mother's uterus in which the fetus develops.

Anemia: A condition in which the blood is low in red blood cells, in hemoglobin, or in total volume.

Anencephaly: A type of neural tube defect that occurs when the fetus's head and brain do not develop normally.

Anesthesia: Relief of pain by loss of sensation.

Anesthesiologist: A doctor who is specially trained to give anesthesia.

Anorexia Nervosa: An eating disorder in which distorted body image leads a person to diet excessively.

Antibiotics: Drugs that treat infections.

Antibodies: Proteins in the blood produced in reaction to foreign substances, such as bacteria and viruses that cause infections.

Antigen: A substance, such as an organism causing infection or a protein found on the surface of blood cells, that can induce an immune response and cause the production of an antibody.

Apgar Score: A measurement of a baby's response to birth and life on its own, taken 1 and 5 minutes after birth.

Areola: The darker skin around the nipple.

Auscultation: A method of listening to the fetal heartbeat during labor, either with a special stethoscope or the use of a Doppler ultrasound device.

Bacterial Vaginosis: A type of vaginal infection caused by the overgrowth of a number of organisms that are normally found in the vagina.

Basal Body Temperature: Body temperature when taken at its lowest point (in most cases, before getting of bed in the morning) used to predict ovulation.

Bilirubin: A reddish-yellow pigment that occurs especially in bile and blood and may cause jaundice.

Biophysical Profile: An assessment of fetal heart rate, fetal breathing, fetal body movement, fetal muscle tone, and the amount of amniotic fluid. Heart rate is determined by the nonstress test. Ultrasound is used for the other four measurements.

Braxton Hicks Contractions: False labor pains.

Breast Implants: Sacs filled with saline or silicone gel that are placed in the chest or breast area.

Breech: A situation in which a fetus's buttocks or feet are positioned to be born first.

Bulimia: An eating disorder in which a person binges on food and then forces vomiting or uses laxatives.

Carpal Tunnel Syndrome: A condition caused by compression of a nerve where it passes through the wrist into the hand and characterized especially by weakness, pain, and disturbances of sensation in the hand.

Carrier: A person who shows no signs of a particular disorder but could pass the gene on to his or her children.

Catheter: A tube used to drain fluid or urine from the body.

Cephalopelvic Disproportion: A condition in which a baby is too large to pass safely through the mother's pelvis during delivery.

Cervix: The lower, narrow end of the uterus, which protrudes into the vagina.

Cesarean Birth: Delivery of a baby through an incision made in the mother's abdomen and uterus.

Chlamydia: A sexually transmitted disease that can cause pelvic inflammatory disease, infertility, and problems during pregnancy.

Chloasma: The darkening of areas of skin on the face during pregnancy.

Cholesterol: A natural substance that serves as a building block for cells and hormones and helps to carry fat through the blood vessels for use or storage in other parts of the body.

Chorioamnionitis: Inflammation of the membrane surrounding the fetus.

Chorionic Villi: Microscopic, fingerlike projections that make up the placenta.

Chorionic Villus Sampling (CVS): A procedure in which a small sample of cells is taken from the placenta and tested.

Chromosomes: Structures that are located inside each cell in the body and contain the genes that determine a person's physical makeup.

Cleft Lip: A congenital defect in which a gap or space occurs in the lip.

Cleft Palate: A congenital defect in which a gap or space occurs in the roof of the mouth.

Clubfoot: A misshaped foot twisted out of position from birth.

Colostrum: A fluid secreted in the breasts at the beginning of milk production.

Conceive: To become pregnant.

Congenital Disorder: A condition that a baby is born with.

Congenital Heart Disease: A condition that occurs when a baby is born with a heart defect.

Contraction: The shortening and thickening of a muscle or muscle fiber—in this case, the uterus.

Contraction Stress Test: A test in which mild contractions of the mother's uterus are induced and the fetus's heart rate in response to the contractions is recorded using an electronic fetal monitor.

Corticosteroids: Hormones given to mature fetal lungs or to treat arthritis or other medical conditions.

Crowning: The appearance of the baby's head at the vaginal opening during labor.

Cystitis: An infection of the bladder.

Diabetes: A condition in which the levels of sugar in the blood are too high.

Diastolic Blood Pressure: The force of the blood in the arteries when the heart is relaxed; the lower blood pressure reading.

Dilate: Stretching of the walls of the cervix so that the opening of the cervix is widened.

Dilation and Curettage (D&C): A procedure in which the cervix is dilated and tissue is gently scraped or suctioned from the inside of the uterus.

Doppler: A form of ultrasound that reflects motion—such as the fetal heartbeat—in the form of signals that can be heard.

Down Syndrome: A genetic disorder caused by the presence of an extra chromosome and characterized by mental retardation, abnormal features of the face, and medical problems such as heart defects.

Eclampsia: Seizures occurring in pregnancy and linked to high blood pressure.

Ectopic Pregnancy: A pregnancy in which the fertilized egg begins to grow in a place other than inside the uterus, usually in the fallopian tubes.

Edema: Swelling caused by fluid retention.

Efface: Thinning or shortening of the cervix during labor.

Electrode: A small wire that is attached to the scalp of the fetus to monitor the heart rate.

Electronic Fetal Monitor: Electronic instrument used to record the heartbeat of the fetus and contractions of the mother's uterus.

Embryo: The developing fertilized egg of early pregnancy.

Endometritis: A condition in which the lining of the uterus is inflamed.

Endometrium: The lining of the uterus.

Epidural Block: Anesthesia that numbs the lower half of the body.

Episiotomy: A surgical incision made into the perineum (the region between the vagina and the anus) to widen the vaginal opening for delivery.

Estrogen: A female hormone produced in the ovaries that stimulates the growth of the lining of the uterus.

External Version: A technique, performed late in pregnancy, in which the doctor manually attempts to move a breech baby into the normal, head-down position.

Fetal Alcohol Syndrome (FAS): A pattern of physical, mental, and behavioral problems in the baby that is thought to be due to alcohol abuse by the mother during pregnancy.

Fetal Monitoring: A procedure in which instruments are used to record the heartbeat of the fetus.

Fetoscope: A stethoscope designed for listening to the fetal heartbeat.

Fetus: A baby growing in the woman's uterus.

Fibroids: Benign (noncancerous) growths that form on the inside of the uterus, on its outer surface, or within the uterine wall itself.

Follicle: The saclike structure that forms inside an ovary when an egg is produced.

Follicle-Stimulating Hormone (FSH): A hormone produced by the pituitary gland that helps an egg to mature and be released.

Forceps: Special instruments placed around the baby's head to help guide it out of the birth canal during delivery.

Foreskin: A layer of skin covering the end of the penis.

Fraternal Twins: Twins that have developed from two fertilized eggs; they are not genetically identical, and each has its own placenta and amniotic sac.

General Anesthesia: The use of drugs that produce a sleeplike state to prevent pain during surgery.

Genes: DNA "blueprints" that code for specific traits, such as hair and eye color.

Genital Herpes: A sexually transmitted disease caused by a virus that produces painful, highly infectious sores on or around the sex organs.

Genital Warts: A sexually transmitted disease that is linked to cervical changes and cervical cancer.

Gestational Diabetes: Diabetes that arises during pregnancy; it results from the effects of hormones and usually subsides after delivery.

Glans: The head of the penis.

Glucose: A sugar that is present in the blood and is the body's main source of fuel.

Gonadotropin-Releasing Hormone (GnRH): A hormone that tells the pituitary gland when to produce follicle-stimulating hormone and luteinizing hormone.

Gonorrhea: A sexually transmitted disease that may lead to pelvic inflammatory disease, infertility, and arthritis.

Hepatitis B Virus (HBV): A virus that attacks and damages the liver, causing inflammation, cirrhosis, and chronic hepatitis that can lead to cancer.

Human Chorionic Gonadotropin (hCG): A hormone produced during pregnancy; its detection is the basis for most pregnancy tests.

Human Immunodeficiency Virus (HIV): A virus that attacks certain cells in the body's immune system and causes acquired immunodeficiency syndrome (AIDS).

Hydramnios: A condition in which there is an excess amount of amniotic fluid in the sac surrounding the fetus.

Hyperemesis Gravidarum: Severe nausea and vomiting during pregnancy that can lead to loss of weight and body fluids.

Hypoglycemia: Abnormal decrease of sugar in the blood.

Identical Twins: Twins that have developed from a single fertilized egg; they are usually genetically identical and may or may not share the same placenta and amniotic sac.

Immune System: The body's natural defense system against foreign substances and invading organisms, such as bacteria that cause disease.

Incontinence: Inability to control bodily functions such as urination.

Induced Abortion: The planned termination of a pregnancy before the fetus can survive outside the uterus.

Intrauterine Device (IUD): A small device that is inserted and left inside the uterus to prevent pregnancy.

Inverted Nipples: A nipple that has pulled inward.

In Vitro Fertilization: A procedure in which an egg is removed from a woman's ovary, fertilized in a dish in a laboratory with the man's sperm, and then reintroduced into the woman's uterus to achieve a pregnancy.

Jaundice: A buildup of bilirubin that causes a yellowish appearance.

Kegel Exercises: Pelvic muscle exercises that assist in bladder and bowel control.

Kick Count: A record kept during late pregnancy of the number of times a fetus moves over a certain period.

Lactation: Production of breast milk.

Lactose Intolerance: The inability to digest dairy products.

Lanugo: Fine hair that sometimes grows on a baby's back and shoulders at birth; it goes away in 1 or 2 weeks.

Let-Down Reflex: A bodily process, triggered when a baby starts to nurse, that signals ducts in the breasts to contract and release milk from the nipples.

Lightening: When the fetus's head moves down into the uterus and presses against the mother's uterus a few weeks before birth.

Linea Nigra: A line running from the navel to pubic hair that darkens during pregnancy.

Local Anesthesia: The use of drugs that prevent pain in a part of the body.

Lochia: Vaginal discharge that occurs after delivery.

Luteinizing Hormone (LH): A hormone produced by the pituitary glands that helps an egg to mature and be released.

Lymph Nodes: Small glands that filter the flow of lymph (a nearly colorless fluid that bathes body cells) through the body.

Macrosomia: A condition in which a fetus grows very large; this problem is often found in babies of mothers with diabetes.

Mammogram: An X-ray of the breast, used to detect breast cancer.

Mastitis: An infection of the breast caused by bacteria in the milk ducts.

Maternal Serum Screening: A group of blood tests that check for substances linked with certain birth defects.

Meconium: A greenish substance that builds up in the bowels of a growing fetus and is normally discharged shortly after birth.

Menstruation: The discharge of blood and tissue from the uterus that occurs when an egg is not fertilized.

Miscarriage: The spontaneous loss of a pregnancy before the fetus can survive outside the uterus.

Multiple Marker Screening: A test in pregnancy that measures the levels of estriol, human chorionic gonadotropin, and alpha-fetoprotein in the mother's blood.

Multiple Pregnancy: A pregnancy in which there are two or more fetuses.

Neural Tube Defect (NTD): A fetal birth defect that results from improper development of the brain, spinal cord, or their coverings.

Nonstress Test: A test in which fetal movements felt by the mother or noted by the doctor are recorded, along with changes in the fetal heart rate, using an electronic fetal monitor.

Nucleus: The center of a living cell that contains the cell's hereditary material and controls its metabolism, growth, and reproduction.

Oral Contraceptives: Birth control pills containing hormones that prevent ovulation and thus pregnancy.

Osteoporosis: A condition in which the bones become so fragile that they break more easily.

Ovaries: Two glands, located on either side of the uterus, that contain the eggs released at ovulation and that produce hormones.

Ovulation: The release of an egg from one of the ovaries.

Oxytocin: A drug used to help bring on contractions.

Pap Test: A test in which cells are taken from the cervix and vagina and examined under a microscope.

Pelvic Exam: A manual examination of a woman's internal and external reproductive organs.

Perineum: The area between the vagina and the rectum.

Pica: The urge to eat nonfood items during pregnancy.

Pituitary Gland: A gland located near the brain that controls growth and other changes in the body.

Placenta: Tissue that connects woman and fetus and provides nourishment to and takes away waste from the fetus.

Placenta Previa: A condition, usually discovered during late pregnancy, in which the placenta lies very low in the uterus, so that the opening of the uterus is partially or completely covered.

Polydactyly: The condition of having more than the normal number of fingers or toes.

Postdate: A pregnancy that extends beyond 42 weeks.

Postpartum Blues: Feelings of sadness, fear, anger, or anxiety occurring about 3 days after childbirth and usually fading within 1–2 weeks.

Postpartum Depression: Intense feelings of sadness, anxiety, or despair after childbirth that interfere with a new mother's ability to function and that do not go away after 2 weeks.

Preeclampsia: A condition of pregnancy in which there is high blood pressure, swelling due to fluid retention, and abnormal kidney function.

Pregnancy-Induced Hypertension: High blood pressure that occurs during the second half of pregnancy and disappears soon after the baby is born.

Premature Rupture of Membranes: A condition in which the membranes that hold the amniotic fluid rupture before labor.

Prenatal Care: A program of care for a pregnant woman before the birth of her baby.

Preterm: Born before 37 weeks.

Progesterone: A female hormone that is produced in the ovaries and matures the lining of the uterus. When its level falls, menstruation occurs.

Progestin: A synthetic form of progesterone that is similar to the hormone produced naturally in the body.

Prostaglandins: Chemicals made by the body that have many effects, including causing the muscle of the uterus to contract, usually causing cramps.

Pudendal Block: An injection given in the perineum that relieves pain during delivery but not labor.

Pyelonephritis: An infection of the kidney.

Quickening: The mother's first feeling of movement of the fetus.

Respiratory Distress Syndrome (RDS): A condition of some preterm babies in which the lungs are incompletely developed.

Rh Immunoglobulin (RhIg): A substance given to prevent an Rh-negative person's antibody response to Rh-positive blood cells.

Ripening: The softening of the cervix that occurs before the onset of labor.

Screening Test: A test that looks for possible signs of disease in people who do not have symptoms.

Sexually Transmitted Disease (STD): A disease that is spread by sexual contact, including chlamydial infection, gonorrhea, genital warts, herpes, syphilis, and infection with human immunodeficiency virus (HIV, the cause of acquired immunodeficiency syndrome [AIDS]).

Show: The discharge, often mucus and some blood, that occurs as labor approaches. It also refers to the mucus plug that pushes out when the cervix begins to efface or dilate.

Speculum: An instrument used to spread the walls of the vagina so that the cervix can be seen.

Spina Bifida: A neural tube defect that results from improper closure of the fetal spine.

Spinal Block: A form of anesthesia that numbs the lower half of the body.

Station: The relationship of the baby's head to a bony landmark in the pelvis.

Stillbirth: Delivery of a baby that shows no sign of life.

Sudden Infant Death Syndrome (SIDS): The sudden death of any infant or young child that is unexpected and in which the cause of death is unknown.

Syphilis: A sexually transmitted disease that is caused by an organism called *Treponema pallidum;* it may cause major health problems or death in its later stages.

Systemic Analgesia: The use of drugs that provide pain relief over the entire body without the loss of consciousness.

Systolic Blood Pressure: The force of the blood in the arteries when the heart is contracting; the higher blood pressure reading.

Teratogens: Agents that can cause birth defects when a woman is exposed to them during pregnancy.

Toxoplasmosis: An infection caused by *Toxoplasma gondii,* an organism that may be found in raw and rare meat, garden soil, and cat feces and can be harmful to the fetus.

Transducer: A device that emits sound waves and translates the echoes into electrical signals.

Transverse: Acting, lying, or being across; set crosswise.

Trichomoniasis: A type of vaginal infection caused by a one-celled organism that is usually transmitted through sex.

Trimester: Any of the three 3-month periods into which pregnancy is divided.

Ultrasound: A test in which sound waves are used to examine internal structures. During pregnancy, it can be used to examine the fetus.

Umbilical Cord: A cordlike structure that forms normally during pregnancy and connects the baby's bloodstream to the mother's.

Urethra: A short, narrow tube that sends urine from the bladder out of the body.

Uterus: A muscular organ located in the female pelvis that contains and nourishes the developing fetus during pregnancy.

Vaccination: To inoculate with a virus to produce immunity.

Vacuum Extraction: The use of a special instrument attached to the baby's head to help guide it out of the birth canal during delivery.

Vagina: A passageway surrounded by muscles leading from the uterus to the outside of the body, also known as the birth canal.

Varicose Veins: Abnormally swollen or dilated veins.

Vasectomy: A method of male sterilization in which a portion of the vas deferens is removed.

Vernix: The greasy, whitish coating of a newborn.

Vibroacoustic Stimulation: The use of sound and vibration to wake the fetus during a nonstress test.

Vulva: The lips of external female genital area.

Index

Note: Page numbers followed by letters *f* and *t* indicate figures and tables, respectively.